The Breastfeeding Café

The Breastfeeding Café

*Mothers Share the
Joys, Challenges, & Secrets
of Nursing*

Barbara L. Behrmann, Ph.D.

The University of Michigan Press
Ann Arbor

Copyright © by Barbara L. Behrmann 2005
All rights reserved
Published in the United States of America by
The University of Michigan Press
Manufactured in the United States of America
♾ Printed on acid-free paper

2008   2007   2006   2005   4   3   2   1

A CIP catalog record for this book is available from the British Library.

Library of Congress Cataloging-in-Publication Data

Behrmann, Barbara L.
      The breastfeeding café : mothers share the joys, challenges, and
secrets of nursing / Barbara L. Behrmann.
          p.   cm.
      Includes bibliographical references and index.
      ISBN 0-472-06875-X (pbk. : alk. paper)
      1. Breast feeding.   I. Title.
   RJ216.B345   2005
   649'.33—dc22   2004020269

Grateful acknowledgment is made to King Features Syndicate for permission to reprint
Rick Kirkman and Jerry Scott's cartoons from "Baby Blues." © Baby Blues Partnership.
Reprinted with special permission of King Features Syndicate; and to Joan McCartney
for permission to reprint her cartoons from *The Other Side Makes Chocolate* and *We
Should Do This More Often*.

This book is intended for educational purposes and should not be used as a substitute
for professional medical advice. Neither the publisher nor the author shall bear responsibility for any negative impact allegedly caused either directly or indirectly by the information contained within it. While every effort has been made to ensure the accuracy
of the information, each person's health needs are unique. For recommendations on your
own particular situation, please consult a qualified health care provider.

To nursing mothers everywhere and to those whose efforts were not and are not supported. And to my former nurslings, Emily Rose and Rachel Joy—my greatest teachers.

Acknowledgments

Like breastfeeding itself, this book benefited profoundly from the support, encouragement, and assistance of others. First and foremost, my heartfelt thanks go out to the incredible women who eagerly and enthusiastically shared their stories with me. Their candor and honesty are the heart and soul of this project, and I will be forever grateful. Probably the hardest task I faced was having to significantly reduce the number of stories in the book and shorten those that are included. (My contributors have my editor's permission to blame her!) Although I regret that I was not able to include everyone's story, each and every conversation and letter deeply informed and enriched this book.

There are two women for whom I have endless appreciation, Diane Wiessinger and Lauren Korfine. Had it not been for Diane, my own lactation consultant extraordinaire, I would never have written this book. Diane not only provided me with ever-ready technical expertise, always-wise counsel, and a generous spirit but unwaveringly believed in this project from its inception. Diane challenged me to think outside the box, and her insight into subtle cultural nuances has been invaluable. Lauren—doula, psychologist, and overall wise woman—shared her critical knowledge of feminism, motherhood, and the politics of the body. She eagerly read chapter after chapter, draft after draft, providing sound feedback on many levels. Her enthusiasm sustained me through many months, and her unexpected presence in my life was a genuine gift of self.

Deepest thanks to Alex Skutt, Gerry Coles, Cindy Gration, and Bryna Fireside for providing invaluable insight into the world of publishing and to Irene "Zee" Zahava, who always was willing to lend an ear, offer advice, and provide ongoing encouragement.

I am grateful to several anonymous reviewers for their insight and suggestions; to Katherine Dettwyler for going above and beyond the reviewer's call of duty; to Karin Cadwell, Henci Goer, Kathleen Huggins, Ruth Lawrence, Nancy Morbacher, Noelle Oxenhandler, Catherine Taylor, Peggy Vincent, and Marsha Walker for reviewing parts of the manuscript and for sound editorial suggestions; and to Linda Ziedrich and Patty Berhaus for helpful comments regarding earlier draft chapters. I am also grateful to the following lactation consultants who provided me with helpful technical information on specific issues: Arnetta Dailey, Ruth DeRosa, Patricia Drazin, Catherine Watson Genna, Lisa Marasco, Linda Pohl, Natalie Shenk, and Linda Stewart.

Heartfelt thanks to the wonderful women who provided me with leads for stories. Space does not permit me to name them all, but this book would not exist without them. Special thanks, also, to Nancy Coffrey, who made it possible for me to include Doua X. Thao's story, and to Ann Allen and the "Sislist" for their ongoing cheerleading and camaraderie.

I am indebted to Ellen McCarthy, the most supportive, enthusiastic editor I could have hoped for, and to the entire staff at the University of Michigan Press, all of whom have made my first publishing experience a delight.

A huge thank you to Annie Campbell for creating the fabulous painting on the cover and to Eric Lindstrom for his brilliantly creative mind. Grateful acknowledgment to cartoonists Joan McCartney, Rick Kirkman, and Jerry Scott for granting me permission to reproduce their work.

Deepest thanks to the wonderful women at the Bunny Trail and the Coddington Road Community Center, who provided outstanding child care when my children were younger, and to Katina Varzos, fast becoming a wonderful midwife.

Last, but definitely not least, I wish to thank my family. Loretta and Arthur Behrmann, my wonderful parents and greatest cheerleaders, have always offered me encouragement, support, and unconditional love. The world would be a better place if there were more parents (and grandparents) like them. Enormous love and gratitude to my clever, analytical, and supportive husband, Mark Fowler, who has lived with this project for many years and without whom this book would not exist. And, of course, my deepest appreciation to my children, Emily Rose and Rachel Joy, whose very lives made this book possible.

Contents

Sources of Information and Support

These organizations and references, all of which offer excellent information and/or support, can be found on the following pages:

Welcome to the
Breastfeeding Café

Stories are not replicable because our lives are unique. Our uniqueness is what gives us value and meaning. Yet in the telling of stories, we also learn what makes us similar, what connects us all, what helps us transcend the isolation that separates us from each other and from ourselves.

Dean Ornish, foreword to
Kitchen Table Wisdom, *by Rachel Naomi Remen*

When I was pregnant with my first child, I read everything I could about pregnancy, labor, and childbirth and eagerly listened to any woman willing to share her birth story with me. But I was so focused on how to get an enormous head out of my body that breastfeeding was completely overshadowed. Besides, what was there to know? I would put my baby to my breast, and she would nurse. End of story. So when my daughter refused to latch on for almost six grueling weeks and screamed whenever facing my nipple head-on, I was caught completely off guard. A dehydrated baby, finger-feeding, supplementing with formula, struggling with nipple shields, and pumping my meager supply of milk every three hours with an electric pump simply had no place in my idyllic prenatal visions. I spent many days in tears, wondering how long I could keep this up. Would my daughter ever be able to nurse?

Somehow, we hung in there and began to make tentative progress. At first we could nurse in only one position, requiring no fewer than four pillows, but little by little we became more comfortable. I clearly remember the miracle of waking up several weeks later to discover her latched on, nursing in her sleep, cheeks gently puckering and releasing.

But even as nursing Emily became more pleasurable, I could not forget the anxiety and heartache of our first weeks together. If I had not had a supportive family, a stellar lactation consultant, and determination beyond belief, I would not have made it through. And I would have missed out on an incredibly rewarding experience.

As I reached out to other new mothers for companionship and camaraderie, I discovered, to my surprise, that I was in good company. Many women weren't prepared for breastfeeding. They received poor information and advice and had little postpartum help. I was astounded at the number of women who had never seen anyone breastfeed or had never even *known* anyone who nursed.

In retrospect, I shouldn't have been surprised. Although current research abounds with the nutritional, immunological, and developmental disadvantages of formula-feeding, the United States has one of the lowest breastfeeding rates among all industrialized countries. In fact, about half of all women who start nursing give it up in the first couple of weeks, a period in which babies leave the hospital and are often not seen by a health care provider.

Although many women consider breastfeeding—or *not* being able to breastfeed—one of the most significant experiences of their lives, it remains one of the most misunderstood, devalued, and invisible aspects of mothering. Our culture is simply not comfortable with breastfeeding. At best, it is ambivalent. In ways both big and small, overt and subtle, our society discourages nursing and undermines our ability to develop a satisfying nursing relationship with our children.

The more I talked with women, both in person and via the Internet, the more I became convinced that mothers need support, validation, and a window into the day-to-day realities of what it means to nurse in a culture where bottle-feeding is the norm. For not only can we sometimes find little support when it comes to nursing an infant, we can find outright hostility when it comes to nursing a toddler, preschooler, or older child. Many women face similar situations—lack of support and appreciation for the ongoing work of nurturing our children and a lack of public understanding that breastfeeding involves more than nutrition, immunology, and health but is also about comfort, security, and connection. And it matters not just to *babies* but to *women.*

I began to visualize a book that would be a collection of women's firsthand accounts of breastfeeding experiences, thoughts, and feelings. I knew how much I had benefited from hearing other women's stories. If others had the same opportunity, perhaps they would be better able to overcome any initial hurdles they might encounter. Perhaps they would feel less anxious and insecure. Perhaps it would enrich their entire mothering experience.

I posed the idea to almost anyone who would listen, and the responses were overwhelmingly positive—such a book was long overdue. So I began more systematically to ask friends, acquaintances, even strangers, about their breastfeeding experiences. I talked with women in person and in cyberspace. I listened to new mothers, experienced pros, and women whose nursing days were far behind them. I spoke with women who bring to their mothering diverse life experiences: they were married and single, in the workforce and out, white- and blue-collar, wealthy and poor, young and old. They had different ethnic and racial backgrounds, sexual orientations, and religious and philosophical beliefs. They gave birth in hospitals, birth centers, and at home and had both positive and negative birthing experiences. They had healthy children and sick children. Some women nursed for a few weeks, others for a few years. Some women wrote about their experiences, but the majority shared them with me via interviews.

For the most part, women did not simply agree to talk with me—they were eager to. Several women even shared their journals with me. They shared their time and some of the most intimate details of their lives and then thanked *me.* I was in awe. And in the end, I was struck by the discrepancy between the image and reality of what it means to breastfeed. Nursing mothers are indeed "patient," "devoted," and "loving," but they are equally strong, determined, and tenacious.

Over time, certain themes began to emerge in women's stories, certain feelings and interactions we commonly experience because of the society and culture in which we live. Understanding this underlying context is as important as the stories themselves—knowing one without the other is partial and incomplete. So in addition to learning from women directly, I read and researched all I could to broaden and deepen my understanding of what it means to breastfeed in a bottle-feeding culture.

The Breastfeeding Café emerged from these interviews, writings, and research. At this imaginary café, women discuss the joys and rewards, frustrations and challenges, sorrow and anger, pride and satisfaction, and humor and poignancy that characterize nursing in the United States today. The stories reveal the many ways in which we create a breastfeeding relationship with our children and show not only how nursing affects our mothering but how it affects our identity as women, mothers, and lovers. But they go even further. "From women's stories," writes anthropologist Penny Van Esterik, "we learn that breastfeeding is about love, ecology, politics, power, women's knowledge and the wisdom of the body. It is about the personal messages and memories that contribute to who we are as people and the way we relate to others" (1994, 73).

In the introduction to her book *Mothers Talking*, Frances Wells Burck writes, "We have a hard time taking ourselves seriously in isolation" (1986, xvii). She is right. We feel comfort and relief when we realize that other women not only understand our experiences and feelings but have been there. And there is great delight when we don't have to hide the facts of our mothering but can joyfully share them with others who won't judge us or call us crazy.

The Breastfeeding Café arose out of my desire to help create a culture in which breastfeeding is visible and valued. Women must begin to talk about it honestly and unabashedly. We need to shatter the myths surrounding it and insist on the right to nurse our children without apology and with dignity. In a society in which pregnancy, childbirth, and child rearing are subject to increasingly sophisticated technology and ever-ready "expert" advice, women have the power to be each other's greatest allies. We can provide each other with wisdom, insight, and inspiration and validate and reinforce each other in the myriad choices we make for our lives.

Nothing can take the place of supportive family, friends, and nursing mothers face-to-face. But *The Breastfeeding Café* can provide the next best thing—a community of nursing women you can visit whenever you are in need of company and support. I hope after reading these stories that you will be motivated to share your story with others and, in the process, help to create a breastfeeding culture. There is power in storytelling, and your story, too, deserves to be heard.

CHAPTER ONE

A Legacy from the Past

STORIES OF DISEMPOWERMENT
& DETERMINATION

I nursed her. They feel that's important nowadays. I nursed all the children, but with her, with all the fierce rigidity of first mother-hood, I did like the books then said. Though her cries battered me to trembling and my breasts ached with swollenness, I waited till the clock decreed.

Tillie Olsen, "I Stand Here Ironing"

It was 1936. After a three-day labor in which she was kept sedated with Twilight Sleep (an injection of morphine and scopolamine—an amnesiac drug that produced a light sleep), my grandmother winced with pain each time she put her newborn daughter to her breast. No one at the hospital helped her with positioning, and the nurses gave her formula to supplement the small amount of milk she produced. Since breastfeeding works on the principle of supply and demand—the more milk removed from the breast, the more milk you produce—this diminished her already meager supply. "Shortly after I left the hospital," my grandmother remembers, "the doctor visited me at home. 'You won't be able to breastfeed your baby,' he declared. 'You don't have enough milk.'" My grandmother, then twenty, was not disappointed. Like many upwardly mobile middle-class women of her time, she found breastfeeding burdensome and distasteful and was more than happy to stop.

Twenty-six years later, her daughter, in turn, gave birth via Cesarean section. My mother's hospital stay was eight days long. "You're not planning to nurse, are you?" the nurses asked matter-of-factly. They bound her chest to prevent engorgement and gave her a pill to dry up her milk supply. My mother didn't think to question it. In the years between 1936 and 1962, breastfeeding had become even less visible and acceptable among white, middle-class women. My mother didn't know a single person who nursed and had no intentions of nursing me. She fed me formula, on a strict schedule, as the male child-care experts typically instructed.

In 1994, at the age of thirty-one, surrounded by my husband, mother, a friend, and midwife, I gave birth to my first of two daughters. I was in the hospital for two days. Although I was committed to nursing her, I needed a lactation consultant to help us through a difficult few weeks. Later, as hard as it had been to get nursing off the ground, it was almost as hard to get my daughter to stop. I never would have predicted that we would nurse for a little over three years (Behrmann 2003).

Breastfeeding is universal, but each of us experiences it within our own cultural landscape and grounded in our own family and personal history. When we are immersed in the daily passions and struggles of parenting, though, we don't necessarily question *why* we do what we do—we just do it. We seldom take time to think about how our behavior has been influenced by history, changing beliefs about motherhood and women's roles, the evolution of medical and scientific ideas, and social and economic change. But all of these factors clearly influence how we care for our children and how we reflect on our experiences. Had the doctor and nurses had an accurate understanding of how breastfeeding works, for example, it is quite probable that my grandmother would have had just the right amount of milk for her baby. And had middle-class culture not viewed breastfeeding with disdain, chances are my grandmother's and mother's attitudes would have been different, too. "With what I know now," my mother says, "I would do it all differently, including the decision to nurse."

My own family experience was part of a U.S. cultural transformation so dramatic that by 1971 fewer than one in four new mothers breastfed. And those who did typically nursed for only a few weeks. Never before in human history were large numbers of babies able to survive without breast milk. (Even the use of wet nurses—popular in various times and places—had involved a breast and a baby!) The introduction of infant formula, of course, was a huge factor. But this alone doesn't explain the degree to which women abandoned nursing and why such a stigma became attached to it.

To recognize the predominant cultural context surrounding breastfeeding today, we must first understand a bit about our past.

Scientific Motherhood

The revolution in infant feeding that we saw in the United States centered around the fact that producers of infant formula, obstetricians and pediatricians, and educators and social commentators all convinced women that their own milk was inferior to anything science and technology could produce. Women learned to hold their bodies in self-contempt, while formula came to be viewed as a perfectly adequate, if not superior, substitute for breast milk. Moreover, throughout the twentieth century, women's magazines made breastfeeding almost invisible and equated feeding a baby with giving a doctor-recommended bottle. As a result, middle- and upper-middle-class women, almost exclusively white, came to believe that only "ignorant" and "lower-class" women nursed their babies. Women with less education and income soon followed suit. "Only peasant women nurse their children," my grandmother said.

These beliefs also influenced hospital practices, which, in turn, perpetuated them. Doctors were taught next to nothing about breastfeeding, and by 1930 it had become routine for nurses to give babies supplemental bottles of formula and to view a baby's initial weight loss as problematic.* Babies were kept in virtual isolation in sterile nurseries, fed on a strict schedule, and separated from their mothers, except for the four or five brief, predetermined periods during the day when the nurses brought them to visit their mothers. The nurses gave the babies bottles at night, regardless of whether their mothers were trying to nurse them.

------

* It is common for babies, both breastfed and formula-fed, to lose weight after birth. For breastfed babies, it typically takes a couple of days for weight gain to occur, while their mother's milk supply develops. The first milk we produce, called colostrum, is a substance rich in protein and antibodies that is just what babies need.

These practices all but guaranteed that women would not be able to build up a sufficient milk supply, and they eroded women's confidence in their bodies. Maternal "instinct" was not enough. Medical personnel and hospitals were better qualified to take care of babies than their own mothers. By the end of World War II, medically supervised bottle-feeding with infant formula was the standard method of infant feeding. It could be measured, regulated, and administered more accurately and efficiently than breastfeeding, and it fit perfectly with "scientific" child-rearing beliefs, in vogue since the late nineteenth century.*

Even women who *did* nurse were influenced by these norms. Reflecting on her nursing experience in 1938, a friend's grandmother recalls, "Of course we had a schedule. It was tough because my baby cried a lot, but whether or not she cried, we nursed at certain times. I had a lot of milk, so there was no reason I couldn't have nursed her more frequently. Sometimes my breasts would be so full, but it wasn't time to take the milk from myself and I'd wait." Instead of listening to her body and her baby, she dutifully suppressed her instincts.

During the post–World War II baby boom, as the marketing of infant formula expanded and *Playboy* magazine began to popularize the sexual aspects of women's breasts, these trends continued. Breastfeeding rates further plummeted, and women continued to seek professional advice in all areas of child rearing. Feeding babies continued to involve elaborate methods for preparing formula, strict schedules, and sterilizing bottles and nipples, and with a few notable exceptions, information on breastfeeding was hard to come by. Women were instructed to simply trust their doctors. Elaine, for example, who gave birth in 1950 and 1952, remembers, "When I asked my pediatrician about breastfeeding he asked me if I was a cow. Not very reassuring for a twenty-one-year-old girl. I felt admonished, and since he was a God figure, a doctor, and the ultimate authority, I caved in."

---

* The phrase *scientific motherhood* refers to the dominant ideology that permeated discussions of motherhood from the late nineteenth century through the 1920s. Influenced by the great reverence and almost religious fervor that surrounded scientific progress, various professionals sought to apply medical, economic, scientific, and technological principles and expertise to motherhood, child rearing, and homemaking. Infant feeding was no exception.

Given the medical and social pressures to use formula and the stigma associated with nursing, it's amazing that any women breast-fed at all! But a minority *did* defy the dominant medical and social messages of the time. La Leche League, an organization that continues to provide mother-to-mother support, education, and encouragement to nursing women, was founded in 1956. Its philosophy was in di-rect contradiction to prevailing beliefs. Frustrated with the lack of breastfeeding information and support, the emphasis on formula feeding, and the imposition of rigid scheduling, the original seven founders challenged the ideology of scientific motherhood and promoted the idea that the mother, not a doctor, could best understand her baby's needs. And what babies needed were their mothers and breast milk—whenever they desired it. Although their philosophy was clearly a minority voice, their message resonated for more and more women. By 1960, four years after the organization was founded, its headquarters averaged three hundred phone calls and four hundred letters a month, and by 1971 there were over twelve hundred groups around the coun-try (Weiner 1994, 1359, 1362).

> *For a fascinating, in-depth discus-sion of the social history of infant feeding and its origins, see* Mothers and Medicine: A Social History of Infant Feeding, 1890–1950, *by Rima D. Apple (1987).*

In Their Own Words:
Scientific Motherhood

From the 1930s through the 1970s, women who nursed did so dur-ing a time when it was actively discouraged and culturally invisible. What did this mean for nursing mothers, for women who chal-lenged the status quo? In this first set of stories, several women—now all grandmothers—reflect on their lives as nursing mothers. Their recollections help us better understand the origins of many present-day nursing attitudes and practices. They also reveal prac-tices and beliefs that have since been discredited, such as giving solid foods to babies as young as several weeks, viewing breast milk as an incomplete food, weaning babies diagnosed as colicky, and preparing one's nipples by cleaning them with alcohol.

The stories that follow also help us to reclaim our history as women and to see our mothers and grandmothers as young women, struggling to become "good mothers."

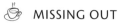 FLASHBACK . . . 1964

I was twenty-one when my first child was born. We were hearing that some hospitals were starting to allow fathers in the delivery room, but even though Larry really wanted to be there, they wouldn't allow it. Nor was he allowed in my room when the baby was there. It was awful. He never held his son until we got home five days later. All he could do was look through a window.

In 1964 feeding was a hospital decision, not a parental one. You could not say, "Do not feed my baby formula." If breastfed babies seemed fussy and it wasn't the scheduled visiting time, they were given supplemental feedings. They were brought to their mothers on a schedule, about every four hours. If I remember correctly, each visit lasted about forty-five minutes to an hour. My son seemed pretty sleepy and not interested in eating. I wondered how much he was fed but had no way of knowing.

My doctor did not *discourage* me from breastfeeding, but he did not *encourage* me, either. Other than my husband—who, like me, thought it was normal and natural—I had absolutely no encouragement from anyone. Most of my friends said, "Oh, how animalistic! You're putting yourself on the same level as a cow." I just laughed and smiled and said, "I think it's wonderful."

Once home, I never had any problems. My doctor encouraged me, at all costs, to give one formula-feeding a day. He felt that formula was complete and convenient, that it wouldn't confine me, and that it would allow my husband to feed the baby.

After six weeks, my doctor told me that breast milk was their *liquid,* but it wasn't their complete diet. He told me to start giving cereal, and by three months my son was eating most anything and everything. The doctors also recommended that I switch over to whole cow's milk. At three and a half months I gradually stopped nursing. I was feeling pretty insecure about whether he was getting enough and had no way of knowing if he was. The doctor was probably very happy when I quit. In 1964, nursing for three or four months was considered to be a very long time.

Nancy Simmons, Ann Arbor, MI

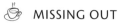 MISSING OUT

In 1968, when my daughter was born, I was twenty, immature, and went from my mother's house to my husband's house. I knew nothing about kids and babies. Remember *The Dick Van Dyke Show?* I thought you just took the babies out when you wanted them and put them back in their rooms when you didn't.

At the hospital where my daughter was born, there were three nurseries full of babies. Only one other woman beside myself breastfed. When the nurses brought my daughter in, they handed her to me and walked away. Back then, you just did it on your own.

By three months, nursing had become easier, it didn't hurt, I was better at it, and I was just starting to enjoy it. But I had to stop. The doctors told me she had colic, and everyone was telling me it would be better for my baby if I quit. If she cried they would say, "We don't know if she's allergic to your milk, if your milk is strong enough, or if she's getting enough." It was easier for them to know the exact formula she was on and how much she got.

I was young enough that I thought everyone else knew better than I, so I stopped. But I had so much milk! Before I went out of the house, I used to take a Kotex, cut it in half, and put Saran Wrap over the top of it so if it got full, it wouldn't leak through. When I came back home, I could squeeze the Kotex out like a sponge. When I bent over in the shower, milk would just run down my body.

Knowing what I do now, I wish I had kept it up. I enjoyed the closeness and feel sad because I stopped just when I could really begin to enjoy it. I missed out on that part. I think I'm envious that women today have all the support they have and that it's accepted.

Bonnie Shifflett, Damascus, MD

Maria, in the following story, recalls her immigrant mother's breastfeeding experience in the early 1960s. As Doua's story in chapter 7 reveals, despite vastly different cultures of origin, immigrant mothers today experience much of the same tension.

☕ CULTURE CLASH

My mother's first two children were born at home, with midwives, in a small town in Italy. The only reason one of my sisters was born in a hospital was because my mother had to have a Cesarean. We were all breastfed. Everybody was. I never saw a bottle until we came to the United States in 1960.

My mother got pregnant two years after we came to this country, and of course there was no midwife. She was told by all the Italian American women she knew that she would have to go to the doctor for prenatal care. And she would give birth at the hospital, not at home.

The nurses expected my mother to feed my brother a bottle, but she started to breastfeed. The doctor told her it wasn't right, that because she was so old—forty-three or forty-four—her milk probably wasn't even good. Somehow, though, she managed to continue to nurse without the nurses or doctor knowing. At the same time, she had her entire family—my father, uncles, aunts—all telling her she was crazy, that this was how things *used* to be done, but they weren't done this way anymore. "Besides, how could you go against what the doctor is saying?" they asked. "Your milk might not even be good!" The entire family regarded my mother as perniciously stubborn. Nobody could understand why she was doing this.

As often happens with immigrant families, the children end up taking on a great deal of responsibility, so when my mother would take the baby to the doctor for postnatal care, either my sisters or I would go to interpret. Rather than simply interpreting, however, we would side with the doctor, telling our mother she needed to stop breastfeeding, even though it was clear that my brother was thriving.

In looking back on it, the thing that horrifies me is that my mother was all alone in this. She had support from absolutely no one. She did not even speak English. I still feel tremendous guilt, given what I have subsequently learned about the medical profession and the issues surrounding child-bearing, childbirth, and infant feeding.

To this day I don't know where my mother found the strength to keep doing what she knew was right. I never had a chance to talk to her about this, and it will be one of my regrets, always. The more I think about it, the sadder I get. It's one of the painful transitional experiences immigrants have gone through—and still go through—in this country.

Maria Coles, Ithaca, NY

Social changes typically start at the coasts and work their way inland. In the next story, Barbara reflects on her experience in 1970 in Hollywood, California.

FOLLOWING HER FEELINGS

The first time the nurse gave me my son, she asked if I had prepared my nip-ples. I told her yes. It was the first time I had ever lied to an authority figure. I had *not* prepared my nipples because that meant washing them with alco-hol. I thought, "Who wants to taste alcohol? Besides, it's drying." Later that day the pediatrician I *thought* I was going to use told me that because my son was such a big baby I would have to give him supplemental feedings of formula. I thought, "We haven't even started breastfeeding—how does she know that? Besides, our whole civilization got here by breastfeeding without supplemental feedings!"

After she left I called my childbirth instructor and asked if she could recommend a pediatrician. The best doctors to go to were those whose wives nursed. They would call their wife at home to ask, "Did our kids do such and such, and what did *you* do?" My instructor wasn't permitted to recommend one, but she did notice that most of the people in her class used Dr. Paul Fleiss. I went, and at my first well-baby checkup he suggested I check out La Leche League meetings.

It was love at first sight. It was a warm and giving environment, very different from other environments I was in. What I most remember was this room full of people who were so connected with their babies.

These were the only people I knew who were nursing. Given how formula was being pushed and mother's milk was not, we were probably radicals. It was a very controversial time, and the meetings gave me the green light to follow my feelings. Women were being put down for nursing and for wanting to be with their babies full-time. I remember hearing statements like, "If you had a brain at all you'd be doing something else"; and, "You certainly don't let your child decide when or how long you're going to nurse him."

I had always wanted to be a mom, and I wanted my baby with me. I felt that the most important job I could do was to take care of a human being, my child. Maybe I'm just lucky that my brain functions that way because it's not for everybody. But I felt I could sit in that rocking chair forever and the whole world could just go on because someday the baby was going to grow and not be there and at that point I would reenter the world. I also remember how wonderful it was to bring my babies into bed with me, rather than doing what society was dictating. (You would never bring your baby to bed with you!) This was very radical, especially for me, who had been raised to follow what people told me to do.

Nursing was easy. The milk was always there, always the right temperature and amount. Because you didn't see mothers nursing in public and it was hard to find a nursing bra and convenient clothes, I nursed under ponchos a lot, especially when my son was little. People wouldn't even know I had a baby with me. Nor did I put myself in situations where I would call attention to myself.

I think it was the time in my life when I felt best about my body. It was working just the way it was designed to work. It was very thrilling to look down at my babies and know that I was completely nurturing and nourishing them. I felt sorry for my husband because he couldn't be pregnant and nurse. I think women really have it over men. We can be replaced anywhere else in society, but we cannot be replaced there. We are so fortunate because there isn't a thing we can't do!

My children nursed for two and a half years. That was also very radical. Other people would see them as *children* and ask, "How could you be nursing a *child?*" But they were my *babies!* What stuck in my mind was something my mother had said when I was pregnant. She told me that my baby would not be found in a book and that I should look to my baby for clues. I also thought, "Everybody makes mistakes. I can't please everybody, so at least I'm going to be comfortable with the mistakes I make."

I just had confidence that babies come into this world knowing what they need. If all of a sudden they were nursing more, I trusted that they were having a growth spurt, weren't feeling well, or needed comfort. I remember people talking about problems they had, such as getting the baby to latch on correctly, and even though I had experienced the same situations, I hadn't thought of them as problems. They were just things to be worked out. Fortunately, my babies knew what to do. They really taught me how to nurse, and I had the confidence to go with them. I didn't worry that they weren't getting enough milk because I was changing diapers, so obviously they were. And they were content. I went with the flow rather than having expectations that at a particular stage, this is what they should be doing.

Nursing remains one of the highlights of my life. I look back with only happy memories and feel grateful that I broke with social expectations.

Barbara West, Ithaca, NY

Challenging the Status Quo

Barbara's story is representative of those of many women who were nursing when the cultural climate surrounding motherhood and women's roles began to shift. In the 1960s and 1970s women were entering the labor force in ever-increasing numbers. Of course, many women had always been part of it—namely poor and minority women—but for the first time, middle-class women with children were seeking an identity apart from "Mom." It is rather ironic, then, that breastfeeding rates began to climb just as women were beginning to spend more time away from their children.

Although the feminist movement typically focused on getting women *out* of the home and *away* from intensive mothering, groups of women began to question the power of a male-dominated medical community to define and interpret motherhood. They desired more control over their bodies and envisioned a new model of parenting that empowered them to trust their own voices rather than those of the medical profession. The revolutionary and seminal *Our Bodies, Ourselves* was published in 1973, and women's self-help groups began to emerge around the country. Women began to share information and experiences about their bodies and their experiences with the health care system.

Growing numbers of women wanted to rediscover the natural processes of birthing and how it felt to nourish their babies with their own milk. Natural childbirth and the woman-centered care of midwives became more popular, and women and their birthing partners worked hard to allow more freedom and participation in the delivery room. They wanted to keep their babies with them, not in a central nursery. They wanted to feed their babies when they were hungry, not according to the clock. In short, while a dominant theme of feminism in the 1960s and 1970s was to make it possible for women to be free from mothering, explains sociologist Linda M. Blum (1993), by the 1980s an equally compelling theme was a true desire to mother.

During the same time period, a growing counterculture also helped to create a nursing revival. Consumers were demanding healthier food, free of chemicals, preservatives, and pesticides. Natural foods proliferated, and a preference for things "homemade" and "old-fashioned" began to compete with the demand for convenience and highly processed foods. Nursing was in. Formula was out.

La Leche League flourished during this time; by the mid-1980s there were well over four thousand support groups in forty-eight countries (Weiner 1994, 1357). Equally significant, the medical community began to recognize the message that feeding a baby was generally not the medical problem it had once been thought. By 1979 the American Academy of Pediatrics had changed its position on breastfeeding from neutrality to a strong recommendation, and for a longer duration than they had ever advised before.

Public attitudes also began to change as people became more aware of controversies surrounding the promotion and marketing of infant formula in Africa, Asia, and Latin America. People learned how deceptive marketing practices, when combined with poverty and a lack of sanitation, clean water, and refrigeration, were causing infant mortality rates to skyrocket. This led not only to the largest support for any consumer boycott in history—of Nestlé—

but also to a more sophisticated understanding of the politics of infant feeding.

The upshot of all these changes was a gradual increase in medical support for breastfeeding and a yearly increase in the number of women who set out to nurse their babies—at least in some communities and within the middle and professional classes—peaking in 1982, when almost 62 percent of women nursed their newborns and 27 percent were still nursing six months later.

For excellent discussions of breastfeeding politics, see Gabrielle Palmer's The Politics of Breastfeeding *(1999), as well as* Milk, Money, and Madness: The Culture and Politics of Breastfeeding, *by Naomi Baumslag and Dia L. Michels (1995).*

Still, medical knowledge and hospital-based practices often continued to promote formula-feeding as the norm. Just like today, new mothers often received mixed messages, and without their mothers to pass on nursing know-how, women had to figure things out for themselves. Many continued to follow the advice of doctors, while some turned to La Leche League, progressive in its critique of medicine and child-rearing practices, even if viewed as conservative by women who were rejecting the cultural mandate to be "stay-at-home" mothers.

This next story is a wonderful example of the revolutionary impact these cultural changes had on women's lives and of how women, in turn, shaped the culture. Not all women had a network of social and medical support for their decisions, but those who did found themselves facing new opportunities to redefine and reconstruct motherhood.

In Her Own Words:
Challenging the Status Quo

 ## A JOURNEY FROM THE BOTTOM UP

I loved nursing in my mother's presence. She and I have not always had an easy time, but breastfeeding was something we had in common. There was a continuity, and she was pleased with it. So was I.

I'm one of five children, and my mother nursed all of us. I was born in 1942, and the others came later, during the late forties and early fifties. She spoke about nursing in very loving terms, and I remember how happy and calm she looked when she was nursing. I knew before I became pregnant that I would breastfeed, and I give credit for that to my mother.

I have three sons, and with each of them I got better at it. I nursed my first son (from a first marriage) for about six months, which I guess was significant in 1965, but even then I knew that it would have been better if I had nursed longer. I was young, though, about twenty-two, and had this sense of these huge, juicy breasts dominating my life! And I didn't have the support from my first husband that I got later with my second. I think our relationship was insecure and unstable enough that I felt more concerned about my appearance. I exercised and dieted immediately back to the size I'd been before my pregnancy, but still none of my clothes fit on top. There were also pressures to go back to work, and I had no role model of a nursing, working mother. Nor do I remember knowing about La Leche League.

In 1970, my second husband, Jack, and I moved to Long Island. I was pregnant with Ian, my second son. During the months before his birth, I was lonely and couldn't get a job. In those days, no one was likely to hire anybody who was noticeably pregnant to do anything! I didn't know a soul on Long Island and had just been through a heartbreaking custody battle over my first son. I went to a few La Leche League meetings, partly out of a desperation to be with people. It was a place where I began to make some friends.

The group I first became involved with, however, had an almost evangelical tone—there was a right way to do it, and if you didn't do it that way, you felt disapproval. That put me off a bit. On the other hand, I learned a lot about breastfeeding on demand, not worrying about schedules, and being comfortable nursing in public. I learned that breastfeeding was more than nutrition, but a whole process of comforting, of mothering.

One of the loveliest things I remember about breastfeeding Ian was how supportive Jack was. He thought nursing was beautiful. I was doing the right thing, and he was loving me more for it. It was great.

Ian nursed on demand, and we enjoyed it very much. He was a good, no-nonsense nurser. But as soon as he was mobile, he began losing interest. I let him use a pacifier, and I think that contributed to his weaning himself at one year—he could get his sucking needs met on the run.

By the time Kyle, my third son, was born in 1973, I had changed a lot. I had become even more comfortable and assured of the real value of nursing. There was a change in the culture, too, an increased emphasis on things natural. There was more research on the benefits of breastfeeding, both nutritional and psychological. On a personal level, Jack's support continued to grow. He loved me being pregnant! He thought I looked beautiful, wonderful, sexy. And he thought nursing was terrific! When you feel honored, respected, and admired for something you are doing, it makes it a lot easier to continue.

I nursed Kyle until he was five years old, partly because of his personality. He was a complex child with strong needs for solitude and independence. In spite of, or maybe because of these characteristics, he also needed to come back to home base, for refueling. He'd run up, get a little sip, and run away. Nursing became kind of secret, not in any shameful way, but we just didn't talk about it. And I think I had the discretion not to nurse in front of people who I thought would be uncomfortable. He was old enough where I could say, "Not now, we'll wait." Or, "Let's go back in Grandma's bedroom." As he approached five, he was only really nursing once or twice a week and usually in the middle of the night.

I don't remember how he stopped. I think I just left it available and one day realized he hadn't nursed in weeks. Baby-led weaning was a hot topic in La Leche League; I bought into it and think it was right. Most babies stop when they don't need it anymore.

Because of the stridency of the first La Leche League group, I became involved with a more accepting group around the time Kyle was born. I met a woman, Betsy, who is still my dearest friend. Betsy was training to be a leader, and I went to her meetings. She had a way of accepting and helping people where they were and of respecting the choices they made.

I was so comfortable with this philosophy that when Betsy asked *me* to become a leader, I agreed. She helped train me, and it cemented our friendship even further. When Betsy retired as leader, I took over the group and led it for the next three years. It was very successful. On occasion we had fifty women with their babies and toddlers—in someone's home! There were more and more of us all the time, and we had to split and have two meetings a month. It was really exciting, and in a way, we felt like pioneers. It was like a little revolution in loving our babies and having our families the way we wanted them.

Nursing became kind of like a crusade for some of us, like guerrilla warfare. We didn't preach or proselytize, but we nursed in restaurants, in the park, on the beach, always discreetly. We always followed the League's suggestions to wear a two-piece outfit and lift from the bottom or drape with a blanket. There was a kind of underground, unwritten list of good places to go with a nursing baby. We wanted to bring nursing out into the air; to minimize the "sexual" connotation and promote the sensual, nurturing, mothering aspects.

At the same time, we didn't neglect the personal needs of mothers and babies. In my own case, Betsy and I cared for each other's infants and, on occasion, even nursed each other's babies. I remember nursing Betsy's two-month-old, Annie, when Betsy had to be away for an evening. Although she looked a little confused, she managed to nurse enough to satisfy herself until her mother got home. Annie is now twenty-six, and I feel especially fond of her.

The "network" was there for each of its members in some very critical ways, as well. One woman had a hydrocephalic baby and needed breast milk. Another woman had a tiny preemie, two pounds. We expressed milk for both of the babies. Some of us also contributed to breast milk banks on a fairly regular basis. I don't know whether or not doctors would support that today, but I hope this kind of sharing and giving is still possible.*

I guess this commitment, this attitude, contributed to the next "phase" of the personal and sociological parenting "revolution." Some of the people from our group formed an offshoot group called Mothershare. It was a support group for us as our babies grew and as we got into other phases of mothering. We met weekly as a play group and later on a monthly basis.

We wanted to do something to improve conditions for families. We did a huge survey of all the hospitals in the five boroughs of New York and on Long Island, fifty or sixty of them, concerning their policies regarding family-centered health care. We asked dozens of questions having to do with birthing, breastfeeding, and visitation policies. If a mother were hospitalized for something noncontagious, could her baby be hospitalized with her? Could a mother express milk and bring it to a hospitalized baby? Could she stay with her child if he or she were hospitalized? We then coded the results and prepared a comparative sheet showing how hospital A's policies compared to hospital B's, and so forth, and then sent them back to the hospitals. When they saw how their policies compared with their competitors, some of them changed and liberalized their policies. We would then revise the comparative sheet accordingly. We distributed this resource guide at health fairs all over Long Island and managed to get some heavy-duty publicity. The project was written up in *Newsday,* and we even wrangled an interview on the *NBC Evening News.* We were pretty pleased with how it turned out!

All this personal and political activity had its start with breastfeeding. I believe that nursing was absolutely crucial in forming the deep physical and emotional connection between myself and my children. And nursing my babies and helping others to nurse theirs gave me a sense of doing something to make the world better. It starts right at the bottom. If you have a happier, healthier child and a happier, healthier family, it stands to reason that society and the world will be happier and healthier, too.

---

* See pages 82–84 for a discussion of milk banks.

I don't mean to sound like such a Pollyanna. There were hard and inconvenient times, times when part of me felt, "I can't stand having somebody attached to my body all the time." The sitting-on-the-john-with-the-baby-on your-lap; not being able to brush your teeth in the early months when the baby is nursing nonstop; when the baby has a growth spurt and is just needy, needy, needy. But mostly it was sensual, pleasurable, natural, and the right thing to do.

Kathleen Kramer, Newfield, NY

Legacies Live On

Fast-forward a couple of decades to the present. After a decrease in breastfeeding rates in the late 1980s, the rates picked up again in the mid-1990s. Unlike in the sixties and seventies, however, the greatest increase occurred among women previously *least* likely to breastfeed—women who were younger, less educated, black or Hispanic, and participants in Women, Infants, and Children (WIC), a federally funded supplemental nutrition program (Ryan, Wenjun, and Acosta 2002, 1106).

During this time, many of the goals of the 1970s social movements became mainstream. Similarly, La Leche League became an internationally recognized breastfeeding authority. Today there are over seventy-two hundred accredited leaders helping women in over sixty countries, and their most widely purchased publication, *The Womanly Art of Breastfeeding* (now in its seventh revised edition), has sold over 2.5 million copies (La Leche League International 2004, 14).

Women today have more options in childbirth, and in many circles, social stigmas no longer surround breastfeeding. Moreover, official medical support for breastfeeding has never been stronger. In 1997 the American Academy of Pediatrics (fifty-seven thousand members strong) strengthened their breastfeeding statement to recommend breast milk for all babies in the United States, including those who are sick or premature.* The U.S. Surgeon General recommends that babies be breastfed for at least one year, while the World Health Organization and UNICEF both recommend nursing

---

* They also recommend exclusive breastfeeding for the first six months, with breastfeeding continuing for a minimum of one year and beyond, for as long as both mother and baby desire.

for a *minimum* of two years. Healthy People 2010, the nation's health agenda for the current decade, is striving for a 75 percent breastfeeding rate among new mothers. At the same time, studies have found that *not* breastfeeding puts women at greater risk for certain breast, uterine, and ovarian cancers, as well as for osteoporosis (AAP Work Group on Breastfeeding 1997).

Within this climate, breastfeeding support and assistance have increased tremendously. Midwives, doulas, and lactation consultants are among the professionals and para-professionals who ease our transition from pregnant women to nursing mothers. Some hospitals are changing their protocols to support breastfeeding, and in 1991 UNICEF and the World Health Organization spearheaded the Baby Friendly Hospital Initiative (BFHI), a global effort to encourage breastfeeding and remove barriers in health care settings. To be designated "Baby Friendly," hospitals and birth centers must implement the "Ten Steps to Successful Breastfeeding." At the time this book went to press, forty-two hospitals and birth centers in the United States had been so designated. According to lactation consultant Anne Merewood, their breastfeeding rates were way above the national average, even in large inner-city hospitals that serve populations least likely to breastfeed (Anne Merewood, personal communication, 2003).

Ten Steps to Successful Breastfeeding (World Health Organization 1998)

1. Have a written breastfeeding policy that is routinely communicated to all health care staff.
2. Train all health care staff in skills necessary to implement this policy.
3. Inform all pregnant women about the benefits and management of breastfeeding.
4. Help mothers initiate breastfeeding within the first hour of birth.
5. Show mothers how to breastfeed, and how to maintain lactation, even if they should be separated from their infants.
6. Give newborn infants no food or drink other than breast milk, unless medically indicated.
7. Practice rooming-in—allow mothers and infants to remain together—twenty-four hours a day.
8. Encourage breastfeeding on demand.
9. Give no artificial teats or pacifiers (also called dummies or soothers) to breastfeeding infants.
10. Foster the establishment of breastfeeding support groups and refer mothers to them on discharge from the hospital or clinic.

All of this is great news. But we merely have to scratch the surface, and things are not as rosy as they appear. We are far from achieving national breastfeeding goals, too few women are nursing, and many who *do* nurse quickly give it up. The majority of women today clearly want to nurse their babies. But many end up feeling discouraged, insecure, and unable to overcome the socially erected hurdles we face. Indeed, most of the women who talked with me about weaning infants revealed that had they received adequate information and support, they would have nursed longer. "To this day it is my deepest regret," wrote one woman.

Many talked about failing their babies and failing as women, and the media is full of stories from women who feel guilty for not being able to breastfeed. Psychologist Harriet Lerner, however, cautions against internalizing guilt. "Try to remember," she writes, "that our society encourages mothers to cultivate guilt like a little flower garden, because nothing blocks the awareness and expression of legitimate anger as effectively as this all-consuming emotion" (1998, 75). Moreover, as anthropologist and breastfeeding advocate Katherine Dettwyler reminds us, guilt and regret are two separate emotions. If we make the best decision with whatever information and resources we have at the time, we have no reason to feel *guilty.*

To avoid the expectation of instilling guilt in women, health care providers often choose to present women with "unbiased" information, assuring us that all will be well if we switch to formula. A first-time mother in Florida told me, "My ob-gyn didn't *push* breastfeeding, but he didn't *not* push it. He gave me a free Enfamil diaper bag with formula inside." While the decision of how to feed our children is clearly *ours,* it is impossible to make accurate and informed choices in the presence of such "objectivity."

Objectivity is also difficult in a culture in which yesterday's norms, attitudes, and assumptions continue to dominate our environment. "I often feel overwhelmed by images of bottle-feeding as the 'normal' way of feeding my baby," bemoans one woman. "As I sit in my living room with my son to my breast, the TV brings many of these messages—via formula commercials and general baby product commercials, for example. Children's books with bottle-feeding babies abound, while ones with nursing babies are a specialty item."

Throughout the following chapters women articulate many of the issues that emerge from a social and cultural legacy of bottle-feeding as the cultural norm: everything from inappropriate medical practice and poor advice to outdated beliefs and a lack of sup-

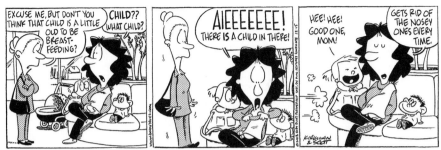

© Baby Blues Partnership. Reprinted with special permission of King Features Syndicate.

port. But they also reveal other legacies centered around a determination and defiance to nurse not likely seen in other times or cultures. If we mothered in a context in which breastfeeding weren't questioned, in which roadblocks weren't erected, a woman would not explicitly express commitment; she would simply *do* it. Instead, as Lori, a strong, passionate woman, asserts, we sometimes have to be "ferocious."

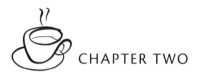 CHAPTER TWO

Welcome to Motherhood

STORIES OF INITIATION,
TENACITY, & ADJUSTMENT

*Ours is not a culture supportive of the English language. We speak
English. This is not a culture supportive of brunettes. Brunettes
just are. If this is a country supportive of gay rights, it means it's
still an issue. As soon as you say a culture supportive of breastfeeding, you've said it's not a breastfeeding culture.*

Diane Wiessinger

During my first pregnancy, my husband and I watched a video
in which a freshly born baby was placed directly on its
mother's stomach.* With no drugs in its system, the baby was alert
and calm. We watched, fascinated, as this baby, with no adult hands
offering assistance, inched and scooted its way toward its mother's
breast, found her nipple, latched on, and began to suck. We were in
awe! This became my goal. I would give birth, my baby would
nurse, we would bond. Bliss.

This vision ultimately turned into a disappointing fantasy—not
just for me but for many new mothers whose first moments of motherhood are far from idyllic. While some women do experience the
wonder of a newborn able to "self-attach," the majority of us do not.

---

*The 1992 video is titled *Dr. Lennart Righard's Delivery: Self-Attachment.*

The stories in this chapter speak to the first days and weeks of nursing when most of us are greenhorns to the world of babies, breasts, and milk. They reveal how our ability to get breastfeeding off to a good start is influenced by the kind of birth experience we have, the early advice we receive, and the involvement of our health care providers. For most of us, our initiation to this new world involves a roller coaster of emotions: everything from delirious joy and love to overwhelming exhaustion, frustration, confusion, and pain. For some of us nursing just "clicks." For others it is a struggle, and the pleasures of nursing seem a long way off. Consequently, these stories may seem dominated by the challenges women face. As you read them, take heart. The fog *does* lift, as does our sense of being lost. It just may take a little while. (Of course, some of us never are able to develop the nursing relationship we had hoped for and reluctantly trade in nursing bras for formula cans. These stories appear in chapter 9.)

The Birthing-Breastfeeding Connection

Imagine going to a pet store and bringing home a potbellied pig. It's a cute, funny-looking creature. You've heard they are intelligent, curious, playful, and quite trainable. With proper care and understanding they can become a welcome family pet. Now imagine bringing your new pig home and realizing you don't know what to feed it. You don't know how voracious its appetite is; the importance of a high-fiber, low-calorie, low-fat diet; and that cat and dog food are too high in protein for it. Imagine how much healthier and happier your pig will be if you know how to take care of it and feed it its own specifically designed food.

Clearly we're not talking about pigs here. But getting breastfeeding off to a good start is really not much different. Studies confirm what may seem obvious: when we are offered reliable information from health care providers, we are more likely to initiate breastfeeding and keep it going (Cadwell 2002, 36). Unfortunately, medical support for breastfeeding does not necessarily mean that women receive consistent and reliable information. Although some obstetricians, pediatricians, and family physicians provide wonderful information and support, scholarly publications that address breastfeeding have often been filled with misinformation and bias, and American medical and nursing students fail to receive the knowledge, training, and experience they need to properly counsel breastfeeding mothers (Dettwyler 1995a, 195–97). Doctors admit this (Freed and Lohr 1995, 472–76).

But access to information and support is only part of the picture, since many of our breastfeeding challenges begin before our babies even take their first breath. To begin with, breastfeeding problems can stem from a disempowering birth. Many women talk about being treated as a machine, rather than as a thinking, feeling woman with a capable body. This can undermine a woman's confidence in her body's ability to nourish a child, creating a double emotional whammy of sorts. Paula, for example, a mother in Pennsylvania, was immobilized during labor, unsupported, and subjected to unnecessary interventions against her will. "I lost a lot of confidence in myself because of my birth experience and my inability to process it," she reflects. "I didn't know I had the right to follow my instincts and demand the kind of birth I had envisioned. I felt I had failed at the birth, so to fail at breastfeeding was devastating."

Moreover, research shows that common obstetrical practices, including medical, technological, and surgical interventions, can adversely impact breastfeeding (Kroeger 2004). Linda Smith, a lactation consultant and well-known lecturer on this topic, notes, for example, that all drugs used to manage labor pains are documented to affect the baby's breathing, sucking, and/or muscle tone. "It's a wonder why any of these kids can suck at all, much less properly," she declares. And the more drugs the mother gets, the more the baby gets, and the more likely its ability to breathe, suck and swallow will be affected (Smith, 1996).

Moreover, internationally renowned midwife Ina May Gaskin points out that using drugs to avoid pain during labor can often lead to pain after the birth (2003, 165). And the less comfortable we are, the more difficult it is to focus on the needs of our babies.

Unfortunately, the connection between birthing practices and breastfeeding success is seldom addressed. Recently, while sitting in a doctor's waiting room, for example, I thumbed through an issue of *Baby Talk Childbirth Guide,* a free magazine from the publishers of *Parenting Magazine.* A two-page chart provided an overview of pain-relief techniques to manage labor. In listing the pros, cons, and possible side effects of various drugs, including epidurals and general anesthesia, the chart failed to mention *any* adverse impacts on breastfeeding.

After-the-birth factors continue to impede our ability to nurse. In many hospitals around the country, medical staff separate mothers and newborns shortly after birth to weigh, measure, and clean the baby. In fact, as documented in a 1990 study published in the medical journal *Lancet,* staff often whisk babies away at about the same time the infants would begin searching for the breast on their own if left undisturbed—fifteen to twenty minutes after birth (Righard and Alade 1990). The authors add that there is "no sensible reason" for this routine separation and that the procedures could easily be postponed.

Medical personnel and hospital policy may further sabotage breastfeeding by giving babies pacifiers and bottles without the mother's consent; by continuing to separate babies and mothers; by not understanding basic breastfeeding mechanics; and by treating women with disrespect and paternalism.* Moreover, in-hospital supplemental feedings have almost doubled in the last ten years (Ryan, Wenjun, and Acosta 2002, 1104), a practice known to lead to shorter durations of nursing. And a recent national survey of women's childbearing experiences found that almost half the babies whose mothers intended to breastfeed exclusively were given supplements (Maternity Center Association 2002, 5).

Many women then leave the hospital before breastfeeding is established and receive inadequate postpartum breastfeeding assistance or follow-up. Biologist Sandra Steingraber asserts, "Given that breastfeeding is a learned art and that few new mothers have lactation specialists waiting in their homes to assist them, this forced expulsion [from the hospital] leaves new mothers in the same position as captive chimpanzees who give birth in zoos and don't have a clue how to nurse their offspring" (2001, 246).

Then add the marketing of baby formula to the mix. Hospital discharge packs may contain formula samples, coupons, and bottles, all suggesting the likelihood of nursing failing. If difficulties do arise, women who receive these packages are more likely to turn to formula—almost always using the same brand (Walker 2001, 24). Formula companies also target their marketing at times when women are most vulnerable, such as when they are pregnant or when breastfeeding is known to be the most difficult (Barbara Heiser,

---

* Babies who receive bottles in the hospital may have difficulty taking the breast later and may need help to learn how to latch on well.

executive director of NABA [National Alliance for Breastfeeding Advocacy] personal communication, 2002).

The obstacles we face in developing a joyful breastfeeding relationship are structural and wide reaching. Yet without an understanding of the bigger picture—and when intellectual reasoning is replaced by sleep deprivation and hormonal upheaval—it is easy to think that *we* are at fault. We take it *personally*. Even those of us who read about breastfeeding ahead of time tend to rely on the particular advice from our own health care providers. And too often we are steered in the wrong direction.

This first group of stories drives home the point that before we can talk about breastfeeding, we must first talk about birth.

In Their Own Words:
The Birthing-Breastfeeding Connection

I still feel my blood pressure rise when I read the beginning of Evelyn's story, a clear illustration of how birthing practices influence our ability to get nursing off to a good start. For many women, as with Evelyn, one intervention typically leads to another, frequently culminating in a C-section. In the United States, where obstetricians—trained surgeons—attend 90 percent of all births, the C-section rate has surpassed 25 percent and is climbing steadily. With the number of *elective* C-sections on the rise, there is a mistaken belief that they are as safe to mother and baby as a vaginal birth. All evidence, however, shows just the opposite. Studies show that interventions and C-sections result in more short- and long-term complications for mother and baby, including a greater likelihood of breastfeeding difficulties (Kroeger 2004). Studies further show that at least one-half of C-sections are medically unnecessary (Coalition for Improving Maternity Services 2003).

For further discussions of this and excellent critiques of childbirth practices in the United States, see The Thinking Woman's Guide to a Better Birth *(1999) and* Obstetric Myths vs. Research Realities *(1995), both by Henci Goer, and* Immaculate Deception II: Myth, Magic, and Birth *(1994), by Suzanne Arms.*

☕ I GAINED CONFIDENCE AND TRUST

Even though the baby was perfectly healthy, it was eleven days after my due date, and my doctor wanted to induce me. I asked for an epidural almost immediately after my first contraction. Nobody in my childbirth class had told me how to relax, telling me instead when I could get an epidural. As soon as I got it, I stopped dilating. Six hours later they did a Cesarean section.

My daughter, Carol Ann, was born with a fever and restricted to the neonatal intensive care unit (NICU) for three days. Her Apgar* scores were nine and nine, she weighed almost ten pounds, and her fever dropped less than an hour after the birth. But hospital policy said she had to have a complete sepsis work-up, and they took samples from every orifice in her body, looking for infection. They wouldn't let her go until after they got the results of a second spinal tap two days later. In the meantime, I wasn't allowed to see her until the third day because I had a fever, too. The doctor said it was a mysterious infection that didn't respond to antibiotics, but I think it was a side effect of the epidural.+

I requested a breast pump to help my milk come in and used it every two or three hours around the clock. The nurses would hold the bottle up, look at my scant ounce of colostrum like it was worthless, and would throw it away instead of taking it to the NICU. Carol Ann was taking plenty of formula, they said, and my colostrum wasn't needed! A lactation consultant came in to see me but didn't want to jeopardize her relationship with the nurses.

I wasn't in any mental state to stand up for what I now know is right, and I spent a lot of time crying. My husband videotaped my daughter in the NICU, and I watched it every time I pumped. But I believed she was in the best of hands, being cared for by professionals—rather than me, who knew nothing—and I was so happy when all the tests came back negative and she was healthy. In retrospect I'm furious that those three days were stolen from me. I am also a bit ashamed. Even a mother rabbit would fight to the death anyone who took her babies, but I didn't even get out of bed.

---

* This refers to two quick assessments, at one and five minutes post-birth, to determine a baby's physical condition. Designed in 1952 by Dr. Virginia Apgar, the Apgar score is based on a scale of one to ten, ten being the highest. Five aspects of well-being are measured: the baby's heart rate, breathing ability, muscle tone, level of response to stimuli, and skin color.

+ Raised body temperatures in both mother and baby are indeed possible side effects of epidurals, which have become so common in some U.S. hospitals that more than 85 percent of women have one (Gaskin 2003, 235). Moreover, studies show that the earlier an epidural is given, the more likely a mother and baby will develop a fever. Evelyn's body didn't respond to antibiotics because she didn't have an infection. And her newborn's spinal tap and other invasive tests were unnecessary, as was their prolonged separation. In fact, separations because of suspected infections are unnecessary, and medical staff should encourage breastfeeding because we make antibodies to whatever organisms we and our babies have been exposed to and transmit them to the baby via colostrum and breast milk.

I finally got to hold my daughter on the third day. My husband had been giving her all her daytime feedings, and by this time he was an expert. He and the nurse would stare over my shoulder, telling me I was doing it all wrong.

We went home later that day, and my daughter had no idea how a human nipple worked. Every three hours for the next week, each meal was totally frustrating. I finally sent my husband back to work because his presence was too stressful. Without him hovering over me, my daughter and I finally were given a chance to know each other! So many people need help after the baby is born, but all I wanted was to be alone with her.

Over the next week she and I were able to calm down and patiently work out our differences. The key seemed to be privacy. And after I gave her two full ounces of bottled breast milk she seemed to realize that it tasted better than formula and was worth working for, so she was more willing to figure out the new sucking scheme. I now know this could have backfired, and she could have preferred breast milk from a bottle, but luckily she didn't.

Carol Ann quit nursing when she was fifteen months old and I was three months pregnant. I learned so much from mothering her that I was eager to do it again. My son was born at home and went directly from my crotch to my chest. He started nursing about twenty minutes later and had a perfect latch-on! While my daughter lost the rooting reflex during the hospital stay, my son could find my nipple easily, and I didn't have to sleep with a night-light on.

J.R. is five months old now, weighs twenty-two pounds, and has never had anything but Mama. I am so proud of his healthy size! And since I am the sole source of his nutrition, I can take full credit for it. The ability to grow and feed a baby without technology, just as mammals have done for eons, has been so empowering for me that I want all women to be able to experience this joy and feel this strength.

I've become a local leader for the International Cesarean Awareness Network (ICAN), and I go to La Leche League meetings to let pregnant women who might be attending know that they *can* overcome initial separations. I also support the work of the Coalition for Improving Maternity Services (CIMS). Successfully overcoming the obstacles I encountered has given me greater confidence to achieve anything I put my mind to. I know that any topic can be researched thoroughly. I read all the different views and then trust my decision of what is best for my family.

Evelyn B. Walker, Coral Springs, FL

As Evelyn eventually discovered, breastfeeding does not have to begin as a set of problems to be overcome. Nursing *can* evolve harmoniously, organically, and holistically. Although this can be the case for women regardless of where they give birth, women who have their babies at independent birth centers or at home are more likely to get nursing off to a good start. This is not surprising. Women in these environments are less likely to be given drugs or be subjected to unnecessary, invasive procedures, both of which can interfere with nursing. They are also more likely to be supported and respected during labor and delivery and less likely to be separated from their babies and offered formula. It is perhaps no coincidence that the primary health care providers in both of these settings tend to be midwives who view birth as a normal, natural, and healthy process and whose mission is, in part, to support breastfeeding.

ICAN, the International Cesarean Awareness Network, is an international, nonprofit, member organization founded in 1982 to help lower the rate of unnecessary C-sections and to encourage positive birthing experiences through education and advocacy. For more information, visit their Web site at <http://www.ican-online.org/>.

CIMS, the Coalition for Improving Maternity Services, is a coalition of individuals and national organizations that promotes an evidence-based wellness model of maternity care. Founded in 1994, its mission is to promote normal birth, improve birth outcomes, and reduce costs. CIMS created a list of ten steps a health care institution must take to become certified as "Mother Friendly." The tenth step is to implement BFHI's ten steps to successful breastfeeding (see page 21). For more information, visit their Web site at <http://www.motherfriendly.org>.

Peggy Vincent is a retired midwife whose book *Baby Catcher: Chronicles of a Modern Midwife* is a captivating account of her career spanning fifteen years and two thousand births. Early on, she describes a woman laboring in a newly created hospital-based birthing center, surrounded by a handful of invited guests enjoying Brie and chardonnay. Vincent recounts the following conversation between herself and an anxious doctor, unsure of his role in a birth that didn't rely on medications, routine IVs, and fetal monitors (2002, 57–58):

Dr. Clark: "What am I supposed to do in there?"
Vincent: "Nothing. She's doing fine. Just catch the baby."
Dr. Clark: "The hell with that. I didn't go to medical school to do nothing at a birth."
Vincent: "But if the birth is normal, then what's there to do?"

Dr. Clark: "Normal birth is a retrospective diagnosis. No birth is normal until after the fact. All births are complicated until proven otherwise."

Their exchange gets right at the root of the distinction between obstetrics and midwifery, between the technical-medical model of childbirth dominant in the United States and the midwifery model of childbirth dominant in western Europe, where C-section rates are lower and fewer women and babies are injured or die in childbirth. This fundamental distinction not only affects how our pregnancy, labor, and birth are managed but also influences how we are treated and what kind of outcomes we have—outcomes that include a greater likelihood of being able to bond with and nurse our babies immediately after birth.

Although their use is rapidly increasing, U.S. midwives attend only 10 percent of births, compared to 80 percent in the rest of the world. This is not in our personal or national best interest. Statistics show that compared to countries in western Europe, as well as Canada, Japan, Australia, and New Zealand, we rank highest in infant mortality, despite spending the most money per capita on maternity and newborn care (Declercq and Viisainen 2001, 274, 277).

Within the United States, the distinction between the *practice* of obstetrics and midwifery is not always clear-cut. Midwives practice in hospitals, birth centers, and homes, settings that greatly influence their ability to provide compassionate, individualized care. Many midwives who work in hospitals struggle to apply their knowledge and skills in domains where medical and technological birth reigns. Others in this setting have become so socialized into the obstetrical model that what they practice is not true midwifery. These challenges are likely to remain as long as midwifery is considered subservient to obstetrics. As Dr. Marsden Wagner, a perinatologist formerly with the World Health Organization, and a specialist in maternity services in industrialized countries, explains: "There is a serious misunderstanding in this country about what midwifery is. Midwifery is not part of obstetrics. It's a completely separate, parallel profession, both of which are essential to good midwifery care" (personal communication, 1996).*

---

* In addition to obstetricians and midwives, about 25 percent of family physicians in the United States provide maternity care, a declining percentage in recent years.

These next couple of stories provide testimony to the quality of care women deserve to help more of us get breastfeeding off to the best start possible.

Petra attributes her smooth introduction to the world of nursing to having given birth at home, where she felt safe and respected. Many women shy away from home births, fearing they are not as safe as birthing in a hospital, where 97 percent of U.S. births take place. Numerous studies in scientific and medical journals, however, conclude that for women considered "low risk," *planned* home births with a *trained attendant* result in equally safe, if not safer, outcomes than physician-attended hospital births (see Goer 1999, 203–7). One needs only to read *Ina May's Guide to Childbirth* (Gaskin 2003) to understand why.

For more information on midwifery or to locate a midwife, contact the Midwives Alliance of North America (MANA) at 888-923-6262 or <http://www.mana.org/>; or the American College of Nurse Midwives (ACNM) at 202-728-9860 or <http://www.acnm.org>.

A RHYTHM ALL ITS OWN

I offered my breast to each of my children within minutes of their births and was amazed at how their little mouths took it. Anthony, my first, was pretty screamy, so while still sitting on the birthing stool, I tickled his mouth with my breast, and he latched on. It was probably not the best positioning, but it stopped him from screaming. He spent the first hour close to my breast, sometimes nursing, sometimes not, and I was amazed at how normal and fluid it seemed. I can't imagine how anxious I would have felt if I had not had him near me, if I had not been in my own home.

Two years later, Eliza, like Anthony, was brought right up to me. She was awake and alert, but so calm that we didn't nurse immediately. "She's obviously dead," I thought, "because babies are supposed to cry when they come

---

Although their practices vary widely, they are typically less interventionist than most obstetricians yet more interventionist than most midwives. Because the obstetrician's patient is the *mother* and the pediatrician's patient is the *baby*, breastfeeding can get lost in the process. By serving the whole family, family physicians potentially bridge this gap in care. "Family physicians provide critical breastfeeding education and support before, during, and after birth," asserts Dr. David Meyers, a family physician affiliated with Georgetown University Medical Center and an outspoken national breastfeeding advocate (personal communication, 2003).

out." At some point I started nursing her, but it was such a natural part of things that I didn't think much about it.

With each child, the midwives checked their Apgars and listened to their heartbeats, but the whole time my babies were in my arms, on my chest. Their exams were done next to me so I could talk to them, hold their hands, or even have them suck on my finger. It was all calm and fluid. I was so pleased that I could maintain that human connection with them in this dry, new world, pleased that my body could continue to comfort them.

In my mind, having a home birth made a huge difference in how we nursed. I didn't have to worry about nurses, doctors, or orderlies coming into my space and distracting me. I didn't have to deal with anyone or anything other than my baby, my midwife, and my husband, with whom I share intimate and trusting relationships. I didn't have to think in terms of protocols and procedures, and I had a sense of being in a protected, sacred environment. This allowed me to do what seemed natural instead of thinking about every detail in a scientific, practical way.

From the start, I felt confident and supported. My midwife and sister would watch me nurse and then make suggestions, pointing out little things that needed slight correction, but they were never patronizing and always gentle. My milk came in about thirty-six hours after giving birth, so neither of my kids dropped a lot of weight. That further built my confidence.

With Anthony I initially lacked discretion and coordination and was topless much of the time. This wasn't a problem with Eliza since I already knew what I was doing.

We nursed a lot lying down. The cradle hold was more difficult for me because you somehow have to support their bodies, hold their heads, and hold your breast. I've often thought it's too bad that we don't grow a second set of arms during pregnancy that would fall off after weaning.

I took to heart what La Leche League says, which is "early and often." Any time my babies seemed remotely interested in nursing and even when they didn't, I would try to nurse them.

Over the next six weeks, I acquired more confidence. Gradually I realized that nursing is not something we learn and do the same way every day. It is more like a dance, constantly changing and moving, with an underlying rhythm all its own.

Petra, Denver, CO

Having a baby at a birth center is another option that facilitates early and successful breastfeeding. As of autumn 2003 there were

160 birth centers, and their numbers have been increasing, albeit slowly (Kate Bauer, executive director of the National Association of Childbearing Centers, personal communication, 2003). The birth center philosophy is in sync with the midwifery model of care and offers a safe alternative for healthy women with normal pregnancies.

For more information on birth centers and how to locate one, contact the National Association of Childbearing Centers (NACC) at 215-234-8068 or visit their Web site at <http://www.birthcenters.org/>.

Vikki gave birth at a free-standing birth center and was home fewer than twelve hours later. Like Petra, she had good follow-up care. Twenty-eight when her daughter was born, she reflects on the commonalties we share with all creatures who nurse their young.

RELATING AS ANIMALS

As a pregnant woman, I felt for the most part quite powerful. For the first time in my life, I felt a raison d'être without angst or confusion. I felt, too, that my breasts were finally going to have a purpose. Sources of life. How I loved that period of time—the anticipation; the space to have philosophical, broad thoughts; not yet being sodden and earthbound by the mundane, wearying, minute-to-minute exercise of mothering.

Breastfeeding was never an intellectual choice for me. It was just the most basic, primal, animal way to be. We were fortunate to have supportive midwives whose entire philosophy and technique is that the baby is given the chance to be on your belly, at your breasts, immediately after birth.

Beginning breastfeeding was not problematic. My sticky-out nipples, of which I was never particularly fond, were well suited for latching on—which is just what Lily did. She was one of those babies who cried ferociously out of the womb and kept crying while lying on my belly, near my breasts. Then, after she calmed down, she discovered my nipples, latched on, and that was that.

Early on we were able to breastfeed lying down so I could be as rested as possible, even doze a bit while she fed. I needed a lot of pillows for support but soon could breastfeed anywhere, even walking around. When I nursed Lily it just seemed right. When she was very tiny, her limbs not yet fattened up, she felt like a newborn monkey, grasping my body, nuzzling my neck when I held her upright, clinging like any tiny infant on any big mama animal. When it worked best, we did not relate as human to human, but as animals.

I remember feeling like a mother pig, lying on my side, Lily suckling at my breast flopped against the bed. This was often time for golden, tender connection. But I also felt like a swollen sow and got tired of myself that way, tired of her pulling at my nipples. Convinced she'd had enough, I would pop her mouth off with my pinky and roll away, conscious of my desire to be comfortable. She'd cry, I'd try to comfort her, she'd breastfeed again, I'd tire of it, and the cycle would begin anew.

Though breastfeeding was easy, I hit one snag when Lily was about three months old. A part of my breast became increasingly tender. It turned out I had a blocked duct, threatening infection.* I was spending a week with a friend, so we went to see her midwife, a vibrant, maternal, British-accented grandmother. Another animal scene. She had me position myself on all fours, my breasts hanging like a cow's udder above Lily's face, and breastfeed there in her office. I was sent home with instructions to orient myself this way so Lily would suck at a certain angle to the blocked duct and basically suck it open. The midwife also suggested two homeopathic potions, plus "the three B's": go to *bed* with the *baby* and a *bottle*—the bottle being beer to relax me and get the milk flowing!

Lily and I ended breastfeeding a little over a year ago. She was seventeen months old, and I was ready to stop. She had become more active, stopping for little bursts of breastfeeding before heading away. And she had developed this exceedingly annoying habit of fondling my breasts, pulling at my nipples, and rubbing and tweaking them. If she had simply sucked for milk, I would have enjoyed it longer.

I really don't miss her as an infant at my breast, in my arms. Yes, we had beautiful moments, but I think also of the grueling boredom of it. Now, at two and a half, she is much more interesting, and our connection seems stronger, more real. Perhaps it is because she made me do the hard work early on, to slow down, learn to take care of her and myself, and learn to accept the mundane chores of meals and the house as being really, truly necessary.

written by Vikki A., Trumansburg, NY

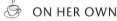 ON HER OWN

My daughter, Jade, quietly slipped into the world in an unassisted, hot-tub home birth. About fifteen minutes later, I lifted her to my right breast. She

---

* Blocked or plugged ducts can occur for various reasons and, as Vikki discovered, are usually easily treatable. If not treated, however, they can lead to mastitis, a breast infection that usually needs to be treated with antibiotics. A good "how-to" book or advice from an experienced board-certified lactation consultant can be of great help.

licked it experimentally. I was nervous and exhausted. But during my pregnancy I had sensed that we would never have problems with breastfeeding. I lowered her back into my lap, and a few minutes later, we tried again. This time she opened her mouth wide and performed what appeared to be a perfect latch. Within a day or two, a friend noticed that her latch could be improved by better positioning her bottom lip to curl out instead of inward. After Jade latched on, I would say "lip" as I untucked her bottom lip. Within a few days she would reposition her lip on her own when I said the cue word "lip." It was one of the many moments of her early days that convinced me that she was so very aware of me and our life.

Bestfeeding: Getting Breastfeeding Right for You, by Mary Renfrew, Chloe Fisher, and Suzanne Arms (1990), contains some of the best photos I've seen of babies latching on correctly and incorrectly.

Diana Greer, San Francisco, CA

Wandering through the Wilderness

Many women who happily nurse for months, if not years, find that the glow of early motherhood is merely a reflection of the night-light burning at three A.M. as we frantically try to figure out what the hell we are doing wrong. While a certain degree of insecurity and angst is to be expected, however, some of us endure far more. Sore nipples, engorgement, nipple-confused babies, and seemingly not enough milk are all common hurdles that with proper support from the beginning could be easily ameliorated, if not prevented.

Along with the impact of birthing practices on breastfeeding, women are often encouraged to breastfeed while applying the principles of bottle-feeding. We may be told, for example, to restrict the number of feedings, feed for short periods of time, encourage nighttime weaning, and offer supplemental bottles of formula. Such advice may create a chain reaction of difficulties. Consider how the common problem of insufficient milk typically develops, for example. The more milk a baby removes from the breast, the more milk a woman produces. When we attempt to nurse at specified intervals, for shorter durations, or offer supplemental bottles of formula, babies suckle less, so our breasts produce less milk. Our babies then become hungry, and we conclude that we don't have enough milk. Voila! "Insufficient Milk Syndrome," a major reason for premature weaning. As lactation consultant Marsha Walker, IBCLC, explains, "Most of it comes from poor breastfeeding management from the start and a poor understanding of a breastfeeding baby's behavior" (personal communication, 1996).

Of course, not all women experience these problems, or breastfeeding rates would be even lower than they are now. But the frequency with which situations like these occur speaks to the degree to which medical mismanagement of breastfeeding contributes to the cultural context of new motherhood. In cultures where breastfeeding is still the norm and one only has to look to one's mother, sister, or neighbor for advice, women may be less vulnerable to medical opinions. In the United States, though, too many of us lack this personal connection to other breastfeeding mothers. And where bottle-feeding remains the norm and the focus is on the birth of a *baby* and not on the birth of a *mother*, we are often left on our own to wander through the wilderness of new motherhood.

It is perhaps not surprising, then, that Cindy Turner-Maffei, national coordinator of Baby Friendly USA, an organization that implements UNICEF's Baby Friendly Hospital Initiative in the United States, points out that the majority of breastfeeding stories we hear tend to center around pain, inadequacy, or embarrassment, hardly themes that make breastfeeding seem desirable (Turner-Maffei 2002). But to pretend that nursing comes easily to all of us does a similar disservice. As Jennifer, a new mother, wrote: "Where were the stories that could have prepared me for this ordeal? Everyone had told me their labor stories, so I knew my labor, while difficult, was 'normal.' But my friends hadn't told me their nursing troubles because they said if I knew how hard it could be sometimes, I'd never have tried. Yet more stories would have kept me from feeling so alone in my journey."

This next group of stories comes from women, like Jennifer, who had a rough time at the beginning. Their stories (almost all of which involve nursing their only or firstborn children) reveal a true sense of wandering into uncharted terrain with no map, compass, or AAA hotline to call. Yet somehow they found their way. Their stories are proof that the benefits and rewards of nursing may not always be evident right away.

In Their Own Words:
Wandering through the Wilderness

The next two stories emphasize the need for good postpartum support, both in the hospital or birth center and after we are back home. Ann, an artist and mother of three, describes several weeks of nursing hell until a lactation consultant finally showed her how to position her baby at the breast. A technical adjustment was all she really needed.

☕ MY LITTLE BARRACUDA

My oldest child was born on Friday the 13th. That was my first clue. She came into the world kicking and screaming, welcomed by two parents who couldn't have been more happy to see her. After checking her fingers and toes, I looked at the nurse and said, "What do I do now?" She informed me that we were going to breastfeed. "We are?" I said in disbelief. My daughter latched on with little assistance, and the nurse gave me the thumbs-up.

"You two make a perfect team!" she gushed.

I was so proud—obviously it was due to the classes I had taken prenatally. I became confident and secure.

Then came the fourth feeding in the early hours of the morning. I was alone in my hospital bed, and my darling daughter wanted to be fed. OUCH!!! When had she grown teeth? It felt like a staple gun on my nipple. OUCH!! No one said that it would hurt like this! In fact, I distinctly remember them telling me that if it hurt *at all* I was doing it wrong! My confidence was withering on the proverbial vine.

I have no clear memory of the eight weeks that followed. Snippets appear like a bad dream. I reached out to many different people and publications and received as many different answers as I asked for. I remember talking to the local La Leche League leader on the phone and wanting her to hang up and come over immediately to personally stuff my "entire areola" into this child's mouth, but I was too shy to ask.

According to *The Womanly Art of Breastfeeding,* my daughter was labeled a "barracuda." But barracudas have teeth—sharp ones. I recall the public health nurse calling to check up on me. She scared the hell out of me when I admitted to having a blister and a crack. "You'll get mastitis if you're not careful," she warned. My husband watched supportively as I cringed and curled my toes while latching her on to my torn and tattered nipple.

In a last-ditch effort I called the lactation consultant at the hospital where my daughter was born. I was convinced she was the only adult woman in the world who hadn't heard my tale of woe. She told me I needed to see her immediately, and I began to cry with relief when she offered to help me firsthand. I packed up the baby, my two-ton diaper bag (since she was my first baby I needed to carry everything I owned with me), and my fatigued postpartum body and headed back to the hospital in the cold Minnesota January. I broke into a sweat under my heavy winter coat as I toted all my accoutrements back to the hospital nursery and got plenty of strange looks from passersby. My paranoid, sleep-deprived mind was convinced they were whispering: "Look! She's returning her baby. What a shame."

Somehow I made it to the lactation consultant's office. I took off layer upon layer and had her, literally, stuff my breast in my daughter's mouth. It didn't hurt. What? It didn't hurt!!! This was great! All I had to do now was heal the wound on my left nipple and learn a slightly different "attack" from that described in the books. I found that "sandwiching" my nipple with a finger above and below the areola instead of on each side allowed me to get more of it in her mouth.

I was home free! I sat in front of a bare lightbulb three times a day to heal that nipple. I wore Madonna-esque nipple shields to allow air to the sore area. I went to lengths that astound me now, and I have no idea where my resolve or stamina came from. But ultimately my daughter and I went on to nurse successfully and blissfully for twelve more months.

Since then I've had two more daughters and nursed them for nearly seventeen months each. My nipples got sore, but I found that going braless to allow air to circulate around the sore nipple helped facilitate healing before any real damage occurred. This, coupled with the latch-on technique I learned from the lactation consultant, helped me to avoid serious problems.

Breastfeeding is the most natural way to feed your baby? Most certainly —but it's important to attach the words, "It doesn't always come naturally."
Written by Ann Allen, Rochester, MN

Latha's story is somewhat long, but the details she provides let us into the private travails of a new mother, particularly one without a partner in parenthood. Because she was a graduate student with no family in this country, much of what she and her baby endured could likely have been prevented had she been given proper support and information from the beginning and not been subjected to a nurse who undermined her self-confidence.

☕ SURVIVING THE BATTLEFIELD

Just now I nursed my two-month-old baby, Viyan, to sleep. I enjoy breast-feeding him, the bonding, the overpowering feeling of love, a sense of accomplishment that my body can provide for him. And these days he looks up at me while nursing with a look of complete adoration that melts my heart. All this was not so in the beginning, however. Until a few weeks ago, breastfeeding was a battlefield.

Having grown up and lived all my life in India (until two years ago when I moved to the United States), I did not even think breastfeeding could have an alternative, so when my midwife asked me whether I planned to or not, I couldn't understand why someone would even ask that kind of question. When I heard about lactation consultants, I almost laughed out loud and thought, "Boy, this can happen only in America. Only here could they professionalize what is natural."

My baby breastfed immediately. He seemed to be doing okay, but that first night, the nurse aggressively pressured me to give him formula. She also offered to take him to the nursery so I could rest. I declined both offers, but she started saying things like, "If you don't feed the baby with formula, he is going to be dehydrated, and I'll have to put him in the intensive care unit with an IV." Finally I told her that if she thought formula was absolutely necessary, I would like to feed it to him myself. I didn't want to be parted from my baby, even for a couple of hours. She turned angry and more aggressive, telling me that my nipples were flat and I would never be able to breastfeed. The first night passed like this, in a series of altercations, but my baby did spend most of the time nursing with me.

This kind of attack continued through the second day, and I was so exhausted from fighting with the nurses that I couldn't pay much attention to what the lactation consultant was trying to teach me that evening. Again that night the nurse told me he was not latching on properly and would be dehydrated, but she never told me that mother's milk does not come in until about three days after birth.

I was home with the baby on the third day. But because the nurses had convinced me that his latch was not proper, I was convinced that I had to teach him. I started to pull my nipple out of his mouth every time he tried to latch on, and that night my baby began a nursing strike. He screamed, mad with hunger but unwilling to try to nurse. The following morning my breasts were engorged and rock hard and my nipples were flat, and he couldn't grab them at all. By now, I was a basket case, haunted by the image of my baby being given an IV, and he really *had* started to become dehydrated by then. My self-esteem and confidence took a real hit.

My friend Sandy, a breastfeeding mom to a sixteen-month-old, saw my pathetic condition and suggested that someone stay with me that night. I phoned my friend Nigel, and he agreed. Looking at him that evening, I didn't know whether to laugh or cry. He had brought some beer, a laptop computer, and a sleeping bag. I realized he had no idea what babies entailed, let alone a five-day-old, but I asked him to hold the baby for a couple of hours so I could take a much-needed nap. After a three-hour reprieve, though, the night was torturous, baby and me crying out of frustration, hunger, and anger.

The next day, Sandy generously offered to wet-nurse Viyan. I accepted, she nursed him, and he seemed to latch on okay. While I was grateful, I also felt personally rejected. My baby was willing to nurse with her but not with me! That same day both Sandy and another friend, Isabel, offered to pump milk for me, and I fed him with a medicine dropper.

That night, I hesitantly asked Mauricio, Isabel's husband, to stay with me for a few hours. Mauricio picked out some tips from *Dr. Sears' Breastfeeding Book* and coached me on different ways to try to latch him on. That book described the mechanics of the breastfeeding process, helped me know how it functions, and told me how I could best try to boost my supply.

By now, the baby was completely dehydrated. When I put my pinkie in his mouth for him to suck, there was almost no saliva at all, he was not getting wet diapers, the spot on his head had gone deeper, and I was scared beyond belief. I tried to schedule an appointment with a lactation consultant but couldn't get one until Sunday afternoon.

Although I was feeling guilty and ashamed, the visit went well. She suggested I rent a hospital-grade breast pump to boost my supply and use the milk to feed my baby. She also suggested herbal teas to enhance my supply and taught me to finger-feed using a syringe and the preemie tube. Each suck would reward him with some milk, unlike the medicine dropper where he was more like a little bird. I came home with the pump and set it on the table where my laptop computer usually sat.

From then on, every two hours, I would try to nurse him, then pump, feed him with the pumped milk—mine and my friends'—and then try to nurse him again. This whole gig would take about an hour, and then in a couple of hours we would repeat it. I remember once being so exhausted while pumping that I didn't know I wasn't holding the bottles properly and all the milk I had pumped spilled on the floor! I started bawling. Not only did I not have the milk, but I also had a whole mess to clean up! Though I followed this routine religiously for a couple of days, I was only pumping about an ounce at a time, and the hardest thing was my dependence on others for milk.

I was exhausted. If somebody didn't bring me food, I had nothing to eat, and I couldn't bear to look around me—clothes, diapers, a couple of breast pumps, bottles, syringes, tubes, books, plants, papers, the works. I couldn't even take a shower unless someone came in for an hour or so. How could supposedly the most beautiful time of my life be so horrible?

On the seventh day, Sandy posted an e-mail on a Web site called YAAPS describing my situation. We received some great suggestions like massaging the breast to assist the letdown and pumping the breast for a couple of minutes before trying to nurse. More than anything, those who wrote gave me encouragement to hang in there and not give up, without making me feel that I would be committing a crime by giving formula.

YAAPS, Yet Another Alternative Parenting Site, can be found at <http://www.yaaps.com>. Among the many subjects discussed on the site are breastfeeding and home birthing.

Their suggestions helped immensely, but in the meanwhile, the milk supply of my friends dropped dramatically. Between that and my supply of eight or ten ounces, he was still not getting enough, and I was going crazy with anxiety, shame, guilt, and fear.

I started to consider supplementing with formula but was getting strong negative messages about this from Mauricio and Isabel. I found it hard to counter the resistance but ultimately decided that my baby needed nourishment. Besides, how could a baby who was dehydrated, hungry, and irritable learn to nurse?

I asked Sandy to bring me some formula and herbal tea, and I started supplementing. With this decision, my anxiety level came down drastically. It suddenly dawned on me that Viyan need not starve. Once his intake increased, he pooped. I did a victory dance around my apartment and called all my friends to inform them of this good news. He pooped!

During this time, I kept my upper body uncovered a lot so Viyan could get a lot of skin-to-skin contact. I held him most of the day and night, and he slept on top of me. Slowly I began to enjoy being with him, holding him, cleaning him, singing to him, even finger-feeding him, and we started building a relationship.

The following Monday we visited the pediatrician for his first checkup. I felt like my performance was going to be judged and the doctor would pronounce a verdict on my "fitness for being a mom." It turned out that Viyan had gained weight and grown in length. The doctor, a warm resident, sensed my anxiety and told me that I was a super mom and had taken care of him well. She was supportive of our current feeding process and asked me to keep trying to breastfeed. I felt reaffirmed and less anxious.

I started to lactate more, and over the next couple of days we transitioned completely to my breast. Although I continued to be anxious, things gradually started getting better. Then suddenly, I started to worry about the coming semester. How was I going to manage the baby, school, and work in the fall? As my anxiety grew, my milk supply fell. I headed back to Dr. Sears, read about visualization techniques, and from then on, every two hours, it was not enough to do everything unthinkingly, but I also had to visualize flowing milk. I also restarted meditating, which helped me reduce anxiety.

But my nipples were killing me. Viyan had learned to suck well on my finger for two weeks, but my nipples were not used to it. It took me weeks to get used to his strong suction. And with growth spurts happening every so often, I felt like he was at my breast day and night. I didn't know if I should be happy that he finally took to my breasts or complain about the fact that he seemed to be addicted to them.

Over the next couple of weeks, we mastered the art and negotiated a working nursing relationship. I cannot begin to describe my pride when I could squirt milk out in jets and not in drops. I had seen Sandy and Isabel do that, so it seemed like the sign of breastfeeding success. Leaky breasts became another badge of breastfeeding. I still thrill when I see milk leaking out of the corners of Viyan's mouth when he nurses.

I discovered that breastfeeding is a mind game and as long as I *believed* I could breastfeed, I could. I also realized that if I hadn't had the humility to ask my friends for help, I wouldn't have received it. In India, it is etiquette to say "No" with the fullest confidence you will get all the help you need, regardless, but in the United States I learned that people appreciate specific requests. So when friends called to ask if I wanted something, I learned to say, "Please bring me some food," or "Can you spend a couple of hours with me today?" so they do not end up bringing a nice card, balloons, and flowers instead.

And I learned that no one knows my baby as well as I. While I did ask for suggestions and support from others, I did what I felt was best, and that's what ultimately helped me focus and build a breastfeeding relationship with my baby.

Written by Latha Poonamallee, Cleveland Heights, OH

Cheli has two children: Brandon, eight, and Alexandra, two. Although she nursed Brandon for three years and was still nursing Alexandra when we spoke (see pages 203–4), her story has a rather unusual beginning. It emerges from the misconceptions that surround nursing and the false assumption that nursing is necessarily painful.

☕ RECONSTRUCTING A LIFE

I'm an only child and knew nothing about babies. My husband's sister has two children and had told me, "Nursing hurts." A friend in New York, an attorney with one child, had said, "Nursing hurts." Everyone told me it was painful and not worth it. But because I wanted my child to get the best nutrition, I was determined to find a way to get breast milk to him without causing undue pain to myself. I decided I would pump and put the milk into bottles. We went to a medical supply store before Brandon's birth and rented a Medela breast pump. And I pumped my breast milk for the first six weeks of Brandon's life because I was so convinced that nursing would hurt.

Because of my husband's job we had recently relocated to Maryland. My husband was at work all day, and I was home, alone with the baby in a new city, in a neighborhood that seemed to empty out during the day. I was spending the entire day pumping milk, feeding him, changing him, burping him, and then it was time for the next round. For almost two months, I was involved in some mode of feeding him for eight hours a day. Aside from my husband, I had no support, and that period of my life was pretty pitiful.

I was also so exhausted, and my child wasn't sleeping. We had borrowed a bassinet, but he wouldn't sleep in it, so we were up all night, pumping and feeding, pumping and feeding. After two months, if not more, of that foggy, foggy period, my husband said, "Can you just bring the baby to bed with us? Then maybe we could get some rest."

So I did. And the baby was next to me and the breast was there and I said, "Okay, let's just give it a try—it can't be that bad," and lo and behold, it didn't hurt at all! Not at all. And although it was almost three months before I started weaning myself off of the breast pump, that was the beginning of my nursing story.

But it was still a lonely time for me. It was the first fall without me being in school or working full-time. My focus was on adjusting from being a full-time career woman to being an at-home mom. By the time I felt together enough to venture out and find people to connect with, it was winter—cold, snowy, and windy—and the parks were empty. I didn't yet feel comfortable nursing in public and was pretty much homebound. We started going to a church, and I tried some Mommy and Me classes and other groups, but I never felt like I connected with any of the women and none were particularly welcoming. I would comb the local newspapers, trying to find a group of women who met during the day.

When Brandon was about nine months old, I saw an ad for La Leche League stating that they met on Thursday mornings. "Oh my God," I thought. "They're home during the day!" Nursing was going fine, but I thought they must be at-home moms and they must be supportive of nursing. I called, got directions, and went.

That was basically when my life as a mother began. They were wonderful women, warm and welcoming, and they became my friends. They were there, they gave me a voice, they were my lifeline. And I am eternally grateful.

Cheli English-Figaro, Bowie, MD

Living in Our Bodies

Breastfeeding, as a physical phenomenon, affects women differently. Here are a few anecdotes that speak to the embodied nature of providing milk.

For the first week or so, I had fairly strong, somewhat painful contractions when my milk would let down, but they only lasted for fifteen seconds or so. After that, I'd feel the letdown as a sort of tingling fullness in my breast. If it had been a long time since I nursed and my breasts were especially full, it would sometimes be kind of painful. Having full breasts, when you feel like you really need to nurse a baby, is a weird feeling. It's sort of like having to go to the bathroom. You can't describe what having a full bladder feels like, but when you feel it, you know that you need to go!

Marie des Jardins, Menlo Park, CA

I eat like I'm in football camp! Nursing's been great! I don't remember eating this much when I was pregnant. I do a little exercise but not nearly as much as I did when I was pregnant, and I dropped back to ten or

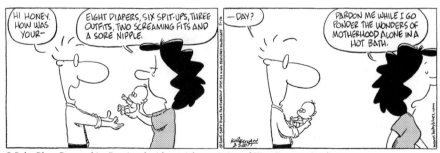

© Baby Blues Partnership. Reprinted with special permission of King Features Syndicate.

twelve pounds below my pre-pregnancy weight within two weeks after giving birth. Nursing helped me drop the weight so fast. In fact, the midwife in my practice wanted me to add another five hundred calories to my diet when I talked to her on the phone before my six-week appointment. I shudder to think of what I'll do when Katie eventually weans!

Stephanie Weishaar, Camp Hill, PA

❍

I had large breasts before I nursed, but not this big. I have to wear two bras to run because they support me in different ways. One is a sports bra with an underwire, but the straps are not strong enough to support me, and the other one fits flat and holds me in place. It's a pain looking for two different sports bras, but at least this way I can run.

Allegra Azulay, Pflugerville, TX

❍

Within forty-eight hours of returning home from the hospital, my milk was dripping out of me, just gushing. I was walking around with only underpants on—to me that was fully dressed—and my two dachshunds would follow, licking the floor behind me. Sometimes my milk would fall on their foreheads, and they would lick each other. It was hilarious! They weren't allowed on the bed, though, even though they would have loved it!

Gwen Shook, Jersey City, NJ

Special Circumstances

Nursing a baby can sometimes draw on our deepest sources of determination, resilience, and tenacity. In *Breastfeeding Special Care Babies,* author Sandra Lang (1997, 15) outlines some of the conditions that may affect a baby's ability to nurse properly. Among them are a cleft lip and/or palate; a short frenulum to the tongue (being tongue-tied); and a small mouth and poor muscle tone, features of some babies with Down syndrome. Babies who are born with certain neurological, respiratory, and cardiac problems may also experience feeding problems. Moreover, separation of mother and child, such as when the baby has to be transported to a different hospital while the mother is recovering from a C-section, clearly makes breastfeeding more challenging.

Other women are blessed with healthy babies but simply have more than one of them! Multiple births are increasing, in fact, due to an increase in the use of fertility drugs and babies born with the help of other assisted reproductive technologies. In such situations, where breast milk may be even more crucial to a baby's well-being, information and support are more important than ever.

There isn't room to include the wide variety of stories that could fit into this section. But the few that follow clearly illustrate the determination and commitment women have to nurse in the midst of especially challenging situations. (Women may also have illnesses or physical circumstances that complicate nursing. These stories appear in chapter 5.)

In Their Own Words:
Special Circumstances

Michelle's story sheds light on the challenges of breastfeeding preemies. Michelle gave birth four weeks early to a six-pound, eight-ounce daughter who did not have a sucking reflex. As challenging as her introduction to motherhood seems, see her story on pages 101–3 to understand why it was all worth it.

BREASTFEEDING A PREEMIE

I gave birth in a large hospital near Seattle, recently given "Baby Friendly" status. But even though the hospital has one of the country's best lactation departments, the nurses in the NICU were not as knowledgeable about breastfeeding as I had hoped. For the first two days, they would often get out a bottle of formula before asking me or checking in the special refrigerator for mother's milk to see if I had any to be used to gavage-feed (tube-feed) my daughter. I had to remind them continually that I had milk. It was only after I had pumped enough for twins and the lactation consultant on call made a big deal about the amount I had that the nurses got the clue. By the last two days of our stay there, they would ring my boarding room every three to four hours or when Taylor woke up, so I could keep trying to establish breastfeeding.

My husband and I quickly began a ritual that went something like this: wake our daughter, change her diaper, and attempt to nurse at the breast. I would then begin to pump, and she was gavage-fed. (A nurse would lay Taylor on her back, fill a two- or three-ounce-size syringe with my breast milk, and attach a long thin tube. This tube was then, as gently as possible, put down Taylor's throat, and gravity drained my milk into her stomach.) After the first full day of this, her voice turned hoarse. Then she lost it entirely, and we could not even hear her cry. I'm sure it must have hurt badly. Even today, four and a half years later, I am almost moved to tears recounting our days in the hospital.

After Taylor was fed, I would hold her for what seemed like several hours, catch a bite to eat or a wink of sleep, then be ready to start all over again. We did this every four hours around the clock. It seemed hopeless some days, especially in the wee hours of the morning.

I became obsessive, counting each and every sucking motion she made. At first she only sucked at my breast five or ten times at a session, but hour by hour, day by day, she became stronger. Soon we began to finger-feed her, using the supplemental nursing system. My husband soon joked that his pinkie had become engorged from feeding her.

Mama Kangaroos

Skin-to-skin contact is one of the best things we can do when our babies are born prematurely. In a practice known as kangaroo care, a baby wearing only a diaper and a head cap—even with tubes and wires attached to its body—is placed on the parent's chest. The baby's head is turned to the side so it can hear the parent's heartbeat.

The idea of kangaroo care first gained attention in 1983 when two neonatologists in Bogotá, Colombia, sought to reduce the high mortality rates among locally born premature babies. Once mothers began to wear their preemies in slings all day the mortality rate fell from 70 to 30 percent. Over sixty studies have since documented the benefits of such care—everything from weight gain, growth, motor development, and relaxation, to increased likelihood of breastfeeding (Luddington-Hoe and Golant 1993, 9). In the United States fewer than 10 percent of mothers of preemies breastfeed, yet according to some studies, between 25 and 50 percent more kangaroo care mothers are able to breastfeed beyond six weeks after discharge (Luddington-Hoe and Golant 1993, 131–32).

An excellent resource is Kangaroo Care: The Best You Can Do to Help Your Preterm Infant, *by Susan M. Luddington-Hoe and Susan K. Golant (1993).*

We were sleep deprived, emotionally drained, and constantly worried about whether our baby would *ever* nurse! The hours and days dragged by. It was such a strange feeling, like the clock was spinning fast, the hours and days were passing, yet each moment was the same.

I tried to keep strong. I knew I had to keep my milk production up, get enough rest, and eat enough calories so my baby and I could go home. There were times, though, when those postpartum hormones and emotions flooded my entire body. When Taylor was five and six days old she was placed in an incubator to help get the jaundice under control (which I later learned was never that bad in the first place). Now I couldn't even hold her.

And I felt like I always had to keep on top of the nurses to make sure they were feeding her my milk instead of formula. Those were the worst two days. "When will we ever be able to leave the hospital?" I wondered.

As the days passed, my daughter began to suck more and more at my breast, and soon she was nursing mostly from me. Then came the day that I got to use the SNS, the supplemental nursing system. It felt like such a big step! Now I would do all the feeding, however artificial it was.*

We continued to use the SNS for two more days and then found ourselves finished with all of the apparatuses and artificiality. I felt like I had just trained for and run a marathon in a week's time and come across the finish line winning the race! I loved looking down at my daughter's beautiful face, and seeing no artificial plastics, tape, tubes, etc., was such joy! It was strange, though. Without having to use all the external devices, I felt a bit naked, like I was missing something. But I also felt a sense of freedom, and the contrast was dramatic.

When my daughter was a week old, we were released from the hospital.+ This may not seem like a long time, but it felt like an eternity to me! Once home we still had to wake her every three to four hours, but we were so much more comfortable. We were finally without nurses, doctors, other moms, and sicker infants around twenty-four hours a day. No machines and beeping sounds, stale smells, and cool temperature. The three of us felt more relaxed, and we could now sleep together in our comfortable bed and be alone, together, twenty-four hours a day!

Our nursing experience was pretty typical after this. Finally I felt like the other moms I had met at the hospital's parent/baby-group weekly meetings.

Michelle Miller, Kirkland, WA

The next two stories are about nursing twins. Jackie not only had to learn how to nurse twins but did so while recovering from a

---

* Michelle is referring to a device sometimes used to transition babies to the breast. One end of the SNS consists of a bag or bottle filled with formula or breast milk and has a tiny tube that runs out of it. This tube is taped to the breast, against the nipple, and while sucking at the breast, the baby gets supplemental milk through the tube. This stimulus of the baby sucking at the breast helps to encourage milk production and enables babies to be fed without resorting to bottles, since the use of bottles greatly increases the likelihood of babies having difficulty nursing from the breast.

+ In one sense, Michelle was actually lucky. In most hospitals she would have been discharged after two days with a vaginal birth and after four days with a C-section.

vaginal birth *and* a C-section. Nursing went well in the hospital (with her adjustable bed, painkillers, and nurses on call), but then she left the hospital . . .

 ## ME AND THE BIG BLUE U

Outside the protective bubble of the hospital a brand-new world waited for us. I never had enough pillows, and my husband kept bringing me these screaming, insatiable little beasts with red faces and gaping mouths. What's more, without the Percocet there was a lot more pain involved in all that gnashing and sucking. And the chewing! For all the gumming they were doing, you would think I was candy-coated. At the same time, the girls had gotten accustomed to a horrible style of latching on when I was on painkillers, and soon I learned the exquisite pain of nipple blisters, after the throbbing pain of engorgement had passed. My breasts ballooned from a pregnancy 36C to a 38DD. All my convictions about breastfeeding disappeared like new snow, and I no longer knew if I wanted to breastfeed at all. In fact, I was pretty sure I would never want anyone to touch my breasts again.

Two things convinced me to keep going. First, we could not afford formula for two babies. Second, my husband remained staunch and stalwart, refusing to give up the fight. He brought me water and food, often feeding me himself over their writhing little bodies. Late at night, he held my head and comforted me as I sobbed through another feeding, telling me about all the wonderful benefits I was giving our little girls. He listened as I ranted and raved about all the horrible people who had never told me it would be this hard, as I swore that tomorrow I was giving up. He nodded and wrote down La Leche League meeting times. As I lay half asleep, babies suckling voraciously, he downloaded songs off the Internet from my high school days and sang them, often with accompanying dances, to keep my spirits up. He would do anything to mitigate the situation, but I was still saying darkly, "Two months. And that's if I make it that long."

Then he found the big blue U.

The big blue U is my nursing pillow, one made especially for twins. It is made out of foam, with a removable zippered cover made out of blue fabric. When I strap it on behind my back, the "arms" of the U are on either side of me, with the bottom forming a shelf across my mid-section. The side of the pillow that faces up is angled so that the babies nestle close to me on either side, their heads in perfect eating position.

Once I got my U, nursing was a whole new ball game, and I finally had a chance. First, I no longer needed to barricade myself with mounds of pillows that constantly shifted whenever the babies moved. This had been especially inconvenient, because we live in a Southern city and didn't get an air-conditioner unit in the bedroom until mid-July. Try covering yourself with pillows when it is 95 degrees and 80 percent humidity. Then press two fleshy little heaters against either side of you for about fifteen hours a day, and you'll begin to know how I felt. But with my beautiful blue pillow, I only needed pillows propped behind me. Second, my hands were suddenly free. Of course, my daughters still had latching issues, so many minutes were spent prying apart their little jaws when they tried to nibble on my nipple, but I didn't have to hold them up anymore. Never very athletic or fit, I simply didn't have that kind of upper-body strength. With the U, however, I didn't need it.

Keeping me and the babies naked most of the time guaranteed us plenty of skin-to-skin bonding, but suddenly I could do things like drink from a glass without using a straw or eat a sandwich with my own hands. Sure, I often looked down to see crumbs scattered through my daughters' black hair, but they were too busy to ever notice. Plus, my free hands allowed me plenty of opportunities to rub their backs, tickle their feet, stroke their foreheads, and run my hands through their hair. Twice the babies means twice the cuteness, and I loved being able to touch my little girls so much, now that I wasn't supporting them with my hands.

The drawback is that the big blue U is anything but portable or inconspicuous. I can throw it in the trunk of the car to go to my mother's house but cannot fold it up and take it into a mall. What it lacks in ease of travel, though, it makes up for in conversation. My aunt wishes she had one when her twins were babies. My mother-in-law took pictures to send to her mother in El Salvador. My father is in awe of it as a feat of engineering, which I think is also a helpful way for him to avoid having to see my nipples pop in and out of my daughters' mouths. He needed something else to focus on, and the big blue U was happy to oblige.

My daughters are three months old now. The blue cover has been pooped on, peed on, spit up on, and dribbled on. Many assorted crumbs, especially of the potato chip variety, have littered its surface. I haven't cried while nursing in weeks, and I don't think I ever will again. My girls still nestle close to me, small fat fists on either side of their mouths, eyes slowly dropping shut, cheeks pillowed on the blue fabric they have come to know so well. Sometimes I catch them holding hands across my stomach, eyes shut tight, nipples slowly falling out of their mouths. I don't know how much longer I will nurse, but I am glad to the bottom of my heart that I did not give up. The images that stand out most in my mind are no longer those of tears and pain and desperation, but rather of the hours I spend staring at my daughters. I am cherishing the time we spend, me and my girls, me drinking them in as greedily as they drink from me.

Written by Jacqueline Regales, Baltimore, MD

Renée co-parents with her longtime partner, Lori. Having conceived through artificial insemination, they eagerly anticipated their babies' births and read up on breastfeeding ahead of time. Renée writes about the challenges she faced getting one of her twins to nurse.

☕ BUILDING AND REBUILDING A NURSING RELATIONSHIP

My earliest recollection of breastfeeding is lifting my shirt to feed my dollies while my mom fed my new baby sister. I was four years old and having fun imitating Mommy, who breastfed all three of her daughters. Years later, as I thought about feeding my newborn, I couldn't imagine using a bottle. And when I learned I was having twins, my convictions never wavered. Two babies, two breasts. It seemed perfectly logical.

After a blessedly uneventful pregnancy, I delivered on my due date. Katherine "Kate" and her sister, Lorin, were both healthy, perfect babies. Kate weighed 7.3 pounds, and Lorin weighed 6.4 pounds. We were blessed beyond comprehension. I kept thinking of that line from a song in *The Sound of Music:* "Somewhere in my youth or childhood, I must have done something good."

One of the night nurses helped me with the girls' first latch, and I breastfed both of them several times throughout the night. The next morning, the pediatrician pronounced them healthy, signed their release papers, and we left the hospital eighteen hours after they were born.

Once at home, I continued to nurse Kate, who was awake much of the day, but Lorin fell asleep, and we did not wake her to nurse—our first mistake. She finally woke up screaming around midnight, obviously starving. I tried to get her to latch on, but she was too frantic to cooperate. In a moment of panic, I broke open a sample bottle of formula I had received from the hospital. She sucked down four ounces and proceeded to vomit it right back up. I spent the rest of the night trying to get her to latch on while rocking her and trying to soothe her upset stomach.

Around midmorning the next day, our doula stopped by for a visit. Lorin was acting listless, and I knew she needed to eat soon or we'd be on our way back to the hospital. Our doula showed me how to put together a breast pump I had previously purchased and helped me express about a tablespoon of colostrum. Since Lorin was having trouble latching on, we spoonfed her the nutrients, and within thirty minutes she was acting much more alert.

Crisis averted, I focused on nursing each baby every one and a half to two hours, even if it meant waking them up. I also continued pumping for Lorin to ensure she was getting enough. Between nursing both babies and pumping when one of them wasn't nursing, I had very little time to do anything else.

By the time they were a week old, sleep deprivation was catching up with me. But after the horror of watching both babies regurgitate formula when they were just over a day old (we fed four ounces to Kate that first night as well), both Lori and I were more committed than ever to making breastfeeding work. Kate was nursing well, but my nipples were sore, and Lorin was taking more and more breast milk from a bottle and less from me. I started to contemplate seeking help from a lactation consultant.

In answer to my prayers, the hospital where I delivered had a woman working on becoming certified. As part of the process, she needed to work with mothers of multiples. I had spoken with her briefly before the girls were born, so I gave her a call. When they were eight days old, she came to our house so I wouldn't have to take the girls out. She charged us nothing and gave me invaluable assistance, like showing me how to ensure the girls were not *nipple*-feeding, but *breast*feeding. The distinction was slight but made a huge difference. She also showed me how to nurse the babies simultaneously since feeding them independently was taking an extraordinary amount of time. To this day, whenever I recall her kindness, I am overwhelmed.

After she left, nursing improved. Kate, a champion nurser before, was now a pro. Lorin, however, still required more monitoring. As a result, I was unable to nurse them simultaneously. And when one was done, it was impossible to burp her while keeping the other one attached. I also found that when I nursed them simultaneously, I missed bonding with either of them. It felt more like a rote, perfunctory task, rather than sharing special time with my babies. So I continued to nurse them independently regardless of the fact that I had almost no time to accomplish other tasks.

On their four-week birthday I awakened in the morning with a dull pain in my right breast, and two hours later, it was on fire. With the exception of back labor, I have never known such excruciating pain. I consulted several breastfeeding books and called my sister-in-law, a La Leche League leader, to confirm what I already suspected; I had a plugged duct.

I followed my sister-in-law's advice and nursed both babies on the affected breast as much as I could. We also stayed home so I could rest, and by midafternoon Lorin's latch finally released the pressure. Unfortunately, this would not be the only plugged duct I suffered. Over the next nine weeks, I endured at least one a week, which was enormously frustrating. I probably would have continued to have them if it weren't for finally attending a breastfeeding support-group meeting when the twins were thirteen weeks old. I learned that when I was pumping, I was pressing the cup of the pump too firmly against my breast, thereby cutting off several ducts. That information alone made all the hassle of getting two babies dressed, into car seats, and out of the house by myself more than worth the effort.

Looking back, I wish I had made the effort to attend the support group long before I did as it probably would have helped to alleviate many of the problems and frustrations I endured. Alone in our house, though, I was immersed in our manic routine. Whenever Lorin stopped nursing, I always tried to latch her back on, but once she became inconsolable, the only thing that calmed her was a bottle. And since I was determined not to give her formula, I continued using my hand pump. I determined that whoever came up with the saying "Don't cry over spilt milk" must have been a nursing mom who'd just spent twenty minutes pumping two ounces only to tip the bottle as she was trying to attach the nipple. That was definitely one of my lowest days.

Shortly thereafter, I caved. It was a Wednesday morning when Lorin was just over six weeks old, and I hadn't had any time to pump. Lorin became hysterical after nursing, so I went to the cupboard to retrieve a can of soy formula we'd received in the mail. I made four ounces, which she consumed with gusto and promptly fell asleep. It was a moment of both success and failure. I couldn't believe I was having to use formula, and at the same time, if it was going to give me some relief from doing nothing but sitting on the couch with either a baby or a breast pump attached to me, I was willing to do it—for the time being.

Over the next ten weeks, Kate continued to be exclusively breastfed while Lorin got about 50 percent of her nutrients from the breast. This was impacting me in two ways. First, I found myself feeling closer to Kate. She was starting to interact with me when nursing, stopping to give me a smile or "talk" while she was drinking. Lorin seemed to view me as a means to an end. And because she was taking a bottle, other people could feed her, which meant I wasn't getting to spend as much time with her. Second, I firmly believe breastfed babies are healthier, with both short- and long-term ramifications, and I had no intention of experimenting with mine. I had never reconciled feeding Lorin formula, so I took several steps in an effort to rebuild our nursing relationship.

First, I got a double-action breast pump with a motor. Expensive but worth every penny. I believe if I'd had one from the beginning, Lorin would not have needed formula for ten weeks. Second, I renewed my commitment to breastfeed her. While this may sound simple, it was actually one of the most difficult things I've ever done, and it remains one of my proudest accomplishments. Because Lorin had been getting so many bottles, she had become quite lazy at the breast. In order to maintain my patience, I would pretend that she and I were leading a breastfeeding class of new mothers and needed to show everyone how it was done. It sounds silly, but it helped me to maintain my sanity. After only a few days, I saw great improvement. And by the end of the first week, she was getting less than half the amount of formula as before.

For more information on nursing more than one, see Mothering Multiples: Breastfeeding and Caring for Twins or More, *by Karen Kerkhoff Gromada (1999).*

By the time she was sixteen weeks old, she was nursing beautifully, and on her four-month birthday, one week later, she was formula free. I nursed her exclusively for another month until we started solids on their five-month birthday. And I will never forget the first time Lorin stopped nursing simply to give me a smile before she resumed. It was one of the magical Mommy moments that no one tells you will flood your heart with such love you think you may burst from the sheer force of the swell.

The girls are now one week away from their sixteen-month birthday, and I am still nursing. But I don't spend nearly as much time at it as I used to, and it's much easier. My biggest challenge now is ensuring they don't pull each other's hair when their busy little hands are looking for something to do.

As I type this, I am sitting in my home office, where I have a picture of myself hanging on the wall. I am five years old, sitting with my legs crossed, intently nursing one of my dollies. I've flanked it with similar pictures taken twenty-eight years later, nursing each of my daughters. The only difference is that my face, while still perhaps a bit intent, also radiates the true joyfulness that only motherhood can impart.

Written by Renée Rocheleau, Peoria, AZ

When I started nursing in the mid-1990s, I had never heard of mothers breastfeeding adopted babies. Since then, I have learned that not only is it possible, but it is becoming increasingly common.

Traditionally, the typical way to induce lactation is to start pumping ahead of time to massage the breast and stimulate the nipple. After the baby comes, a supplemental nursing system is used to feed the baby. (See page 50 for an explanation.) Some moms produce a lot of milk; some don't get much at all.

Another way to induce lactation is relatively new. Dr. Jack Newman, a pediatrician in Toronto, has developed a protocol using a high-progesterone birth control pill (which, in some ways, mimics a pregnancy) and a medication called Domperidone. Used in other countries to treat gastrointestinal conditions, Domperidone has a side effect of raising the level of the hormone prolactin. Used in a certain order and combination, these medications trigger the production of milk. Neither medication is available in the United States (because other drugs treat the same conditions for which the drugs were originally created), and women must order them from overseas pharmacies where they are available without a doctor's prescription. The protocol is untested, however, and no studies have examined whether there are potential adverse effects on either mother or child or whether the medications could interact with other drugs.

This next story is of one woman's experience of following this protocol.

☕ PLAYING THE WAITING GAME

"Breastfeed Your Adopted Child." What the hell? I'd never heard of that before, but this headline on the cover of *Mothering Magazine* caught my attention! I firmly believe in natural parenting and that "breast is best," but I didn't think that would ever be a choice for me. I have severe, debilitating eczema and have to take high dosages of steroids throughout the fall and winter. Even though my husband and I wanted to start a family, we didn't feel my health was good enough to be able to carry a pregnancy, and I would have felt a lot of guilt if I were taking medication that could be potentially harmful to a fetus. So we decided to adopt. Having spent a year in Beijing in the mid-1990s, we chose an agency that has programs in China and Vietnam. We thought we would get a referral early this year.

It was during this time that I came across the article on adoptive breast-feeding. I was amazed and decided to do it. I've always been fairly proactive with my own body. I have a long history with the medical profession, and I tend not to trust them very much. But I read about the interactive effects, and very few women have any side effects. I did send an e-mail to Dr. Newman when I started to do this, and he was extremely supportive. There is also an active on-line board with many moms who have successfully nursed their adopted children, both with and without interventions.

I took this birth control pill for sixty-three days, during a time when I was taking steroids. I gained twenty-five pounds in sixty-three days, exhibited various symptoms that people associate with pregnancy, and was snooty. According to the protocol, the longer you stay on the birth control pill, the better, but I stopped because I couldn't handle it anymore. Before stopping, however, I started taking the Domperidone to trigger my milk supply because I was expecting this referral from Vietnam.

Quite a few Web sites provide information on breastfeeding adopted babies. One good place to start is the Adoptive Breastfeeding Resource Website at <http://www.fourfriends.com/abrw>. Another good site, primarily for the links on the second page, is <http://adoption.about.com/library/weekly/aa072400a.htm>.

I made up my mind that if I wasn't successful, I would still nurse with a supplementer. I believe that it's not the *milk* that makes the nursing relationship, but the psychological closeness, the physical bond that comes from a mom and a baby who are in sync. The milk is a great bonus, but, for me, the most important thing is the nursing relationship.

I started out pumping every two to three hours around the clock to bring in my milk, waking up in the middle of the night to do it. I didn't know what would happen because every woman responds differently, but four days after going off the pill I was making four ounces of milk a day. Using a double, electric pump, my supply gradually increased to twenty-five ounces a day. It was amazing! Once I started producing a lot, I started dropping down, and now I pump only three times a day. My supply has dropped to about eighteen ounces, but it's become a lot more manageable.

Gradually I filled up two deep freezers with little bags. When I ran out of space, I shipped a bunch in coolers to my in-laws' house in another state. I also ended up donating seven hundred ounces of milk to two other mothers who needed milk for adopted babies.

In the meantime, the agency in Vietnam started to have problems with U.S. immigration, and the INS shut down adoptions from the Vietnamese agency that our domestic agency used. We realized there would be no referrals forthcoming, and, more than a month after I began taking the birth control pills, we decided to switch countries. It was really sad to abandon our plan, and it felt almost like losing a child.

Our dossier has now been in Colombia since March, when I started pumping. They told us we would have a referral in May. It's now August. The agency keeps telling us we're first on their list, and we're supposed to have a referral any day.

We're desperately hoping for one by the end of the month. We're moving to another state, and it's getting down to the wire for us. If we move, we'll have to redo the home study, and it would set us back probably another three months.

If I had it to do all over again, I probably wouldn't have started to pump as early as I did because it has taken an awful lot out of me. And if we don't get our referral soon, I don't know if I will continue. I hope we get it soon. My body and brain are ready; my home and husband are ready. Now we're playing the waiting game. They tell us everything is fine, but every day that passes is like a knife through my heart. On some days, every time I pump makes me realize that I don't yet have a baby. On other days I feel that at least it's keeping me connected to the process. But the agency has a high success rate with placements, and that's what matters.

Sondra, Southern United States

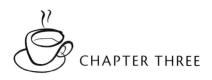 CHAPTER THREE

No Mother Is an Island

STORIES OF FAMILY,
COMMUNITY, & SUPPORT

Being in a breastfeeding relationship with another human being is not an officially recognized association in the same way that, say, being married, incorporated, employed—or even pregnant—is. The idea that there are women walking around in the world whose bodies are the sole sustenance for other living beings has not inspired new working, travel, urban planning, or business arrangements. . . . In a nation that venerates autonomy, breastfeeding is a largely unacknowledged ecological bond between interdependent individuals.

Sandra Steingraber, Having Faith

The lactation consultant who spoke at the childbirth education classes my husband and I attended repeatedly told us that the mother's first job is to feed the baby. Everything else could wait. She encouraged us to prepare meals ahead of time, not to worry about dishes or housework, not to rush to get out thank-you notes. As it turned out, her advice was right on target. If I had not had ongoing help from my husband and mother, I don't know how my firstborn and I would have survived.

Even the most well-intentioned and loving of family members, though, may be clueless when our breasts suddenly triple in size or our babies become too sleepy to latch on properly. As important as family support is, studies confirm it is often not enough (Locklin 1995). You've heard the saying, "It takes a village to raise a child"? Well, in some cases, it takes a village to get a baby to nurse. As many of the stories in chapter 2 reveal, nursing may indeed be natural, but it doesn't always come easily. For many of us, technical assistance and emotional support mean the difference between breast and bottle, between developing a satisfying nursing relationship and weaning in frustration and defeat. Many women who spoke with me stopped nursing precisely because they lacked such support. Studies back this up (e.g., Lawrence 1985, 475; Locklin 1995). Low-income women, for example, are more likely to quit nursing during the first two weeks, when no one is available to take over housekeeping responsibilities, help care for the baby, and offer breastfeeding encouragement (Bove 1996).

Unfortunately, there is much less mothering of the mother in our culture than in many preindustrial societies. As Jane Swiggart asserts in *The Myth of the Bad Mother* (1991), we focus so much on the needs of the child that we often neglect the needs of the mother. Consequently, many women feel misunderstood, bewildered, isolated, and exhausted. When we combine this with a 50 percent weaning rate in the first two weeks, a lack of social support for new mothers in the workplace, and a lack of quality affordable day care, it's no wonder the United States has the highest postpartum depression rate in the developed world.

It Takes a Village

Fortunately, recent years have brought some positive trends in postpartum care, including help with breastfeeding. Along with midwives who offer an array of postpartum services, a growing number of women are finding help from doulas (pronounced DOO-las), women who "mother the mother." Although the idea has been around for centuries, doulas today are para-professionals who offer emotional and physical support to women and provide various combinations of support before, during, and after the birth. Although studies of labor doulas illustrate the positive medical and psychological benefits they bring (Hodnett et al. 2003), no randomized, controlled studies have yet examined the impact of *postpartum* doulas, explains Penny Simkin, longtime doula, childbirth educator, and an original founder of DONA, Doulas of North America. Still, as virtually any woman who has hired a postpartum doula will attest, their presence can make a world of difference.

Others offer help specific to nursing. Lactation *consultants* offer "top of the line" clinical expertise; lactation *counselors* provide clinical help and support for women with easily overcome difficulties; and lactation *educators* educate the public on breastfeeding-related issues. They all play valuable roles. But hospitals and other health care facilities don't always make careful distinctions among the services they provide, and mothers rarely understand the different levels of expertise the titles carry.

For more information on how to find a doula, visit the Web sites of DONA, Doulas of North America, at <http://www.dona.org> (888-788-DONA); CAPPA, Childbirth and Postpartum Professional Association, at <http://www.childbirthprofessional.com/> (888-548-3672); or ALACE, Association of Labor Assistants and Childbirth Educators, at <http://www.alace.org/> (617-441-2500).

The only *official* title for breastfeeding professionals is that of International Board Certified Lactation *Consultant*—IBCLC. To become an IBCLC, an applicant must have spent thousands of hours working with nursing mothers, have certain educational qualifications, and pass an internationally certified exam. Lactation *counselors,* who participate in a one-week forty-hour course and pass their exam, may offer wonderful help to women encountering common and easily corrected problems but may be unable to recognize when women need greater intervention. The risk, of course, is that we may think we've gotten as much help as possible and give up if our problems continue, without realizing there are people with more knowledge and experience who could have assisted us.

To locate a lactation consultant, visit the International Lactation Consultant Association Web site at <http://www.ilca.org> (919-861-5577).

Along with clinical expertise, women need contemporary role models and emotional support. Mother-to-mother support groups—whether based in hospitals, birth centers, or community organizations—offer nursing mothers the chance to meet face-to-face. La Leche League, of course, is the largest and most well-known of such groups. While some women come seeking answers to specific concerns, others are attracted to the friendship and camaraderie of other nursing mothers. Meetings are free, and the organization remains a source of information and assistance, with trained volunteer leaders available around the clock.

Since 1987, in response to the need for breastfeeding support in underserved areas—typically in low-income and minority communities—League has also offered a nonaccredited, certificate-based program to train women to become volunteer peer counselors, providing information and support to those who otherwise might not have any. Statistics show that in communities with peer counselor programs, more women begin breastfeeding and stick with it longer.* Peer counseling programs may also be available through WIC, a federally funded supplemental nutrition program that operates out of state health departments and local clinics.

Along with face-to-face support groups, the Internet, too, has become a way for women to network and support each other without having to leave the comfort of home. Wired but tired, keyboard-to-keyboard, such forms of twenty-first-century community can be a godsend.

A Note about League

Despite its respected reputation and profound impact on breastfeeding and Western culture, La Leche League has not been without criticism. As is the case with health care providers, women sometimes encounter a leader who offers inappropriate advice or appears judgmental, and leaders may differ in their expertise. The organization has also been criticized for maintaining a middle-class bias and a narrow-minded view of what constitutes family, "good" mothering, and appropriate breastfeeding (Blum 1999).

In recent years the organization has worked hard to change these perceptions. For example, despite an arguable bias in The Womanly Art of Breastfeeding *against mothers who work out of the home and are separated from their babies, League, as members often call it, has recognized the growing need for relevant information and has created an abundance of helpful material.*

Visit La Leche League on the Web at <http://www.lalecheleague.org> or call 847-519-7730.

Despite such sources of support, though, women may be reluctant to seek it out. In a culture that places a high value on independence and self-reliance, some of us learn to feel embarrassed or ashamed if we cannot solve our own problems. As one young mother told me, "I felt like I needed to prove myself. I had read a lot about breastfeeding and lined up support, but when I had sore nipples and was engorged, I didn't use it. I guess I felt pressure to show my mom

---

* For more information on La Leche League's peer counseling programs, see <http://www.lalecheleague.org/ed/PeerCounsel.html>.

that I knew what I was doing. I also felt like my problems were so normal and trivial that I didn't want to bother anyone."

The stories in this first section come from women who *did* seek help and emphasize the impact that professional, para-professional, organizational, and group support can have on our breastfeeding experiences and in our lives.

In Their Own Words:
It Takes a Village

Jennifer and her husband are high school sweethearts who married at eighteen. Now twenty-eight, Jennifer has six children, including two sets of twins. All six were born prematurely. Her last child, Andrew, is the first one she's been able to nurse the way she always wanted to, thanks in part to an on-line support group. She is one of many women whose lives have been positively transformed by on-line "sisters."

One of the main issues Jennifer faced was difficulty in generating a full milk supply. Many reasons can be given for this. Some have a research basis; many do not. Moreover, it's hard to know cause and effect retrospectively. Jennifer's story, however, demonstrates the importance of persistence, of never saying never.

☕ KANGAROOS, AT LAST

Andrew and I were like kangaroos. He needed to nurse all the time, and to keep up my supply, I did just that. I even nursed him while bowling, babe in one arm, ball in the other. I actually bowled the best game of my life with him attached to the breast!

I don't think there's anywhere I haven't nursed—even on the gynecologist's table. My son came off long enough for the breast exam and then went right back on. "Yep, they're working," my obstetrician said.

Nursing him has been great! I feel like I missed out on so much with my first five. But I had the same problem with all of them—I couldn't keep a supply up. I had never imagined myself a bottle-feeding mother and I was—five times over. I was mourning the loss of not being able to nurse the first five and desperately wanted to try again. Everyone told me I would never be able to nurse enough, no matter what I did, but I did a lot of research before I became pregnant again and joined an on-line support group—Mothers Overcoming Breastfeeding Issues, or MOBI. I was relieved to discover that regardless of what the problem was, someone else had had it and could help. I found all kinds of support on the list. I learned that certain things in one's diet can affect supply, and I needed to avoid certain foods, drinks, and medications.

Not only did the ladies of MOBI help me deal with my grief over having failed at nursing my girls, but they cheered me on and calmed my fears. They listened to me when I had doubts; shared our joy in the conception of our son; and gave me a wealth of information, ideas, and encouragement. I learned so much from them.

My son didn't latch on immediately after birth, but when he finally did, twelve hours later, he didn't have any problems and calmed right down. I felt like crying I was so happy! I set small goals: four weeks, a month, then a few months. I kept waiting for nursing to fail, and when it kept working I was ecstatic. I set longer and longer goals and felt proud of myself. And it was much easier than I thought it would be with so many kids at home. I never let him go too long between feedings when he was little, and I nursed on demand. We've been fine! He's never had a bottle or formula, and he didn't take a cup until fourteen months. Still, I've had to work for every drop of milk I make. Nursing my son has made me realize that had I been more informed and had more support I could have breastfed the girls. They all had allergies to formula, so their bottle-feeding experience was pretty bad. I feel that they were a bit cheated.

I'm still on MOBI and will probably never leave. It's like a sisterhood. We share problems, successes, birth stories, milestones in our kids' lives—pretty much anything is open for discussion. If it weren't for that group of women, I would not have been successful nursing my son. He is now just over two, and we are still nursing. My dream has come true. It was hard to achieve, but we did it!

There are occasions on which a nursing mother may need medication, but that rarely means the end of breastfeeding. Nor do most medications affect milk supply. Our individual experiences, however, may suggest otherwise. The ultimate resource on this is Medications and Mother's Milk *by Thomas Hale (2004), a leading expert in the use of medications in breastfeeding women. This book is updated yearly. Visit <http://neonatal.ttuhsc.edu/lact/>.*

As stated on their Web site, MOBI is an organization that provides a safe place "for women who are/were unable to breastfeed, feel unsuccessful in breastfeeding, are/were experiencing severe breastfeeding problems, or experienced untimely weaning." The Web site and e-mail support group can be accessed at <http://www. internetbabies.com/mobi/>.

Jennifer Gardner, Yamhill, OR

Although Amy is recently married with a two-and-a-half-year-old daughter, this excerpt from her much longer story takes place six years earlier, when she was a single parent whose baby's father was out of the picture. Amy's son was on the verge of failing to thrive when she met Linda, a lactation consultant who turned her life around.

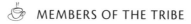 A JOURNEY OF DISCOVERY

"Don't listen to anything else," Linda had told me. "Follow your heart and your baby, and you will do fine." It was as if one day I felt wrong about everything I was doing as a parent, struggling with what my baby was telling me he needed, and the next day I felt encouraged, supported, and able to connect with my child and to a part of me that was confident about what I needed to do. Ian was a difficult, colicky baby with high needs. I had been lost, struggling to adjust to this little person in my life, and the only way I felt I could meet his needs was somehow to control them. My poor child only wanted *me,* and all I could do was stick that pacifier in his mouth, wrapping elastic around the back of his head to try to hold it in place.

Linda owned a store for breastfeeding moms, and whenever I went for my appointment I got to chat with all of these nursing mothers. It was the beginning of my journey into learning about breastfeeding and trusting myself. I was introduced to slings, started carrying Ian around all the time, and made sure we had lots of skin-to-skin contact. Even though he remained high-need, he turned into a much more contented child. I learned that what he really wanted was to be with *me;* to suck on his *mother,* not on a pacifier. Once that was established he started to thrive.

Amy Comte, Tempe, AZ

Studies show that racial and ethnic prejudices of the dominant culture can affect breastfeeding among women in minority cultures (Turner-Maffei 2002, 109). Lisa, a legislator for the Chickasaw Nation, speaks to this in the next story.

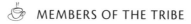 MEMBERS OF THE TRIBE

Government boarding schools are a part of our family history. Historically, these were schools where children as young as five years were separated from their families and sent by the government to be "civilized." Unfortunately the children were often embarrassed and humiliated. They were taught that being dark skinned and speaking a language other than English were inferior. Some of these attitudes about our people persist today. It's almost like we have to do more than the average person in order to be accepted by the dominant society. So when it came to nursing, I didn't want to do anything out of the ordinary that would draw attention to my baby or myself. Many of my colleagues and acquaintances who had children thought of nursing as passé. And my mother recalls that here in Oklahoma in the 1960s, breastfeeding was the last option. It meant you were poor and had no other means of feeding your baby.

But every time I went in for a prenatal appointment, a nurse, who has since become a good friend of mine, gently encouraged me to breastfeed, telling me she had nursed her three children. "I could never do *that*," I thought. "It doesn't even sound normal!"

Because I know the challenges my people have faced in relation to white people, developing trust in a white person about my baby would have taken time. But Sherri, the prenatal care nurse, was a member of my tribe. This was very important to me. Not only did she help me during my pregnancy, she actually came and checked on me after my child was born! She even gave me her phone number so I could call anytime I needed to—and I did, quite often. Because she led me by example she set the stage for me to nurse all three of my children.

Sherri would give me bits of information, but never too much. Instead she would bait me to get me to ask more questions. I started learning about how breast milk changes with your body and with babies' needs. My body is the perfect temperature and offers perfect nutrition all the time. I had no idea. I just knew it was easy. I didn't have to clean bottles, and it just made sense, especially at night. I could just roll over, and as my son got older he could pull my gown up all by himself.

I nursed my son because Sherri talked about the convenience of nursing and about how much money it would save. But once I started nursing, I did it because it was comforting and we both enjoyed it. I didn't know then how nurturing, healing, and nutritional breast milk is.

Now, having nursed three children, it's pure enjoyment. It's helped me to become more connected to my children, and I know when they need to be fed because my body tells me—I can feel my milk coming down. I know a lot of the *facts* about breastfeeding, but I don't even think about them anymore. It's just the most comfortable thing to do. There's nothing in the world like nursing and having that baby look up at me and make a little whimper sound. It's like they are saying, "Thank you, Mommy, for giving me the very best."

My youngest is now nine months old. I breastfeed on demand, when she's hungry, when she cries, when she needs to be comforted, when she's hurt. She loves it, I do too, and I don't care how long I nurse.

Lisa Johnson-Billy, Purcell, OK

L'dia, forty, has four daughters ranging in age from twenty-one to seven. Pregnant with her fifth when we spoke, L'dia talks in the next story about her decision to nurse her first and how she found support for her style of mothering. For another aspect of L'dia's experience, see pages 150–51.

 TAKING IT BACK TO AFRICA

Some black women I know think about a "mammy syndrome" when they think about nursing. They think about the mammies who nursed the babies on the plantations or went into the white homes and nursed the white children.

But I took it all the way back to Africa. I had some African friends who nursed, so as a black woman in America, I thought of breastfeeding as natural, and I expected it to be a beautiful experience.

I was eighteen and living in Columbus, Ohio, when I became pregnant with my first daughter. I wasn't breastfed, and my family and most of my friends thought I was crazy. They said, "How are you gonna be on the bus and pull out your titties and nurse this baby?" And my friends were *older* women, some with six children.

I said, "There's ways you can dress and cover up. This is the natural way, and this is what I want to do."

I sought out La Leche League even before my daughter was born and went to their meetings. By the time she was three weeks old I had moved to Kansas City, Missouri, with my husband, who was in the military. One of the first things I did was to look up La Leche League again. I was the only black woman in the meetings, but it never bothered me. I have a strong black awareness, but I'll go wherever necessary in order to get information I need.

Because such a small percentage of African American women breastfeed, the African-American Breastfeeding Alliance (AABA) was founded to help educate African American women about breastfeeding and to increase the percentage of nursing women in the African American community. AABA, in collaboration with other organizations, provides valuable resources and ongoing support. They also offer a peer counselor training program. Visit their Web site at <http://www.aabaonline.com/> or call 410-225-2006.

La Leche taught me well, and when I moved to California after my second daughter was born, I got involved with a chapter that had a black women's group. The information was basically the same, but it was nice to have something else in common besides babies. We talk differently when we get into our own groups. It's more relaxed. We have similar ways. Although the black community has much diversity, it's nice to look up into someone else's face who looks like you.

I've always looked at my breasts as being there to nurture my children, and I enjoy nursing because I know I'm using my body for what it was made to do. I haven't had to rely on cows or the formula companies. I could nurture and feed my babies in a way no one else could. They were healthy, plump, and robust, and people would look at them and say, "That's all breast milk?" It made me feel great.

L'dia S. K. M. Muhammad, Berkeley, CA

To say that our society does not hold single, teenaged mothers in high esteem is an understatement. Lauren's story, however, shows the amazing potential of young mothers when they are given appropriate and meaningful support.

CONSTANCY AMID CHAOS

I was seventeen when I got pregnant, young and really scared. A woman at my high school, Melody, was starting an empowerment program for teen mothers. We'd go there after classes and talk about parenting skills, self-esteem . . . everything. Melody talked about the benefits of breastfeeding, and right away I thought, "There's no way I'm giving my child a bottle." With her help, I even became certified as a lactation educator and peer counselor while still pregnant.

Early on, Melody seemed like the kind of person I could trust and talk to. I got really close to her. So when my mother kicked me out, after I had graduated but a month before I was due, I went to stay at Melody's friend's house for a couple of weeks. After that I moved in with my daughter's father, who was living with his mother at the time, and I had the baby the next night.

Taea was tiny—five pounds, five ounces. I tried to nurse her as soon as I could, but it didn't go well at first. That night a nurse brought Taea to me, saying she was crying in the nursery and wouldn't take a bottle. I laid her next to me, started nursing her, and she went right to sleep. I thought, "I'm a real mother!" I felt close, happy, and warm.

After leaving the hospital, my boyfriend and I moved around a lot. Finally we got our own basement apartment, but things were falling apart between us. He was physically and emotionally abusive, and if his friends called and said, "Let's go out and party," he'd be like, "Forget y'all," and he'd just leave. And he wouldn't come home for maybe four days.

I got really depressed, and we were broke all the time. My boyfriend worked as a cook for Red Lobster, but the money barely kept a roof over our heads. There were days when we didn't have enough money to eat. Sometimes I was just too depressed to eat. But I was so grateful that I didn't have to worry about Taea being hungry! I would just nurse her, and it made me feel better because she was close to me and warm.

Nursing Taea was the one thing that remained constant during the chaos of not having a place to live, of moving from place to place, of having huge problems with my boyfriend. Nursing was our comfort zone, the one thing we could rely on. I learned quickly to get her in any position that worked with my daily life. I could do whatever I needed to do and still be able to nurse her whenever she was hungry or tired.

During this time, Melody helped me a lot with breastfeeding. I was also still involved with the Teen Empowerment Program. We started to talk about how we were going to organize our lives and get everything together to be successful parents. We set and accomplished goals. That was a big help, to have other people push us, and we became each other's support.

When Taea was nine months old I left my boyfriend and went back with my mother. (We had made up after the baby was born.) I realized I needed to set goals for myself; things weren't going to just fall into my lap. I got tired of relying on other people to do things that I knew I should be doing for myself—finding a place to live, finding food. I decided to get my own apartment and find a job. I became more in tune with Taea's needs and more playful. We were able to communicate better because I was able to focus on her.

Just after moving back with my mother, I got into a two-year program that helps low-income single mothers get on their feet. We get rental assistance, child-care vouchers, and have classes twice a week—parenting, budgeting, cooking—pretty much everything to help us become better parents and to work toward self-sufficiency so we don't have to rely on social services.

Through this program, as well as through the Teen Empowerment Program, I've learned that I'm not invincible. I'm no longer that typical seventeen-year-old, thinking I can do anything I want. I've become a nicer person. I'm more patient. I attribute this to nursing. If I can do that for such a tiny, little person, why can't I help somebody else out and sacrifice something for them?

Eventually Melody asked me if I wanted to run one of the Teen Empowerment groups. "Of course," I said. I'd been through it. I knew what it was all about. Currently I oversee the program in Montgomery County and facilitate all three groups. There's a big focus on breastfeeding. I try to get the barriers out of people's heads, to explain how amazing it is that women can carry another human being around and then feed them with something our own bodies make! When I see a young woman breastfeeding and I know I'm the one who told her she should do it, that makes me feel great!

I'm now nineteen, and Taea is two and still nursing. I thought she would be done before now, and I'm kind of surprised. She nurses about three times a day, and she'll continue until she weans herself. It would be nice to have my body back and not have a child hanging off of my chest, but I'll let her continue for as long as she wants. My mother said I might as well savor this time because we won't be this close again.

Taea and I now have a nice, little apartment. I'm in my fourth semester of college, studying psychology and working two jobs. I waitress and do data entry for the police department. Eventually I'd like to get my Ph.D. in psychology, have a private practice, and work with schizophrenic people. But my main goal is to raise my daughter to be healthy, happy, and well taken care of. It's difficult, but I'm getting there.

Lauren Leigh Humphrey, Kensington, MD

A Family Affair

In an era in which women are being discharged from the hospital earlier than ever before, all of us should have the right to decent postpartum care, including breastfeeding support. Not surprisingly, our families play key roles, both positive and negative. Kristina, for example, a mother from San Antonio, Texas, recalls: "My mom told me, 'You're too thin. You can't do that. You'll be tired all the time. It's not good for you.' I didn't let her influence me, but I was a little afraid that if it didn't work out, she would say, 'See, I was right!'"

Overall, it's a lot easier to nurse when your family isn't giving you incorrect information or making fun of you, when your mother isn't telling you to stop so your child can be away from you for a night, and when family members don't give your baby formula on the sly.

The stories in this next section illustrate some of the ways in which families both help and hinder us. The first few illustrate some of the ways in which they can make nursing more challenging and provide a striking contrast to the stories that follow.

In Their Own Words:
A Family Affair

Patti's story, following, could easily have fit within the chapter on weaning. I include it here, though, to emphasize the ways that families can influence our experience. Her story is representative of many that I heard.

THE FAMILY ODDBALL

My entire family thinks breastfeeding is "gross." My mom doesn't even like to hear the word *breast*. So I'm kind of the oddball. I waited the longest to get married and have children, I've nursed them, and I don't spank them. "That's just Patti," the family says.

During my pregnancy I read enough to know that nursing was best. I thought I would do it for three months or so, but I never expected to like it. Once I started, though, I loved it. I didn't know I could feel that close to a baby—it was overwhelming!

Beyond a year my family really started giving me a hard time. "When are you going to stop nursing that child?" "He's got teeth." "He's going to be five years old and coming up to you, saying, 'Mommy, give me my breast!'" I stopped nursing sooner than I would have liked because everybody was making fun of me. At that point, I was more vulnerable. I didn't want to be the different one—I wanted to be like everyone else. It was the same thing with Jeffrey, my second, and I weaned him between twelve and fifteen months, too, for the same reasons.

With both the boys, nursing was as special the last time as it was the first time, and after I weaned each of them, I cried. I missed it. It felt like all of a sudden they were getting away from me. Next thing I know they'll be in college, getting married, and having their own kids. In retrospect, I wish I had nursed them until they stopped on their own.

Erin is my third baby. As she's my last one, there's something in me that wants to hang on to it a little longer. She is seventeen months old now, and I plan to keep nursing until she weans herself. But my family is still giving me a hard time, and it hasn't been easy for me. In fact, until Erin was born, I never even nursed in front of them. Instead I would go into the bedroom, and everybody would kind of laugh at me.

Today I'm more comfortable about nursing and not as influenced by my family. I've realized over the years that my parenting style is quite different from theirs. And it's okay because I've enjoyed nursing immensely, more than I ever thought I would. I like cuddling up in the bed, putting a pillow on my lap, turning on some music, and nursing. When I used to nurse Jeffrey, Christopher would sometimes climb in bed and lie down beside me. Now when I'm nursing Erin the kids are constantly climbing up on the bed and lying with me. It makes me feel more like a *mom*. These are my children. This is my family. The cavewoman nursed her babies, animals nurse their young, and I know that I'm one of them. I feel more connected to the planet and more a part of the whole world.

Patti Murray, San Francisco, CA

Those of us in loving, supportive relationships may have little insight into what life is like for nursing mothers whose family relationships are more adversarial. Sometimes one parent leaves the other and steps completely out of the picture. Other times separation paves the way for battles over visitation rights and custody battles.

Juanita was a high school sophomore when she found herself pregnant at fifteen. Her mother wanted her to attend a school for pregnant women and young mothers, one and a half hours away, but Juanita continued to attend the public school in town. Although she and her boyfriend have since reconciled and their relationship has improved, her story sheds light on how nursing can be affected when parents don't get along and the legal system becomes involved.

☕ VISITATION RIGHTS

I got pregnant at the end of August with this guy I'd been dating for several months. I told my parents a month later. After that, my dad only let me see my boyfriend at my house, with supervision. By the end of October, we broke up.

My boyfriend never tried to get back together with me and started seeing another girl who went to my school. Then, when I was eight months pregnant, he mailed me a letter telling me that he had gotten an attorney and wanted fifty-fifty parental rights. So my family found an attorney, too, and a whole court process started concerning where the baby would live.

Our attorneys agreed that when the baby was born, my boyfriend could come to see her at the hospital. He and his mom stayed for a few minutes and left. Over the next two months, he wanted to see Lucinda, but the times he wanted to come weren't good because my parents didn't want me to see him alone. Then he and his family wanted to take her for the entire weekend. Lucinda had never seen them before, and how did they expect her to eat?

The attorneys took forever, but we went to court when Lucinda was two months old. The judge decided she could go two and a half hours without eating. As of the next week, her father and his family could take her for that amount of time. I didn't like it. I didn't want her to leave the house, and she was only comfortable with people she knew well. We offered to let his family come and see her at our house, but they wanted her at *their* house. So they got to take her for two and a half hours every Tuesday, and for one and a half hours every Sunday. Her father also came on Mondays and Wednesdays for two hours each.

My plan was to feed Lucinda before she left and when she got back, but she would be full when she got home. I could tell they were bottle-feeding her because she would come home and throw up. She hardly ever even spit up when she was with me. But her father denied it. "You can't do this," I said. "It's messing up my supply of milk." Since she wasn't hungry, I had to wait longer to nurse her, and instead I would pump the milk that had been waiting for her. Later, when she wanted to nurse, I didn't have enough and had to give her what I had pumped.

I offered to work my feeding schedule around them, telling them they could bring her back when she was hungry and then take her back again. I tried to send him with breast milk, but both he and his mom laughed in my face when I gave it to them.

Another time she came home burping, with a smell on her breath. "Did you feed her?" I demanded to know. "Did you give her formula?"

"Yes," he said.

"I *told* you not to."

"I can't come all the way over here just for you to feed her again," he replied.

I told my attorney this wasn't right, they can't be doing this. She told me the judge would get upset with me if I ran back to the court for every little detail, and nursing was not considered a big deal in the courtroom. Basically she told me I should deal with it; there could be bigger problems than this.

So that's what I had to do. It didn't get easier until she was five or six months old, when she started to eat baby food.

Lewis still thinks the only reason I nursed was so that they couldn't take her for more than two and a half hours. And so many people told me I didn't have enough milk or that I shouldn't nurse. The director at my daughter's day care always bragged about her son, a six-foot-tall, record-setting athlete. "Formula never hurt him," she said, "so it wouldn't hurt yours." The day care even printed out four or five pages on why formula was good for a baby.* "See," they said. "It's not so bad. We don't know why you're so against it."

But despite all this, nobody else was sitting in my shoes. They didn't know how much milk I had. They didn't know my daughter like I did. And I loved nursing! It was easier at night because I didn't have to get up to make a bottle, and I *liked* holding her that way. She would sleep with me, starting out on the other side of the bed, but within an hour she would wake up and make her way right up against me. Only then would she fall back to sleep. It was also easier to put her down for a nap, and I felt we were closer to each other.

If a teen mom wants to nurse, people should work with her. Just because somebody else doesn't do it doesn't mean they have to be so against it.

Juanita, Southwestern United States

The rest of the stories in this section are from women who have supportive partners or who come from families where nursing is the norm. Many women receive help in ways you might expect. Lisa's story represents the more typical ways in which our partners help us.

☕ A SUPPORTIVE SPOUSE

I come from a computer-science background where things are systematic and analytical—nothing like babies and breastfeeding! I was used to checking things off a list, but with a daughter who wanted to nurse ten to fourteen times a day, I never had a feeling of closure. It was definitely *not* what I was used to!

My husband's support was critical. I'm convinced I would only have nursed for three days if it hadn't been for Stan. He gave me the encouragement and confidence to stick it out. He never suggested that I didn't have enough milk and that perhaps that was why the baby wanted to nurse all the time. His attitude was, "If she's hungry, feed her." It didn't matter if she'd just eaten thirty minutes ago. We understood that because breast milk is di-

---

* This, of course, is blatantly untrue.

gested more easily and quickly than formula, babies need to feed more often. Stan also encouraged me to nurse in restaurants if the baby was hungry. Everyone else was eating—why shouldn't she, too? We figured it was better than having to listen to a screaming baby or having to leave the restaurant.

I can see where a dad might feel left out if a baby is breastfeeding, but Stan found other ways to become involved. He changed her diapers in the middle of the night, brought her to me to nurse, gave her most of her baths, and cut her fingernails. And as Kelly continued to nurse, he never commented that I should wean her. "It's so wonderful to see you two sharing such a strong bond," he said.

Everyone thinks that nursing makes life easier on the husband, but he has to be willing to take up the slack. I'm thankful my husband has been wonderful!

Lisa M., Chandler, NC

In this next story, Renee reveals another way our partners can help us. This kind of help is much less visible than, say, helping us comfortably position our pillows. Still, it may be more common than we think, since Renee was not the only woman to share such a story with me.

RELIEVING PRESSURE

The day before my thirty-first birthday we had gone to an annual party at a friend's house, two hours away. My son was staying with my mother, and I would be back the next day by four o'clock. I pumped before I left, and I wouldn't need to pump again until the next morning. It wasn't until that moment, however, that I realized I had accidentally left at home the charger that connects my breast pump into the wall.

It was eight thirty in the morning, and my breasts were getting painful. There was no way I could wait until we got home. I tried to hand-express in the shower, but they were so huge I couldn't get any milk out. I woke my husband up. "LaMont," I said, "you're going to have to help me because I'm going to explode before I get home. I need you to come into the bathroom to get this milk out. I need you to suck."

I sat on the toilet, and my husband knelt between my legs, holding one of those red, cold-beverage, plastic party cups. He sucked out the milk and spit it into the cup, but after the first cupful, he said, "I'm not wasting this, this is good stuff," so he drank maybe a quarter of a cup. "Wow, Renee," he

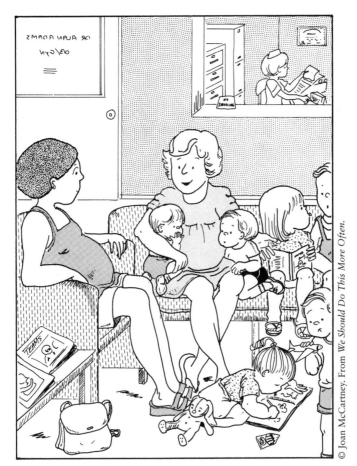

YOU'RE IN GOOD HANDS...HE'S AN EXCELLENT DOCTOR
AND EASY TO WORK WITH. I'VE SPENT A NUMBER
OF YEARS TRAINING HIM MYSELF.

said, "it's really sweet." He said it was like a little spigot, and he hardly had to suck at all.

We had a good laugh over this. I know some women who would never let their husbands do that, but for us, it was just par for the course.

Renee, Washington, DC

Teal's story offers a picture of how we might experience nursing in a culture in which breastfeeding is both an expectation and a norm. A thirty-year-old pediatric physician's assistant, Teal is tandem-nursing two children—Cameron, two and a half, and Graham, six months.

FROM GENERATION TO GENERATION

Breastfeeding has become a tradition in our family. Back in 1969, when breastfeeding in the U.S. was near an all-time low, my mother successfully nursed my older brother through his first year. Three of my mother's five sisters were bottle-feeding their firstborns, but after witnessing my mother's breastfeeding experience, the bond it created and the relationship it nurtured, they all wanted that for themselves and their children. The next time my mother nursed, she was one of four sisters breastfeeding at the same time.

I have many memories of being nursed. Mom nursed me on demand, wherever and whenever I wanted or needed to. Eventually I developed some kind of understanding that other people didn't understand I still nursed and that it was more comfortable to do it at home. This met most of my needs at that point in my life: bedtime, nap time, cuddle time, fix-my-ouchie time, bad dreams, or when I was sick. I remember Mom nursing me, on more than one occasion, in the croup tent in the hospital. Nursing always made me feel safe, secure, and loved. It made the world a reassuring place and seemed to make everything better.

Because I was nursed for so long, I am able to relate to the feeling of comfort, closeness, and happiness that nursing provides. Today, my sister-in-law, Victoria, and I each have two children, and it has been interesting to watch our family tradition continue. Not only have I nursed her children and she nursed mine, but even my mom has nursed her grandkids to comfort them. Before my eight-month-old niece's christening, my parents flew into Texas from Colorado, and my sister-in-law left Diana with them while she picked my husband and me up from the airport. When we got back to the house, there was my mother, standing in the middle of the room with Diana cuddled up to her dry breast. Diana was sound asleep, but my mother was still standing there, rocking her. Diana had been crying and wouldn't go down to sleep. "I couldn't just listen to her cry anymore," my mom said, "so I nursed her!" I think my mother-in-law's mouth had to be picked up off the floor, but it's fine with us. If our mother's watching the kids and they wake up, she'll nurse them back to sleep. She knows that's what they want.

I know so many mothers who don't have anyone to turn to. But my sister-in-law and I have each other and a mother who understands. There was no question about *whether* it would be done or *how* it would be done, and there was always someone to turn to for support and understanding.

That's what we all need—families where mothers can help their daughters nurse without this breakdown where women have to learn how to do it all over again. If we breastfeed *our* children, they will be more likely to breastfeed *theirs*.

Teal Peck, Torrington, CT

Judy, the mother of two, had a hard time getting nursing established the first time around. Her story speaks to the fact that sometimes what we need more than professional help is another set of breasts or someone else's milk.

LACTATING SISTERS

I was in absolute agony by my second trimester. Something was going on with my breasts, but I didn't know it. My sisters and midwives told me that this was just part of pregnancy. Once I was in labor, though, and they saw my breasts, the midwives exchanged a look, and I knew something was wrong. My sister's jaw hit the floor. She told me later that she thought I was never going to be able to nurse. What happened was that all the blood vessels in my breasts had expanded, and my breasts were like huge, hard balloons, swollen, with blood vessels popping out of the skin.

Even though my daughter was born at a birth center, she was hospitalized immediately. Her temperature was low, and they feared she had an infection.* She was put on several strong, intravenous antibiotics for three days, the time it took for the results to come back—negative. She was taken off the drugs and sent home.

During those three days in the hospital we never really nursed. My nipples were sore, and my milk was streaked with blood. The hospital staff freaked out and told me to stop nursing. I called a lactation consultant and found that the blood vessels had ruptured during pregnancy and it was okay to feed her. They actually call this rusty-pipe syndrome, from the brownish, rusty-colored, old blood.

My daughter was little, didn't have a rhythmic suck, and my breasts were like rocks, and she couldn't latch on. Her bilirubin was high, and she desper-

---

* According to world-respected midwife Ina May Gaskin, lower body temperature is not a sign of possible infection—*higher* body temperature is. And it is important to keep both mother and baby warm after the birth (personal communication 2003).

ately needed breast milk. I would hold her to my breasts, and one nurse would think she was nursing, but the next would think she wasn't. My sister said, "Just tell them that she's nursing and get the hell out of the hospital!" So that's what I did.

Nursing didn't go well at home. Amanda would take two sucks and fall asleep at my breast. We constantly had to wake her up. We rented an industrial breast pump, and I started pumping, but very little milk would come. I tried using an eyedropper, but half the meager amount of milk would run down her chin and we'd lose it on the floor.

My lactation consultant told me to keep pumping and spoon-feed her or use an eyedropper, but I was getting too fatigued. I was sitting at a pump all day long and not getting much into her. My sister had gone home, my husband was working, and I couldn't hold the baby and pump at the same time. I had people begging me to give it up. Alan was saying, "Judy, it's not worth it, just give her formula." But my attitude was that my child's start in life was the opposite of what I wanted. Her first "food" was major drugs, and I wanted to give her something healthy and natural. I was also afraid of nipple confusion because Amanda had never established nursing.

One night, my lactation consultant called me and I burst into tears. Then she told me that formula didn't have to be my next step. "You have three lactating sisters," she said. "You need a break and a chance to chill out and let your breasts heal a bit. And the companionship, too."

Could I ask them for that? They live three and four hours away from me. I called them up. One of my sisters was able to come for three or four days, and another was able to come after her. My third sister, who couldn't come, looked into sending her milk by Federal Express on dry ice.

So Nancy came. I had the pump set up, and I could see by the look on her face that she hated pumping. All of a sudden it dawned on me how stupid this was. Why should we do this intermediate step? Besides, Amanda needed practice. I said, "Here. Nurse her. It makes no sense for you to pump and then lose part of it as it runs down her chin."

So she did. And Amanda latched on without a problem. When my other sister came, Amanda latched right on to her, too. I was so grateful. My daughter was getting to nurse, I was getting a break, and I had company. After a week or so, I got enough rest, my breasts healed, and Amanda got enough milk so that she became a little bigger and stronger and her suck got stronger. By the time they left I put the pump away and was solely nursing. By three months we were a normal nursing couple.

Societal pressure says we aren't supposed to let other people nurse our babies. I was concerned about what other people were going to think. I was supposed to be territorial that this was my baby and I was the only person who should nurse. Instead, I was so grateful! And it was special for my sisters. My sister Catherine later bemoaned, "I'm the only one who didn't get to nurse Amanda."

I think breastfeeding was the best thing I could have done for myself because I don't know if my breasts would have been able to heal without that cleansing process. And my daughter went on to nurse for three and a half years. As hard as it was to start nursing, it played a big role in my decision to let her wean on her own. I worked so hard to do it, I couldn't imagine ending it before I had to.

Judy Wagner, Ithaca, NY

Bosom Buddies

Stories like Teal's and Judy's illustrate that even within a culture as "modern" and technologically oriented as the United States, some women are rediscovering that when we don't let the dominant culture dictate our actions, we can ease the work of mothering and discover wonderful ways to help one another.

Too often, though, our decisions are met with shock and scorn. Just as we are supposed to be monogamous with our sexual partner, we are supposed to have a monogamous relationship with our babies and children. Only the *mother* is supposed to nurse her child. Only the *mother* is supposed to supply the breast milk. Perhaps, given our sexually charged society, people may mistakenly think of a woman nursing another woman's baby as strangely analogous to wife swapping.

I experienced this kind of derision firsthand. Knowing how long it had taken my milk to come in after Emily's birth, and remembering too well her refusal to latch on, I was fearful of enduring a similar experience with my second child. Shortly before my due date, I asked a friend if she could spare several ounces of breast milk. She was nursing a three-month-old and kindly obliged. The presence of this small bag in my freezer gave me the security that even if my milk didn't come in right away, my daughter would still have breast milk and likely be more alert. When I left for the hospital, I took it with me.

The nurses were thunderstruck! Why would I want to use another woman's milk, to expose my baby to another woman's smell? This was not hospital approved! But *they* did not know my breastfeeding history and the angst it had caused me. *I did!* And this was what I needed to do for peace of mind and the confidence to prepare myself psychologically for nursing another newborn.

As it turned out, my fears were not realized. Nonetheless, it still took Rachel about a day to successfully latch on, during which time I could not relax. When, in the middle of the night, I asked one of the nurses to please bring me an eyedropper and the milk, she was appalled and replied that she didn't have authority to do so. I realized I needed to go home to work on establishing nursing in a supportive environment in which *I* was the authority.

These attitudes are in sharp contrast to much of human history. Wet-nursing, for example, has always been around. It can be exploitative (as in the United States, when black female slaves became nursemaids to their master's children), but it really began as a way to save babies whose mothers could not (or would not) nurse them (Baumslag and Michels 1994, 39–40). Similarly, in family-oriented cultures, it is not uncommon for women to nurse each other's children when one of them is working or unavailable. (See Doua's story on pages 209–11.) It is largely with the advent of commercialized formula that these practices have become less popular.*

In the United States, the only medically acceptable way for a women to express milk for another woman's baby is via one of a handful of milk banks across the country. Carefully screened women donate their milk according to specific instructions concerning how to collect, handle, and transport it. The frozen milk is then thawed, pooled, cultured, pasteurized, cultured again, and made available to sick infants upon a doctor's prescription. Milk banks are a lifesaver for sick babies, babies unable to tolerate formula, and babies with medical conditions requiring them to consume human milk.+

Unfortunately, the number of milk banks declined during the 1980s, partly due to lack of funding and the advent of formulas for premature babies. Many neonatologists mistakenly view formula as the

---

* Contrary to popular belief, formula is not the second-best choice for babies. According to World Health Organization recommendations, the ranking of feeding choices after a mother's own milk is as follows: the milk of another woman; pasteurized donor milk from a milk bank; and finally, coming in fourth place, infant formula. Nonetheless, providing our babies with breast milk other than our own meets with great cultural resistance.

+ According to Mary Tagge, coordinator of the Mother's Milk Bank in Denver, Colorado, women donate for several reasons. Some have stockpiled a lot of milk before

equivalent of human milk and prefer knowing all the ingredients that make up formula compared to not knowing all the components of breast milk, asserts Lois Arnold, former executive director of the Human Milk Banking Association of North America (HMBANA). This does not have to be the case. Elsewhere in the world, Arnold explains, human milk is considered the "gold standard" and formula and cow's milk substandard.

Concerns about the possibility of HIV and other diseases is another reason milk banks have closed, despite the fact that pasteurization kills HIV. Moreover, according to Naomi Baumslag and Dia L. Michels, authors of *Milk, Money, and Madness*, there have been no cases of HIV being spread through donated breast milk (1995, 100).

For more information about milk banks, including how to donate or order milk, visit the Web site of the Human Milk Banking Association of North America at <http://www.hmbana.org> or call 919-861-4530.

In addition, HMBANA has established guidelines to prioritize who gets the milk first when the supply is low. Because a milk bank's first priority is sick babies who cannot tolerate formula, not all babies who need breast milk are able to receive it. Gretchen Flatau, the executive director of the Mothers' Milk Bank at Austin, explains that they get many requests for milk where it would be *beneficial* to babies but is not considered a medical necessity. It is not mothers who define this, however, but doctors. Even if breast milk were available to all who desire it, the expense makes it prohibitive for many women. Processing fees are high—an average of three dollars an ounce—as is the cost of shipping frozen milk over long distances. Although HMBANA guidelines clearly state that no one should be denied access to donor milk for financial reasons, the reality is less straightforward. Furthermore, medical insurance may or may not cover the cost, and Medicaid coverage of processing fees varies from state to state.

returning to work and discover they have more than their baby needs. Others are home with their babies, have an abundant supply, and choose to help women who can't provide milk themselves. And sadly, some women have babies who didn't survive but have stored a lot of milk their baby was never able to use. Similarly, women may lose a baby but choose to express and donate milk to help them through their grief. (See Jacqueline's story on pages 254–56.) Tagge reports that donor women often comment that they wish they had started sooner or could have done it longer. Regardless of whether they give ten ounces or over five thousand (yes, there are some women who donate that much over the course of months!), this is the typical response. "We've all been given gifts," says Tagge. "For these women, it's the gift of an ample milk supply."

Some women, desperate to provide their babies with breast milk, make independent, unofficial arrangements to receive donated milk outside of milk banks. Some rely on family and close friends. Others, particularly those who need large amounts for an extended time, may construct their own network of women from around their community or even from around the country.

To be sure, these practices today are highly discouraged by the medical community, largely because drugs and various diseases—including hepatitis, herpes, and HIV—can be transmitted through breast milk. Clearly we should not be cavalier about these things, and no woman should nurse another woman's baby without the mother's knowledge and permission! Even those we may trust the most—our families—may end up being the same people who have the most to hide from us in terms of their sexual history or health status. But in our cultural and personal desire to protect our babies, judgment and common sense can still prevail. All judgments involve some degree of risk. The question is, who has the power to assess those risks—individual mothers or the medical and legal community?

Women who take these social risks are not trying to jeopardize the well-being of their babies. In fact, it is just the opposite. I spoke with several women, for example, who went to incredible lengths, doing whatever possible to ensure their babies' health. That some women are willing to do this speaks to the importance of finding ways to make breast milk available to *all* babies. Blood banks are common. Sperm banks are common. Milk banks, too, must become not only common but affordable and accessible.

A lot needs to change for this to happen, especially involving education, explains Lois Arnold. Until the medical community understands breastfeeding not simply as an individual choice but as a public health issue, prescriptions for banked milk will remain few and the supply of milk banks will not grow. "We need to know exactly why physicians don't prescribe human milk," Arnold explains. "Is it because they're unaware that it exists, they don't know how to access it and they are embarrassed by that, or do they really have valid safety or nutritional concerns? If so, how do we address those issues? Or is it that breast milk is simply thought of as a yucky female body fluid, with women's breasts being fine to sell beers and cars, but not to nourish a child?"*

---

* In a conversation with Arnold shortly before this book went to press, she stated that there is a growing interest in starting new milk banks. Success will depend, at least

In the end, whether we are talking about pasteurized donations from milk banks, a sister's kind offer to share her breast, or a variety of situations in between, they all reflect human milk as the gold standard for babies' health and well-being. Making this possible is more than a public health issue; it is an ethical one. In the meantime, some mothers will find ways to "go for the gold" and develop new (and renew old) possibilities for mother-to-mother help.

The stories in this next section look at some of the less visible, embodied ways in which women provide mother-to-mother support, helping us to nurse our children and/or provide them with mother's milk.

In Their Own Words:
Bosom Buddies

 A HELPFUL FRIEND

My son, Patrick, was four months old when I started pumping for my best friend. Her milk supply had been fine, but once she returned to work, at six weeks postpartum, her supply went down quickly, and she didn't have enough to pump. She was shy about this, too embarrassed to go to a lactation consultant, and felt like a failure that she was unable to provide enough.

For several days, her baby stayed with us while she was at work. This helped me increase my production. A couple of times I nursed them both at the same time. My son had no problem sharing and thought it was kind of fun. Physically, it felt very different. Her mouth was smaller, and she was a slower, daintier, more gentle nurser, who took smaller mouthfuls.

Ultimately, I pumped for about four weeks, giving my friend time to build up a store of her own milk, without feeling pressured. I was flattered that she asked me, and I liked being able to help her out. We've been friends for close to twenty-five years, and now I feel like I have this extra closeness with her daughter.

Rebecca McClay, Houston, TX

Barb is the mother of six: three grown biological children and three adopted children. She and her husband are Latter-Day Saints

---

in part, on whether a given community has an interdisciplinary task force backed by a broad base of community support.

—Mormons—and "find intense joy in raising children." At the time of our interview, they had been foster parents for two months to Savannah, a nine-month-old baby whom they are hoping to adopt. Savannah was born with a rare genetic skin condition called epidermolysis bullosa. Here, Barb talks about the importance of donated breast milk in Savannah's life and reflects on how providing Savannah with breast milk has helped her to heal from three unsuccessful attempts to nurse.

☕ SAVANNAH'S LIFELINE

When we got Savannah and they told us she was being fed with donated breast milk, I was absolutely amazed that there are women who will do this and so grateful to them for giving this life-supporting substance for our daughter. I hadn't even known that milk banks exist.

Savannah was born without enough collagen in her skin for it to adhere properly on her body. She was born without skin on one foot and part of both hands. Friction causes blood blisters or clear blisters that have to be lanced after they appear, and if she even scratches her face, she gets them. She even has them in her mouth and esophagus. She experiences pain, but boy, is she a trooper! She's a happy little baby.

Before we got her, when she was a few weeks old, the blisters in her mouth and throat were so bad that she wouldn't swallow anymore. The doctors put a tube into her stomach to feed her and put her on donated breast milk. It is the only thing that gives her enough of the antibodies she needs to fight this terrible skin condition.

This is still how we feed her. Four times a day we put breast milk through a tube, to which we add human milk fortifier, a product that adds calories and vitamins. Children with this disease tend to become very thin, and nutrition is key for them to be able to heal their wounds. Savannah is also on a continuous feed all night long, a pump that feeds her breast milk through the night. Even though she is beginning to eat solid foods, the doctor would like her to stay on breast milk until she is at least a year old, so that she can receive the antibodies. I don't know what will happen then.

In the meantime, every other Wednesday I go downtown to the milk bank, about twenty-five miles away, to pick up frozen breast milk. I put it in my cooler and bring it home to the freezer. I must say, the first time I put some milk in my sink to thaw out, it felt strange. I thought, "Wow! This belonged to somebody else!" It took my breath away. Some of it spilled on my hand, and while I don't want to say it was gross, it was almost like when someone sneezes on you and you don't want it to land on your hand. I just wasn't sure what to do. It was very foreign to me.

But we don't think anything of giving blood to help another person, of giving time, or comfort, or food to a neighbor who is sick. This has taught me the same thing. It's the same principle of caring for another human being. And if I had the ability, you bet I would now do this for someone else!

Taking care of Savannah has been a healing process for me. It's helped me to feel better about myself. I felt very much of a failure with my own three nursing attempts. In some strange and warped way, I feel that I'm giving the milk to her. Other women are making it possible for me to give this very life-supporting substance to her. Without the milk, I don't believe she would be as healthy as she is.

Barb, Western United States

Julie, thirty-nine, is an energetic woman who runs a unique program out of her mobile home, voluntarily matching women who have excess milk with women in need of it. Arguably one of the most controversial stories in the book, it speaks to the urgency of making milk-banked milk available to all who need it. Happily married for twenty-three years, she and her husband are the parents of three adopted children—two older teenagers and a four-year-old. Despite the controversy her story may arouse, she was clearly acting out of kindness and good intentions.

PROVIDING A SERVICE

My last daughter, Meagan, was allergic to everything. She spent her first year with stomach cramps, diarrhea, constant congestion, you name it. It didn't matter what kind of formula I gave her, she would throw up no less than fifteen times a day. The only thing that would have worked was breast milk, but at the time I didn't have access to the Internet. It was terrible.

Meagan has been adamant that she wanted a baby sister, and we decided to adopt another baby later this year. This time, I was determined that the baby would have breast milk. I started searching for donors, beginning with an on-line adoptive breastfeeding support group. One of the moms was getting donor milk for her baby and had talked quite a bit about the donors she had. The more I read, the more I thought about it. I contacted her, she told me more about it, and I started right then.

I went to an on-line board for women who, for various reasons, don't *breastfeed* but exclusively pump their milk, asking if anyone knew anyone who had extra. An adoptive mother contacted me because she had such an oversupply. She was my first donor. My second donor was giving her milk to a milk bank, as well as exclusively pumping for her baby. She was pumping sixty-five to seventy ounces a day. After she gave her baby his milk, half the milk went to me; the other half went to the milk bank. She ended up sending me one thousand ounces a month! I purchased two fourteen-cubic-foot freezers that are now full of breast milk. One of the freezers is in my bedroom, and the other is in my son's bedroom.

This experience just lit a fire under me! I thought about what Meagan had gone through, and I had read on-line about babies who were having a hard time. I thought, "Gosh, it wasn't that hard to find donors for me. Why don't I offer it as a service to other mothers?" I just didn't want to see any other kids go through what Meagan went through.

So now I match mothers up with donors. I have the recipient send the donor a cooler and money for dry ice, the Gerber storage bags, and her FedEx number. The donor then fills up the cooler with milk, puts dry ice on the top, seals it, and sends it overnight, guaranteed delivery by ten thirty A.M. If the mothers want the donors to be tested they can request it, along with the paperwork. I've never had a mom refuse to have testing done. In fact, they'll ask me, "Where do I need to go? What do I need to be tested for?"

It is amazing how many people are willing to do it. Once the word got out about what I do, mothers began contacting me. I have surrogate moms who haven't delivered yet but contact me because the adoptive parents aren't interested, but the surrogate moms want to give their milk to a baby. Even the ones who were paid to have these babies still contact me. They don't get anything for this—they're doing it out of the kindness of their hearts. Other women are exclusive pumpers and milk-bank donors. One lady has never been pregnant and is producing twenty ounces a day. She doesn't have a baby yet, but from the herbs, drugs, and pumping, she has thirty-five hundred ounces in her freezer. She wrote to me, saying, "My freezer is about to overflow. Do you have someone I can donate my milk to?"[*]

I've been doing this for over a year now, and it goes by word of mouth. I don't have a Web site, but I get about twelve to fifteen inquiries a month,

---

[*]Lois Arnold, former executive director of HMBANA, cautions that the herbs and drugs some women take to establish a milk supply may have an adverse effect on the health of the baby who receives the milk. In addition, it is a situation that raises enormous liability issues for the donor, in this case, the middle (wo)man.

mainly from prospective donors. Recipients contact me, too—women who can't get milk from a milk bank. A lot of them can't afford it or can't get a doctor's prescription, and others don't like that it's pasteurized. I had one baby whose adoptive mother was nursing and providing him with almost 50 percent of his breast milk. He started bleeding from his bowels, she contacted me, I got her donors, and his bleeding stopped. I can't shut it down. If I don't have donors, I go looking for them.

It's really rewarding, what I do, and I've always loved children. I know how helpless I felt when Meagan was sick and there was no place for me to go. When I hear mothers asking, "What do I do, my baby is throwing up, she can't handle anything?" or hear from a woman who had to take chemo and now her baby is sick from the formula, it just rips my heart. I can't explain it, but nothing compares to the feeling I get from being able to help these babies.

Julie, anywhere, United States

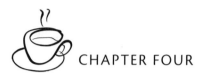

CHAPTER FOUR

Becoming Wiser

STORIES OF EXPERIENCE,
INSIGHT, & DISCOVERY

*Because there is so little interest in what care givers actually ex-
perience, mothers deny or hide much of what is real and vital
about the complexity of the tasks. This cultural silence about the
emotional realities of child-rearing creates such anxiety, guilt, and
feelings of inadequacy that it is too threatening for many people
to examine their subjective states as they care for their children.
It is as though care givers do not have permission to speak openly.*
Jane Swiggart, The Myth of the Bad Mother

One of the surprising discoveries along my parenting journey
was the realization that every baby is unique. This should have
been obvious to me, but it wasn't. By the time Rachel, my second-
born, came along, I figured I knew everything about nursing. I knew
the mechanics, of course, but I also knew how nursing was a source
of comfort, a way to help my child relax into sleep and keep her
content. For as much as Emily initially taught me what it means to
struggle with nursing, she subsequently taught me how nursing is a
baby's lifeline.

Or could be. To my surprise, I discovered that nursing was *not*
the answer to Rachel's every need. Instead of nursing her when she
was fussy, I had to wear her in a sling and walk with her. I came to
realize that she liked to suckle but not necessarily eat. As redundant

as it seemed, she would sometimes fall asleep with her head in the crook of my arm, her face near my breast, a pacifier—something I never thought I would use—securely in her mouth.

Rachel was never a calm and relaxed nurser. While Emily *needed* my breast, Rachel *kneaded* it. Instead of lying contentedly, she went back and forth, flip-flopping over my body, like a self-propelled pancake. She was constantly distracted, popping on and off my nipple, leaving me exposed and frustrated. For about six months, I found myself seeking private places as I had never done with Emily.

Like other parents, my mothering evolved in response to the unique personalities of my children. By paying attention and through trial and error, I gradually became familiar with what worked and what didn't. I developed what is commonly thought of as "maternal instinct." Contrary to those who assert that this is an inherent quality women possess because we are female, or because of our brains' biochemical response to the hormone oxytocin, I believe it is an intimate knowledge we *acquire* through the day after day, night after night experience of tending to our children.

This does not happen, of course, without cultural influence. Meredith Small is an anthropologist who studies how biology and culture intersect with each other to influence how we parent our children. Each of us makes parenting decisions based upon our personal experience, knowledge, and values, Small explains, but we seldom notice how we are influenced by dominant cultural ideologies and economics. It is only when we contrast our own culture with others that we understand how standards of normality are culture bound. Research into this new field of ethnopediatrics shows not only that different caretaking styles affect the health and well-being of babies but that biology and culture do not always mesh well. "Nowhere," writes Small, "is the interface of culture and biology more at odds than in the area of breastfeeding" (1998, xxi).

Small refers to "the prominent Western care-taking package," a style of caregiving designed to foster early independence and self-reliance. According to this "package," babies feed on schedules and sleep alone and through the night. By contrast, she explains, in much of the world, babies sleep with their parents (or at least their mothers), are carried in slings, nurse frequently throughout the day and night ("on cue," she calls it, as opposed to the American phrase "on demand"), don't cry very often, and tend not to develop colic (Small 1998, 227–28).

Although midwives and natural-childbirth advocates had long been emphasizing this alternative approach to parenting, in the late 1980s Dr. William Sears and his wife, Martha Sears, coined the phrase "attachment parenting" (AP). They popularized the basic premise that, if we listen and respond to the needs of babies and young children and develop strong physical and emotional bonds with them, our children will gradually venture into the world with greater security and confidence.

Among other things, AP typically consists of wearing one's baby (in a sling or cloth carrier), co-sleeping, and extended breastfeeding (which, in the United States, is often incorrectly assumed to mean nursing for longer than a year when it actually refers to nursing for longer than three years). Taken to the extreme, this means rejecting any sort of artificial nipple, including pacifiers, and avoiding infant carriers that keep the baby separate from the mother (e.g., strollers and cribs).

Within a country such as the United States, attachment parenting can be thought of as both traditional and revolutionary—traditional because it has existed for thousands of years and across myriad cultures and revolutionary because it contradicts the more recent approach to child rearing in which babies' needs are often subordinated to the needs of adults. In a culture that treats babies as afterthoughts in the lives of adults, and in an economy based on the presumed invisibility of babies and young children, AP offers a radical departure based on connection over autonomy and listening rather than silencing. On the flip side, however, it can also present the challenge of responding to our babies with sensitivity and compassion without simultaneously neglecting our own needs to a consistent and sometimes dangerous degree.

In trying to explain the overarching social context in which Western women nurse today, lactation consultant Diane Wiessinger offers the following analogy: Take two magnets and hold them far apart. There is no tension between them. This is similar to bottle-feeding. Now, stick the magnets together. Again, there is no tension. This represents attachment parenting. Now hold the magnets a little distance apart, but don't let them snap together. There is a *huge* tension between them. It's exhausting to keep the magnets at that close-but-not-too-close distance, and you're glad when you're finally allowed to keep them farther apart. This is what it means to breastfeed like a bottle-feeder: breastfeed, but don't fall asleep together; breastfeed, but only when you perceive that the baby is hungry; breastfeed, but don't carry the baby much of the time; breastfeed, but pump daily for "relief" bottles. It's hard work, a kind of martyrdom, not a kind of joy (personal correspondence, 2002).

These tensions provide insight into some of the struggles we may experience throughout our nursing relationship. To be sure, many find that AP practices work well. But our society is not designed to support this kind of attachment. It's pretty darn hard to wear one's child, for example, when we have no choice but to return to work at six weeks postpartum. Some of us try to compensate when we return home by getting in as much nursing, baby-wearing, and co-sleeping as possible. In many ways this makes our mothering work easier and more enjoyable, but even among women who consciously choose to follow AP practices, it can still be hard to give oneself over to the needs of one's child. That doesn't mean that women want to abandon nursing for formula, though. Lauren, a doula and psychologist friend of mine, points out the lack of safe spaces where nursing mothers can give voice to the darker side of nursing without validating those who tout formula as women's best friend. "In this culture," she says, "whenever something is hard the answer is immediately, 'Then don't do it.' It's hard to be in labor, so take the labor away. It's hard to have a fever, so take the fever away. It's hard to mother your child in a conscious, attached way, but people are afraid to say that because the reaction from others would be, 'So put the kid in a crib or give the kid a bottle.'"

The stories in this chapter, as well as the next, center around what it means to make authentic parenting choices and the insights and discoveries that unfold as we come into our own as mothers. Many of them shed light on the process of moving away from "the prominent Western care-taking package" that Small describes and what happens when we embrace some—if not all—of the ideals of attachment parenting.

The Discovery Zone

In her book *Woman to Mother: A Transformation* (1989), author Vangie Bergum describes the "inner journeys" women undergo as we move through pregnancy and childbirth. It is through this process, Bergum asserts, that we transform ourselves into mothers. We become "caught by life." That is, we don't necessarily make deliberate, rational choices ahead of time, but the sudden presence of our child causes us to think in ways we can't understand until we are actually the mother of that child. Seldom do we realize the depth and extent to which having a child changes our priorities and way of thinking.*

This is certainly true when it comes to breastfeeding. I vividly remember the first time I saw a woman nurse a child of about three years. I was in graduate school and knew as much about babies and child rearing as I did about performing heart surgery. As this woman put her articulate child to her breast, I turned to my husband and whispered with disgust, "I will *never* nurse a child who can ask for it in words!"

Years later, after my older daughter had gone from a babe in arms to an active, verbal toddler, I remembered this moment with chagrin. I had never counted on having my own little one who could not only tell me which breast she preferred but practically chanted mantras in honor of them. "Nummy, nummy, num, num, nummy, nummy, nummy," she would sing, pointing her chubby index finger first to one exposed breast, then to the other, and back again.

My experience was not unique. Women repeatedly talk about how nursing challenges their expectations and assumptions. This is particularly true regarding two aspects of breastfeeding: *why* we nurse and how *long* we'll nurse. Despite our initial plans, many of us discover that we can't come up with a good reason to stop. But we receive little cultural support.

As anthropologist Katherine Dettwyler has written, outside of La Leche League circles nursing is typically thought of as a feeding method only, appropriate for young babies, and carried out within the private world of the home (1995a). But I can't count the number of women who talked about how they don't simply *feed* their children, they *nurture* them at their breast. Mother's milk doesn't simply nourish; it soothes, pacifies, sedates.

Given the narrow parameters within which breastfeeding is viewed, misperceptions abound. Several years ago, when I was giving a talk on breastfeeding, a woman, five months pregnant, asked me why someone would continue to nurse a two-year-old. Were there

---

* In a later book, *A Child on Her Mind: The Experience of Becoming a Mother* (1997), Bergum expands her analysis to include the experience of women who become mothers through adoption.

any benefits? She was not antagonistic, just astonished. (As an aside, I ran into this woman two years later. She eagerly approached me, reminded me of her question, and somewhat sheepishly informed me that she was still nursing. "I totally get it now!" she exclaimed.)

According to Katherine Dettwyler, studies document that the longer a child nurses, up to two years of age, the better his or her health. (Although no studies have compared the health of children who nursed for more than two years versus less than two years, no studies have been able to claim any *detriment* to nursing beyond this time [Dettwyler 2000, 124].)

Anecdotal evidence also points to many benefits not likely to make it into a documented study. When my first daughter was two, for example, she fell and hit her mouth on a car's metal door frame. Her hysterical cries quickly turned to rhythmic whimpers as I put her to my breast. I held a cold washcloth against the cut on her chin, while the pressure from her sucking stopped the blood from the cut on the inside of her lip. Before long, she had soothed herself to sleep. Magic. But how do you quantify this? How do you measure the benefits that come from knowing you are providing your child with what she loves most in the world?

Moreover, in interview after interview, women admitted to feeling differently about the children they nursed compared to those they didn't. "My love for my son is steady and true, and I will love him until the day I die," asserts a mother in northern Michigan who had used formula with her first, "but I feel so much closer to my daughter. Every time we nurse I feel like we become one again, like I could melt into her. It is the deepest love I've ever felt, and I have never loved with such ferocity before."

"I have found that I am closer and feel more of a bond in proportion to how long I nursed a child," adds another mother. Even grandmothers in their seventies talked about how they still have a closer relationship with the children they nursed compared to the children they did not.

I admit this makes me feel uneasy. I would never want to suggest that bottle-feeding women don't feel close to their children. I was not breastfed and share an extremely close relationship with my mother. I can hear other mothers and daughters defensively saying the same. On the other hand, not a single woman talked to me about feeling closer to her bottle-fed children than she did to her breastfed children. It seems easier to dismiss comparisons between women who *nursed* all their children and women who *bottle-fed* all their children—if we've never done anything else, on what basis do we measure?—but it is harder to discount the experiences and perceptions of a woman making this comparison on the basis of her own mothering experiences.

The point, though, is not comparisons. It is that nursing promotes a certain kind of closeness, a "tuning in" to one's child in an intimate and profound way. This next set of stories addresses this.

In Their Own Words:
The Discovery Zone

Many women discover that books and experts don't have the answers we need and that only by responding to our babies are we able to get through some rough times. In the following story, Marsha shatters the myth of angelic, sleeping babies and illustrates how the idiosyncrasies of our children may be present from the beginning.

DOING THE BABY DANCE

My son, Griffyn, was very high-needs and in the earliest months insisted on being held—by me—at all times. He would only nap if I held him and would fuss if I didn't. But holding him was not enough. I needed to remain standing and in motion. If he sensed me attempting to sit he would awaken and cry. Of course, I could not nap *with* him. How could I lie down when I wasn't even allowed to sit?

It would literally take Griffyn hours to go to sleep at night. I was often up watching late, late television; vacuuming an already clean carpet; running the hairdryer or clothes dryer—anything to persuade him to sleep. People suggested I drive around with him, but as soon as the car stopped he would wake up.

I finally learned that what worked best was to bounce Griffyn (the "baby dance") and nurse him at the same time—standing, of course. It was so much work!

Most of those early nights I would get Griffyn to sleep while walking around downstairs; then I would creep upstairs and ever so gently slide into bed with him. One wrong move and he would be awake, and I would have to start all over. Fortunately, he did not fully "wake up" during the night but would rouse just enough to nurse and fall back to sleep. This was the advantage of having him in bed with me. He would wriggle a little or I would notice him making sucking sounds, and I would put him to my breast. He would sleep with me until about ten o'clock A.M.—a good thing since we had been up until two or three in the morning. Eventually I learned to nurse lying down, and we fell into a comfortable if somewhat sleepless (for me) routine.

During those first several weeks of nighttime feedings I got no more than two hours of sleep at a stretch and sometimes no more than four hours for the whole night. It was exhausting. I cried a lot, more than my baby did. I lived for those moments when I would be alone with my child and he would finally fall asleep with his warm, sweet-smelling head on my shoulder.

Soon, however, I became a breastfeeding pro, even once or twice nursing my baby in my sleep. I will admit there were times (like when he'd pinch or bite me or pick at my skin) when I would wish he would just leave me alone, but I was persistent and continued breastfeeding until the day my son decided he'd had enough. I cannot imagine a finer way of caring for my child, assuring his good health, and sharing with him my endless love.

Marsha C. Hudson, Seattle, WA

IDIOSYNCRASIES

I called my son my little wildebeest pup. He'd bob his little face on my nipple until he could latch on. I wanted my husband to take a video of it because it was so hysterical! Today, he refuses to nurse if anyone is talking. If somebody says anything, he'll actually get off the breast and look at them, waiting for them to finish. Only when they are quiet will he resume breastfeeding. It keeps it our *moment. I'll miss that, someday.*

Deborah Daly, Wilton, CT

As soon as my son could babble, he would sing to me. He used to hum to me while he nursed.

Jami Lee Wiercioch, Harpers Ferry, WV

 ## BECOMING LESS RIGID

My daughters are almost exactly two years apart. I was a lot more rigid with Kelsey, my first. "I'm not going to nurse you any more often than every two hours," I said, because I had read a book that recommended this. I had some friends who said it worked well for them, and I had this big fear of having a daughter who was constantly nursing. I didn't want to be a human pacifier.

When Kelsey fussed, I would walk her around outside, play with her, or bounce her. Sometimes distraction worked well, but sometimes it didn't, and I would say, "Oh, it's only been an hour and forty-five minutes, but I'm just going to nurse her." Then I would feel guilty about not following the schedule.

I've been a lot more relaxed with Larissa. I know now that nursing her at night is mostly to get her to sleep and less for nutrition or hunger. I don't know if she is more mellow because of that or if it's because we're more relaxed in general, but I wish I hadn't been so rigid about schedules with Kelsey. I just didn't know enough the first time around to use my own judgment or to sense when she was or wasn't hungry. I'm better at picking up on Larissa's cues when she's hungry, tired, fussy, or has a dirty diaper.

I wonder if part of the reason I've been a little more easygoing about the schedule is because I *can* be. I went back to work when Kelsey was four months old. Because *I* was on more of a schedule, *she* had to be, too. But since Larissa was born, I've been home full-time on a year's leave of absence. It's worked out okay, and we're all less stressed about it.

Joan P., Loveland, CO

Joan also has a story about nursing and pumping while working (see pages 163–64).

These next two stories reveal that when we trust our judgment and acquire the knowledge we need to make informed choices, we open ourselves to more authentic experiences of motherhood and to the possibility of more satisfying, intimate relationships with our children. They help us understand the centrality nursing can have in our lives, and they expand our understanding of what it means to mother at the breast.

Elisabeth found that nursing completely changed the way she mothers—both her biological children, as well as the child she adopted.

BEING A MOTHER IS WHO I AM

The first six months of Louisa's life were a big adjustment for me, and my view of parenting shifted 180 degrees. "My kid's going to nurse every three hours, sleep in her own bed, and take regular naps," I thought. I expected to be able to put her on a schedule, and a little loving firmness would bring things around to what I thought they should be. That's how I was raised, and that's the kind of mother I assumed I would be.

Well, Louisa wanted to nurse a lot more than every three hours. From day one, she craved stimulation and fought sleep to the bitter end. She needed to nurse to sleep and didn't sleep well alone. I had been programmed not to be manipulated by a child and was bound and determined not to give in. She really knocked the superiority out of me and made me realize I needed to start at ground zero, figuring out my own answers to things. Right about that time, somebody mentioned the book *Nighttime Parenting* by Dr. William Sears, and it changed my life. It validated my feelings about what was right and what kind of mother I wanted to be.

Now I thank God Louisa was like that because if I had had Amelia first, I could have put her on a schedule, taught her to comfort herself to sleep, and thought, "Oh, aren't I a wonderful mother." Having Louisa first made me take all the puzzle pieces and shift them around. It was hard at the time, but it was the best thing that could have happened to me.

Nursing was Louisa's lifeline. It calmed her down, brought her into sleep, and woke her up when she couldn't transition. She was a voracious nurser, and it was such an intense thing with her. When she was maybe eighteen months old she caught strep throat and could hardly swallow. I'd lie down with her, and she couldn't nurse because it hurt too much, but she'd say, "See nurnies, see nurnies." She just wanted me to take my breast out so she could see it.

When I became pregnant with Amelia, Louisa was still nursing a lot for a three-year-old. One morning I said to her, "You can nurse as long as you want this morning." Two hours and fifteen minutes later, we were still in bed. Finally I had to say, "I know, Honey, that I said you could nurse for as long as you wanted, but we've got to get up!"

Over time, Louisa cut down, and I found ways of limiting her. By the time Amelia was born, she would nurse for about three minutes, then turn over, and we'd kind of spoon, and she'd go to sleep like that. That was a big change and made things easier.

We had Amelia at home, and Louisa cut the cord and gave the baby her first kiss. She didn't show any jealousy, I think partly because she was nursing and wasn't excluded.

From the beginning things were radically different with Amelia. Her temperament was very different from Louisa's, and she was much easier to parent, but I think a lot of it had to do with the fact that I now felt confident in my mothering and my ability to make my own choices.

We adopted Millen when Amelia was two. Amelia was still nursing, and I didn't think I'd have much success nursing Millen. Many kids with Down syndrome have a lot of trouble nursing, and by the time we brought her home she was already ten weeks old.

Millen had a terrible time drinking from bottles. It would take her an hour to drink three or four ounces. She had a very ineffectual suck and couldn't really form closure around the nipple. Eventually I tried to nurse her, and she latched on and sucked beautifully. I couldn't believe it! The feeling of looking down at this child and seeing my white breast and her deep brown skin, with dark eyes looking up at me, was beyond description. But I didn't think she could be doing it right, so I continued to give her formula. Gradually, though, she drank less and less of it. After I'd been nursing her for about a week and a half, I started to panic. She was on this super-high-fat, high-calorie formula, but now she was only drinking about an ounce a day. I took her to the doctor and found that she had gained about a pound. This was unbelievable! When we got her at ten weeks, she'd only weighed about an ounce more than when she was born.

Before I started nursing her she used to get high fevers about once a week. But the first week I nursed her exclusively, she didn't. Still, I wasn't able to trust that my body and Millen were able to do it. I called a friend of mine, a La Leche League leader, and said, "Mary, I gotta have you take a look at this." She watched her nurse and was flabbergasted. "I can't believe it," she said. "She's nursing beautifully. If I didn't know better, I'd think you had given birth to her. She was meant to be your baby." From then on, we didn't look back. She was completely breastfed. And she didn't have any more fevers.

I nursed her for a little over a year, not as long as I would have liked. But when she got close to a year I was concerned that she was not getting enough stimulation because she needed to nurse a huge amount of time to get the milk she needed. I decided to start supplementing—something I'd never done with my other kids. By then she was a little older, could suck a little easier, and started to drink more from the bottle.

But she started getting sick. She got a stomach virus that hardly affected the rest of us, but she was so tiny and her immune system so sluggish that it really overtook her. Once she got hospitalized I let myself get pressured into weaning her. I look back and wonder how I could have been so stupid. Obviously breast milk was what she needed. But I still think her year of being completely breastfed helped her so much. Even now, the therapists are amazed that she has such good tongue control, and I think that's from breastfeeding.

Being a mother is what I am; it's *who* I am. And the pure, emotional nurturance of being a mother was crystallized in nursing Millen.

Elisabeth Shiffer, NY

I always have a hard time when I hear people say, "Oh, toddlers only nurse for comfort." That's like saying "You're only eating Ben and Jerry's ice cream for comfort." You get caloric intake whether you like it or not. I've talked to women who tell me that their doctor wants to know how many nutritive nursings their child has and how many non-nutritive nursings they have. How do you differentiate? You can't keep your body from having a letdown. Even if the baby only gets a little bit, it's nutritive. I think of it as his vitamin.

Petra, Denver, CO

Michelle's story begins in chapter 2 (page 48), where she talks about trying to nurse her daughter, born four weeks early. Her payoff appears in the following story.

 NURSING MEANT EVERYTHING

Looking back on four and a half years of nursing my daughter I have many favorite memories:

- One night when my daughter was three months old, I awoke to see my beautiful baby cuddled next to my body, latched on to my breast, sleeping. She had found my breast all by herself, nursed herself to sleep, and I had not even been awake for the feeding.
- One day when she was about nine months old, we were lying on the floor, nursing and listening to music. I assumed Taylor was finished when she stood up next to me, but then she bent down and began nursing while bouncing up and down to the beat of the music.
- Quietly nursing her at eighteen months, during an hour-long IMAX film where she remained quiet and awake through the whole thing. I am sure most people were unaware there was even a baby there.
- The first time she described what my milk tasted like: "Sweet, yummy milk. The best!"

- Having her ask me, when she was three and a half, if I wanted to nurse from *her!*
- Taylor's idea of a shower often included nursing. I would hold her, and in between having her hair and body washed, she would gravitate to my naked breasts and begin nursing. When she was around two and a half, she began standing by herself in the shower, playing as I washed myself. Often I would bend down to reach soap or shampoo, or to clean her, when she would grab hold of one breast and begin nursing. Occasionally I would pick her up, and while she nursed I would sing "You Are My Sunshine," as I had done when she was a baby, and we would share a quiet moment, swaying with the warm water showering us. Those tended to be our best days, the ones with fewer temper tantrums.
- Nursing, cuddling, and always, at any age, seeing her soundly sleeping at my breast. She seemed to be the most peaceful person in the world.

Nursing has been an important and integral part of my daughter's life, and she often plays out the nursing relationship with others. Once, while playing doll babies with my mother-in-law, she informed her that the babies were too young for solid food. My mother-in-law went to get a bottle to feed the doll, and my daughter said, "Let me pump some milk for her." Another time she had my mother (who never breastfed) nursing twin dolls.

At eighteen months, she asked her daddy if she could nurse from *him.* At two, she asked my mother-in-law if she could nurse from *her.* At four, she requested a squirt of milk in her hot cocoa to make it taste "even better," and she pretended to squirt her own breast milk onto her daddy's back while giving him a massage, saying, "There is my love for your back to make it feel better."

I often think of my relationship with my own mother. We are not close emotionally nor terribly connected to each other. She did not breastfeed me, often left me to cry myself to sleep alone, didn't hold me much, and later used physical punishment. I quickly attached to my favorite blankie and learned how to soothe myself to sleep by rubbing my feet together, which I still do today. I constantly sought her attention to be held and played with. Could I say that all of this is related to her not breastfeeding me and not listening to my cues? Not with absolute certainty, but maybe. The bottom line for me is a feeling that my basic biological and physiological needs were not respected and I wasn't loved enough. I definitely feel that breastfeeding has improved my mothering and that I would have been a different mother

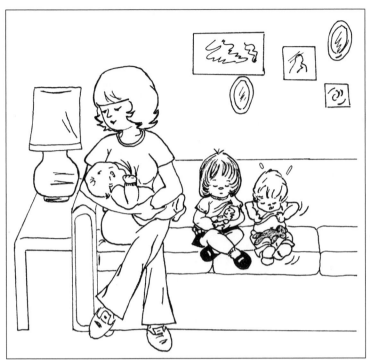

© Joan McCartney. *The Other Side Makes Chocolate.*

without it. It has taught me to listen to my child's cues. I became so in sync with her that it naturally flowed into other areas of my parenting.

My daughter knows we are planning to have a new baby someday soon. The other day, she bent over, kissed my nipple, and said, "I put enough love in here to last for the baby when it nurses." Why is it that children instinctively know what nursing is all about? And how did society get so far removed from the simple idea of nurturing and love?

Michelle Miller, Kirkland, WA

Humor and Antics

One of the discoveries we make on our parenting journeys is that nursing, particularly past the baby stage, provides endless opportunities for laughter. Some of the greatest rewards of an extended breastfeeding relationship come from the words and antics of our children. Here are excerpts revealing some of the tender and lighthearted moments taking place under the cultural radar.

A ROSE BY ANY OTHER NAME . . .

◖

We always called nursing "num-nums," and my son started calling it nummies on his own. After my son is done nursing, he'll pull down my shirt and say, "Bye-bye, nummies." We were at the park one day, and there was an older woman there with her two grandchildren. Damien started playing with them. She offered him a cookie, saying, "Do you want some nummies?"—her word for cookies. He started running over to her, and I shouted, "No! No! Wait! That's not what she meant!"

Alexis Weinstein, Hillsdale, NJ

◖

When Kelly was about three years old, she called my breasts her "bow-bows" (rhymes with wow-wow) as a derivation of "boo-boo," which came from "boob." One day her daddy asked her, "What are Mama's bow-bows for?"

"For getting milk," she responded.

"And what are Daddy's bow-bows for?" he asked.

Kelly chuckled and then said, "Daddy's bow-bows are just for decoration!"

Lisa M., Chandler, NC

FAVORITE MOMENTS

◖

I loved the first time that my son smiled while he was latched on and I could see the corner of his mouth. It was the first time I knew he was looking at me in the eyes, and he actually flipped off the nipple because his smile was so wide. That was just delicious!

Now we have a routine at night where my partner carries him upstairs while I get ready for bed because once he goes down, I'm down for the night. When she hands him over to me to nurse and his head is coming toward my breast, he gets all excited and giggly and then sighs the minute he latches on.

Nina M. Panzer, Ithaca, NY

◖

Because I have somewhat flat nipples and the twins are so little, the lactation consultants have me using nipple shields. They are thin, flexible plastic and shaped like big pointy breasts. They fit over the nipple and kind of draw it out as the boys nurse.

When Steven was three or four months old, Elizabeth, four, wanted to nurse him but told me she needed to find something to help him eat. I didn't realize what she was doing until she sat on the sofa with Steven on her lap and produced the lid from her toy teapot—a lid shaped sort of like a giant nipple shield.

She put it against her chest and actually got him latched on to it! My husband ran to get the camera for a hilarious picture while I tried to explain to Elizabeth that the nipple shield is temporary and soon the boys will not need something on my breast in order to eat.

Theresa Hemingway, Charlotte, NC

My number-one wonderful nursing moment was when my daughter would lean back, grin, and then plant a tiny, delicate little kiss right on the end of my nipple—complete with little smacky, kissy noises!

DeeDee Farris-Folkerts, Columbia, MO

FUN AND GAMES

Megan has been really entertained by the fact that my milk sprays around. I had mastitis once and was really engorged because she wasn't nursing—I guess she was teething or something. I was lying on the bed, and she pulled my shirt up and took a couple of sips. Then she sort of stepped back and touched my breast, and suddenly the milk sprayed right up in the air and she started laughing! So she developed this little game where she would push on my breast if it was really full, and every time she poked it, my milk would spray up in the air.

Vicki Duncan, Columbia, MO

My daughter was about one and a half years old when she came into bed one morning to snuggle. "Nummies?" she asked. She started to nurse, but she wanted to talk at the same time. Milk was going everywhere. "Stop the nummies, Mommy!" she said.

"I can't stop it!" I said, laughing. "You've got to stop sucking!" The milk was spraying her all over, and we both ended up in giggles.

Danielle Haven, Bessemer, AL

I discovered one morning while lying naked in bed that if I kneel over my son and shake my breasts back and forth, kind of slapping him in the face with them, he loves it! My breasts are everything to him, sometimes even toys.

Nina M. Panzer, Ithaca, NY

◗

My son will practically hang upside down and still manage to nurse. "Mommy," he'll say, "I want nummy one or nummy two," depending on which breast he wants. He'll flip on his own and say, "I want this way nummy," and when he wants me to sit in the rocking chair to nurse, he'll say, "I want rock baby." When I was teaching him not to bite, I would tell him to be soft. Now while nursing, he'll sometimes talk to me. "Soft nummy num," he'll say, and he pets it. I wish I'd never had to miss out on these things with my oldest.

Tamara Mercer, Van Wert, OH

◗

I'd intentionally squirt my husband once in a while, saying, "You're getting on my nerves!" He'd say, "Oh, gross," and go away.

Susan A. Keen, St. Louis, MO

◗

I remember when my sister's son was just learning to crawl, my sister used to lie on the floor and flash him her breast. He'd start coming over really quick, and then she'd cover it. Once my kids understood the concept of object permanence, after about ten months, we played the same game. David or Susan would go to latch on, and I'd whip the nipple to the side. They go to latch on again, and I whip the nipple up or down. They begin to squeal and giggle with delight when the breast reappears and disappears. After a couple rounds we settle down to nurse. You couldn't do that to a six-week-old, of course—it would be torture to the child. But with older babies and toddlers, it's very funny.

You can't talk to people about this, though, because they see it as being too teasing, too tied to sexuality. Perhaps someday we can all look at nursing as just another part of nurturing our children and can relax and have some fun with it.

My kids also become little Pavlovian dogs and want to nurse when-

ever I'm on the phone. Never fails. As soon as they see that phone at my ear, they start to salivate. In fact, once I needed to go somewhere for a lengthy period of time, and I wanted my son to nurse before I left. He was too busy playing, so I asked my husband to bring me the phone. I didn't even dial. I just put the phone between my shoulder and ear, and literally, within thirty seconds, my son was latched on and nursing away.

Andrea, Denver, CO

Grace has been developing a sense of humor. The first time she made up her own joke was when she started to nurse and then stopped, saying, "Hot!" Then she blew on my nipple and started laughing!

Ida Bettis Fogle, Columbia, MO

The Warrior Within

As we come into our own as mothers and our insecurities give way to growing confidence in our ability to make decisions for ourselves and our families, we become less susceptible to the opinions and judgments of others. This theme occurs throughout the book whether it involves having our children in bed with us, nursing them in public, letting them decide when *they* are ready to wean, or making various parenting decisions that have nothing to do with nursing. In the process, we become more comfortable questioning, confronting, and often resisting what may be thought of as "conventional wisdom."

This next set of stories comes from women who learned to speak up to doctors, challenge hospital protocols, and become less susceptible to the unsolicited advice and opinions of others. Some of the stories come from women who endured breastfeeding difficulties that were either created or exacerbated by poor medical advice and health care providers who failed to respect their wishes. I could easily have put together a whole book on the impact inappropriate advice and medical protocol have on breastfeeding. Frustrated with their experiences in the hospital and angry at their health care providers, women vowed to do things differently with their subsequent children. Their stories serve as lessons to all of us.

In Their Own Words:
The Warrior Within

Lori, twenty-nine, failed to receive the support and assistance most new mothers need. But in her case plenty of reading and research before she gave birth to her first of four children, along with a strong dose of determination, enabled her to overcome the hurdles she faced in the hospital.

AGGRESSION IS A FEMININE TRAIT

I haven't been incredibly successful being a female the way society thinks you ought to be. Throughout my life, even in junior high school, people would say, "This isn't the way you're supposed to act. You should be more ladylike, more feminine." I was always being told I was too aggressive, too boisterous, too overwhelming. I never felt like I met people's expectations.

It's true—I'm not ladylike. I'm loud. If I had been a teenager in the nineties instead of in the eighties, I would have worn combat boots, purple hair, and a nose ring, but in the eighties, those options weren't that available. A lot of times I'm overwhelming, even domineering, and take over conversations and relationships. When I was younger I was aggressive, sometimes to the point that I might hurt someone's feelings without even knowing it. I was completely obtuse.

I was very young, twenty, when Bishop was born. As soon as I saw him I became the she-wolf from the Amazon. I didn't feel immense, incredible love—that came later—but as soon as I held him in my arms I felt absolute protection. The nurses had to pry him out of my arms to get him away from me, and when they did, I made my husband go with them every second. I had no idea that I would feel like that, so intensely and so quickly.

I was fighting with the nurses over the most mundane things. Breast-feeding? Forget it. I had to be an absolute asshole to get what I wanted. The nurses would say, "It's not going to hurt him to have a little water out of a nipple." And I would say, "Well, my understanding is that it *could* be harmful and set back my chances of success, so I don't want you to do that."

I'm not sure where my *urge* to breastfeed came from because none of my relatives or friends had done it. I'd never been to a La Leche League meeting and never saw anyone else do it, but damn it! I was going to do it! I don't think it was an intellectual thing. It felt very primitive. If I had followed my brain, instead of my instincts, I never would have done it. I'm not very demonstrative physically. I don't do a lot of hugging, and it's difficult for me to be physically touched all the time. I also like schedules. I don't like to play it by ear, and I only like surprises if I *know* about them.

But breastfeeding Bishop was the most absolutely satisfying relationship I'm ever going to have, and I know that for the rest of my life I'll think back on nursing him and my three other children and know that those moments were the oomph, the core, the reason for me to be alive. With Bishop, we might as well have been one person. I remember feeling the most intense, overwhelming, incredible joy that I'll ever feel. I may have great moments ahead of me, but not that intense, that close together. Even if I become a Supreme Court justice and do wonderful things for the country, the absolute most important thing that I have ever done was to be available for those babies, to feed them and care for them with the intensity that I did.

Breastfeeding, for me, was absolutely feminine. It was the first time I ever felt comfortable in my own skin. When I gave birth and started using my breasts to produce milk and make a difference in a baby's life, I acquired incredible respect for my body. Breastfeeding was an *accomplishment*. Having never felt comfortable as a woman before, I suddenly couldn't deny that I was a successful woman. And it was undeniably feminine because only women can do it.

Aggression is considered a masculine trait. But it takes a great deal of aggression to actually push a person out of your body, to push a person out into the world. And if I had not been absolutely determined to breastfeed, I don't know that I would have been able to. It was one of the few times in my life where aggression came in handy, when it worked for me.

I had to fight a lot of battles. I had to fight all the "medical authorities" in the hospital, to stand up to the attitude of, "We know what's best, Honey. Just get back into bed." My obstetrician was not supportive of breastfeeding, and nobody in my family had ever done it. So I had to fight that battle of being different. But I'm someone who researches all the issues beforehand; reads everything; and then, based on the information I collect, makes a decision and follows through with it. It doesn't really matter what people think of me. I don't need superficial support.

I'm a powerful person and always have been. Breastfeeding helped me pull in the power of my own presence. It's helped me use that power better, to make it a tool for me. When I need it, I use it. When I don't need it, I don't. It's not part of every interaction I have now. And because it took so much aggression for me to breastfeed, it said to me, "You're fine. You can be female and be this way. And not only is it okay, but it's appropriate."

Lori Bishop, Jacksonville, FL

When Emma's third son was born, she was forty years old, had two children under the age of four, worked full-time, and had a one-hour subway commute each day. She also had a new job and found out she was pregnant just before starting it. She talks in the next story about her battles with the NICU nurses and the tensions that arise when breast *milk* is emphasized over breast*feeding*. (See pages 268–71, where she talks about having to wean her firstborn, and page 49, for a discussion of caring for preemies, kangaroo style.)

CONFRONTATION IN THE NICU

The doctors and nurses in the NICU were extremely pro–breast milk. I barely got to see my baby before I got a speech about how important it was to pump. A pumping room was available in the NICU for mothers to use after they had been discharged and were coming back to visit their babies. Every mother I saw was bringing milk with her. Perhaps that's why I was so taken aback when the staff proved to be so unsupportive of *nursing*. They were delighted when feeding the babies bottles of breast milk. But when it came time for me to try to nurse my baby? Forget it. Only looking back did I realize that, for all the talk of breast milk and pumping, I never saw anyone nursing, or even talking about nursing, except me. The breastfeeding *mothers* got in the way of the nurses.

My son was born at thirty-five weeks. He was admitted to the NICU with breathing difficulties and soon developed intestinal bleeding. I was devastated. I felt guilty, wondering if I had inadvertently caused him to be born prematurely because of how hard I had pushed myself during my pregnancy.

I felt lucky that I was going to get three months of maternity leave, even though I wasn't covered by the Family and Medical Leave Act. On the other hand, I felt that I couldn't stop working early, because I wanted to be able to spend all the time nursing my baby at home after he was born. I had successfully nursed my older boys after returning to full-time work, and I knew that those months establishing our nursing relationship would be crucial to our success.

While I wanted to nurse this baby because it was best for him, I had also loved nursing my older boys and greatly anticipated nursing again. In my distressed and hormonally chaotic postpartum state, I wondered if my drive to nurse had been selfish and if *that* had caused him to be born prematurely. Because of the guilt I felt, it became even more important for me to nurse him.

For the first five or six days, my son was fed with an IV, after which the nurses gave him some of my milk through a feeding tube in his stomach. They also liked the babies to do non-nutritive sucking and encouraged them to suck on a pacifier. My son didn't like them but loved to suck on my little finger. This made the nurses crazy! Everyone had to scrub like they were going into an operating room before entering the NICU, and my hands, I'm sure, could not have been cleaner. Nevertheless, they thought it was disgusting that I was sticking my finger into his mouth. "What's so terrible about it?" I asked. "He likes it, it calms him when you're drawing his blood, he breathes better, and it's non-nutritive sucking." I also thought it would enable me to do some of the oral-motor stimulation exercises I had done with my firstborn, who, three years earlier, had been born with a weak suck and had all sorts of problems latching on.

Rather than have him get bottles, I also wanted to cup-feed or finger-feed him when he was ready to go off the feeding tube. I said, "I'm here for seven of the eight feedings each day. I'm not asking *you* to do these unconventional feeding methods. Just let me do them when I'm here." It turned into a real battle. The hospital lactation consultant and the NICU feeding therapist both agreed with me and saw that my son had some problems with his suck and swallow coordination. They agreed that the exercises would help him. But the NICU nurses adamantly fought them. "That's not how we feed our babies," one of the nurses actually said to me.

"Well, it is how I feed *mine!*" I replied, outraged.

I kept saying to the NICU staff, "I don't want to do anything that's going to be detrimental to him, but I *know* it's going to be an uphill battle to teach him to nurse. All I'm asking is that we not do things that are going to make it any harder than it already has to be." I had to be in their faces the whole time! I even called the patient representative and the chief of neonatology. Finally, whether it was because of my insistence or not, I got permission to try to nurse.

Like most New York City hospitals, ours caters to a diverse multicultural patient population and prides itself on rendering culturally sensitive care. The hospital serves a huge Orthodox Jewish clientele. As an Orthodox Jewish woman myself, I'm not comfortable nursing in front of other babies' fathers, until nursing is well established and can be done with a fairly high standard of modesty. Since I obviously couldn't take the baby into another room, because he was hooked up to various monitors, I asked for a screen to be set up for this much-anticipated first session. I also had to explicitly ask for a chair with arms, but pillows were out of the question. The nurses were resentful of the extra effort it took, and by the time they got everything set up it was a half hour after the baby should have finished his feeding, and it threw their schedule off. "Sorry, guys," I thought. "You should have started setting up earlier."

By this time, his breathing problems had resolved, and he could swallow what dripped into his mouth from a bottle, though he didn't suck well on either bottle or breast. It quickly got to the point where they "advised" me that if I bottle-fed him my milk for twenty-four hours, he could be discharged, and then I could take him home and feed him however the hell I wanted. Since he wasn't taking a bottle terribly well, I was skeptical of taking him home but couldn't bear to fight with the staff any longer.

Within twenty-four hours after we were discharged my son had a weight check at our pediatrician's, a visit to the lactation consultant, and a visit with the feeding therapist from a community-based early-intervention service provider. We used finger-feeding to give supplements of expressed breast milk, in addition to nursing, and began a program of oral-motor stimulation exercises to improve his latch, suckling technique, and strength. It took six weeks before my son could nurse exclusively. He is now sixteen months old, still going strong, and I'm delighted.

My son was a wonderful, unexpected little miracle to come into our lives. But it continues to amaze me that this NICU that was so pro–breast *milk* was so unsympathetic and uninterested in doing things that could help promote breast*feeding*. My concerns were treated as if the matter were a medical issue about which I should have no input or a trivial matter I was giving too much importance to, especially since the bottles they wanted to feed him contained my milk. But how we feed our children is not purely a medical issue. Nor is whether the milk is expressed or the baby nurses a trivial difference. Maybe someday the staff of that NICU will learn that lesson.

Emma, Brooklyn, NY

People, including those in medicine, don't understand that breastfeeding entails a certain amount of physical closeness between mother and baby not based on standard child-rearing practice in this country. Medical schools educate on the anatomy and physiology of breasts, but they don't teach us about breastfeeding behaviors. Changing the perceptions of those in the medical profession would be a good starting point for other changes.

Catherine L., internist and mother of three, MD

🍵 BAD ADVICE

I didn't realize at first that my son wasn't getting enough to eat. But when he was about eight weeks old, a friend who was also breastfeeding came over and told me that he looked hungry. After she left I made him an eight-ounce bottle. He drank it all, slept for about six hours, and I sat down and cried. I felt really, really depressed. I had been starving my baby and didn't even realize it. "How can this happen to me?" I thought. "I'm so pro-breastfeeding!"

I had wanted to breastfeed exclusively, but my pediatrician had told me it was no problem to supplement through the night or when I felt I needed a break. A lot of my breastfeeding problems were directly related to her advice—I had no idea what supplementing would do to my supply. Here I was a nurse, I'd been telling people how to breastfeed, and I didn't know anything about it! And in the end, I only breastfed my son for thirteen weeks.

The second time around, I was not about to start supplementing when my milk was just coming in. My pediatrician was adamant that I use formula before leaving the hospital. She felt that I *couldn't* breastfeed and thought I was going to need to supplement. But I was adamant, too. I talked to the lactation specialist, who spent almost a full day with me, and I pumped like crazy from the start and supplemented with my own milk. The pediatrician had a public health nurse come to my house every day, and for the first couple of weeks we had to take Henry in for weight checks.

Henry is now six months old and has had no formula at all since he was born, even though I went back to work three months postpartum. I feel so much more successful and confident in my abilities, and I'm so happy!

Several years before I had Raymond I lost a baby with fetal abnormalities, so I was pretty devastated about my ability to be a mother. When the feeding problems happened with Raymond I felt really bad. Now, with Henry, I feel that I've come full circle.

Laura P. Burke, Syracuse, NY

◖

My daughter nursed almost exclusively for a year, but I had to fight my pediatrician and ended up changing doctors. He told me to stop nursing her at six months because there was no benefit to nursing and that anything after a year was not necessary or beneficial. As soon as a child was old enough to say "nurse" it was time to stop. They also told me my child was iron deficient because she wasn't eating solids, even though I had her iron tested at nine months and she was perfectly normal. I didn't want to fight this battle anymore, so I switched doctors, and I now have one who supports nursing until the age of two years.

Leslie V., Phoenix, AZ

In the next story Susan talks about her experience with thrush, a fungal or yeast infection that can make nursing quite painful. As a baby nurses, the infection can be transmitted back and forth, so both mother and baby should be treated. As in Susan's case, however, health care providers may be reluctant to treat it in the absence of obvious signs, such as milky white spots inside a baby's mouth.

While Nystatin, an antifungal agent, has frequently been used to treat thrush, current studies show that Nystatin resistance has been increasing. Almost 45 percent of *Candida* strains are now resistant (Hale 1999, 83). (This is not unlike infections becoming increasingly resistant to antibiotics.) When used carefully, gentian violet, an antifungal and antibacterial agent, provides one alternative, among others, that enables treatment without a prescription.

    MOTHER KNOWS BEST

The thrush went undiagnosed. There were no visible signs, none of those cheesy-looking things in my son's mouth. But after Christopher had been nursing for about one month, we both came down with a severe case. I told my pediatrician several times, but he refused to take a culture. He would look in the baby's mouth and say, "There's nothing in there."

I said, "My nipples are very painful when he nurses. It feels like they're on fire, like I've got glass coming through them. My husband has to rub my back to soothe me while my son latches on because it is so initially painful."

He said, "Well, all women get sore when they breastfeed."

I told him he was *wrong.* I'd been to a lactation consultant, he was latching on properly, and I wasn't sore before. I simply didn't understand why I was getting sore now. I called my obstetrician, but his wife hadn't had any trouble, and he didn't understand there could be problems. He told me to talk to a lactation consultant. Eventually I did. She told me that even without physical and visual signs, it sounded like a case of thrush.

I went back to the pediatrician. "I know my baby has thrush. I'm not *asking* you. I'm *telling* you. I want you to take a culture of his mouth and test for yeast."

He said, "Well, your insurance company's not going to pay for it because it's not going to come back positive."

I said, "That's *my* problem and *my* business. You take the culture. We'll deal with payment later."

So he did the culture, and it came back with yeast. He gave me a prescription for Nystatin, and I assumed it was for both Christopher and myself. I realized later that while he gave Christopher some Nystatin liquid, he didn't give me anything. I called him back and asked him where *my* prescription was.

He said, "What do *you* need a prescription for?"

I said, "I've been infected with this yeast. My nipples are full of it." I had to explain that we were going to pass the thrush back and forth unless we were both treated.

He wanted me to use the same liquid on my nipples, rather than a cream, and it was very messy. I finally told him that if he ever wanted to see us again, he would call me in a prescription for Nystatin cream.

Well, by this time, the thrush was so far gone that after using Nystatin for about three weeks, we were still suffering from it, though less than before. I finally went and got gentian violet, a powerful germicide available without prescription but kept behind the counter. You are only supposed to use it once or twice—it can be lethal or poisonous if used incorrectly—but I read the directions, used it carefully, and treated Christopher twice and myself once. The thrush went away the next week, and we had no more trouble.

My son is now twenty-six months old. Except for one ear infection, I had no reason to take him back to the pediatrician. But on our last visit he made us wait in a small examining room for forty-five minutes—which I didn't think was acceptable with a two-year-old—and then paid little attention to what was going on with Chris and dismissed all my concerns. We are currently in search of another pediatrician.

Susan A. Keen, St. Louis, MO

According to Roman mythology, the goddess Juno, wife of the supreme god, Jupiter, was nursing her baby Hercules when he let go of her breast just as her milk was letting down. Streams of milk poured out of her, but instead of being swallowed by her suckling infant, they spurted upward into the heavens and became stars. This mythological interpretation of how our galaxy came to be named the Milky Way may not be as far-fetched as it seems. A friend of mine relayed an experience that happened to her when she was a young nursing mother in the 1970s. Had she felt that the medical community was open to working with her, her experience would likely have been resolved quite differently.

☕ THE MILKY WAY

My husband and I were sitting in our parked Dodge Dart with our nine- or ten-month-old daughter between us. The front piece of the car seat was attached by hinges. Since we were parked for quite a while, we had unfastened the car seat, and I was sitting with my left arm draped around the back of it. Our daughter was happily lifting it up, putting it down, lifting it up, putting it down, when my left breast got squished in the side hinge. It was exquisitely painful. Immediately I lifted my shirt to assess the damage and discovered that a blood blister had instantly formed.

I didn't know what to do. I was living in New York City but vacationing in upstate New York and was terrified to go to the local hospital because the political climate for breastfeeding in the 1970s was not at all supportive. I had heard many stories of women being told they had to stop nursing because of mastitis or plugged ducts, so I was afraid to seek any medical attention because I didn't want to wean my daughter.

That evening, my breast became harder and harder. I tried to get my daughter to latch on to the affected side, but no matter how much she tried to nurse, no milk was coming out. In looking at my nipple more closely, I realized it was completely covered up by this blood blister and there was no way the milk was going to get out. I also tried putting hot compresses on it all evening, but they didn't work. My breast was getting harder and larger. I realized my only hope for any kind of relief was to break the blood blister. It was so painful, but with the nails of my thumb and forefinger, I broke it.

You can't even imagine the force that had built up behind this hard, painful, overfilled breast. I was lying on my back on a futon, and as I broke the blister, the milk shot completely up to the ceiling and sprayed all over it. It just erupted upward with a tremendous ejaculation, and I thought to myself, "Well! It's the Milky Way."

Of course, I felt an immediate sense of relief. The bad news was that the blood blister kept reforming, and I had to break it several times, which was really painful. But at least I was able to keep the milk ducts open enough for my daughter to nurse and for me to get relief, and eventually the paths through which the milk flowed kind of rerouted themselves in a different way.

Gail L. Birnbaum, Ithaca, NY

Benefits and Rewards

Fewer ear infections. Reduced incidence of asthma. Fewer digestive problems. Most of us are familiar with these kinds of benefits of breastfeeding.* But there are myriad benefits and rewards of breastfeeding that have little to do with nutrition and health. Unfortunately, they seldom make it into typical how-to books. Here is just a sampling.

❍

A few weeks ago, Grace came down with an intestinal virus. She was throwing up, couldn't eat, and wouldn't even try to drink water. But she would nurse. I had horrible visions of what could happen if she weren't breastfeeding, things I knew other parents had gone through: dehydration, frantic efforts to force-feed electrolyte solutions, even hospital IV drips. Fortunately, nursing both comforted her and kept her adequately hydrated. I was extremely grateful we got through her illness so easily without having to take drastic, unpleasant measures. On the other hand, when I was hit with the same virus a few days later, I wasn't particularly happy about nursing her. But we managed to survive.

Nursing has also made it easy for me to rinse shampoo out of my daughter's hair. We bathe together, and I put her in standard nursing position. This way I can use one hand to take a washcloth and rinse the shampoo off so it doesn't go into her eyes. It's the only way I've been able to convince her to lean her head back.

Ida Bettis Fogle, Columbia, MO

❍

When Haleigh was six weeks old we had a snowstorm, and the power was out for four days. We have a well, so no power meant no water.

---

* Lactation consultant Diane Wiessinger emphasizes that the risk of stating these facts as benefits is that it takes formula-feeding as the biological norm, the standard against which babies' health and well-being should be measured. If *breastfeeding* were the standard, however, we wouldn't hear that breastfed babies tend to be *healthier*. Instead we would hear that formula-fed babies tend to be *sicker*.

Without water or power I would have had no way to mix or warm formula. A couple of years later, when Rebecca was five weeks old, we had an ice, snow, and windstorm that knocked the power out for twelve long days! If I hadn't been nursing, feeding my babies would have been very difficult, perhaps impossible.

Peggy Olsen, Elma, WA

❍

We traveled a lot by plane. Whenever the plane took off or landed, I would breastfeed, and it helped with their ears.

Opal Palmer Adisa, Oakland, CA

❍

I remember a distinct difference in the diaper odor when I stopped nursing and switched to formula. Even the day-care workers noticed!

Veronica M., Indianapolis, IN

❍

I discovered that you can use breast milk for everything. A mild case of diaper rash? Breast milk. Pinkeye? Breast milk. It was amazing. I like that I can nurture my children in a way that no one else can.

Danielle Haven, Bessemer, AL

❍

After several months of calmly easing my way into mothering my second-born, I suddenly experienced a temporary period of depression and anxiety during which I doubted my abilities as a mother. Breastfeeding Emma served as a constant reminder that I was, in fact, able to satisfy my daughter's most basic needs for nurturing and sustenance, and it was one of the most important factors that influenced my rediscovered peace of mind.

Amy C. Condra-Peters, NH

❍

I didn't want to put icing on my son's cake for his first birthday because I thought it was too sweet, so I pumped out about eight ounces of milk, whipped it with sugar and a little vanilla, and iced a small cake. My husband thought it was the best whipped cream he had ever eaten. We have

*this on the video camera—my husband eating finger-fulls off the cake
and commenting on how sweet and wonderful it was. And he had no
idea until maybe five months ago.*

Susan A. Keen, St. Louis, MO

Memory and Connection

*Growing a baby inside, as well as mothering a newborn, puts a
woman in closer touch with her own childhood experiences, allowing old, deeply buried thoughts and emotions to surface.
Hopes and fears from the past and for the future merge at the surface of her daily consciousness, as time compresses in the physical experience of pregnancy, and past, present and future together
are carried in her womb.*

Robbie E. Davis-Floyd,
Birth as an American Rite of Passage

Before we are mothers, we are daughters. When we have our own
children, it is this first, primary relationship we revisit. The insight
and experience we acquire throughout our nursing relationship not
only cause us to reexamine our preconceptions of parenting and our
interactions with health care providers but also help us to gain new
insights into our relationship with our own mothers. It is only natural, for example, to compare and contrast the similarities and differences between how we mother *our* children and how we *ourselves* were mothered. For those of us who were breastfed, nursing
our own children becomes one of the ways in which we experience
continuity and connection with our mothers. For those of us who
weren't, it can become part of the basis from which we differentiate ourselves. In either case, some of us discover that nursing not
only causes us to revisit our childhood but may affect our *current*
relationship with our mothers.

The next few stories speak of insight and discovery within the
powerful context of intergenerational connection.

In Their Own Words:
Memory and Connection

Annette was one of several women who talked about the unexpected impact nursing had on their relationship with their mothers.

Originally from Mississippi, she describes herself as having over-come low self-esteem, a lack of confidence, and an inability to make deep connections with people. "Because of what I went through with my daughter," she said, "I'm a much stronger person than I thought I was. I feel that I can handle anything that comes along."

FINDING RESPECT AND INTIMACY

My mother is very critical and usually negative. I never felt I met her expectations, even though I didn't know what they were. She's not emotional, she doesn't express her feelings, and she's not very demonstrative. I would never have called her my friend.

But ever since my daughter was born, our relationship has improved. She arrived the day Tammy was born and came to help for a week. I was having a difficult time breastfeeding, in part because my milk didn't come in for at least a week. Although I had a doula helping me, my mom commented that, as my mother, *she* should have been able to help. But she had never breast-fed and had no experience with it. She felt useless not being able to help. Of course, I told her that just having her there was encouraging and supportive.

Since this time, my mom seems to have a respect for me that I never felt before. I think that came from her seeing the kind of sacrifices and effort I made to provide Tammy with the best thing for her. It's amazing that the only benefits I anticipated from nursing had to do with my daughter's health and an intimate start for the two of us. I never would have predicted that it would bring my mom and me closer. And my mom has become a big breast-feeding advocate. She'll tell anybody now why breastfeeding is best.

Annette, Houston, TX

After overcoming cancer in her late twenties and years of failed efforts to conceive, Debbie gave birth to her son when she was thirty-eight. Her story illustrates the discrepancies that can exist be-tween what we know intellectually and what we feel emotionally. In Debbie's case, much of what she struggled with was the direct re-sult of what she learned as a child.

BATTLING OLD MESSAGES

As soon as I peeked in the door, a feeling came over me, like a physical force hitting me in the face at ninety miles an hour. It felt very ancient, very primal. I saw my son, six weeks old, comfortably taking a bottle. I had expressed milk that morning and left it for the doula to give to him while I worked in the other room. I knew when he woke up she would give him a bottle for the first time. I had kind of hoped I would hear a lot of screaming, but I didn't, so I was checking in.

"How's it going?" I asked.

"No problem," she replied. "He's drinking from the bottle just fine."

I burst into tears and started sobbing. I realized in that moment there was something really wrong with someone else feeding my child. I thought, "Oh, my God. I could be replaced. I'm not needed anymore." It was like getting stabbed in the gut.

I come from a large family where people took things away from you. Everyone struggled to be seen, and any type of recognition was sought after, craved. My parents had four kids within five years. If one of us did something wrong, we all got in trouble. We were seen as "the kids," lumped into one group, instead of as individuals. There was nothing you could ever claim as your own. We weren't allowed locks on our doors, and our diaries were read. Our boundaries melted into one another.

My father was an alcoholic and very abusive. His driving message to us was, "You are not good enough. In fact, you are the worst there is." Any time he knew that you really wanted something, he would take it away. So when I saw how easily my son took a bottle or when I thought about going out for the night, I saw how easily I could be replaced and have things taken away from me. It brought up the "I'm not good enough" tape: "He doesn't like me, and he'll like somebody else better."

I've struggled with low self-esteem all my life. A lot of times, instead of having this overwhelming feeling of nurturance when I'm nursing, either I'm hoping I'm making enough milk or hoping that chemicals and pesticides aren't going through the milk. To this day when I look at my son, I can't believe he's mine. He's so incredibly beautiful and pure, and it's so hard for me to believe I had something to do with it.

What little self-esteem I did have growing up came from an intense drive to be the best, to master every task. But when I had my son, I had no clue how to breastfeed. I felt there was something wrong with me that I didn't intuitively know how. But Kyle latched on perfectly, and I took my cues from him. We figured things out together, rather than me having to seek help. That would have been worse because growing up, we never went to others for help, and we didn't go to doctors. My father wouldn't allow it. That meant you weren't good enough or smart enough.

My son is seven months old now. If I see him reaching out for somebody else or playing with someone else's face, my heart breaks. I think, "He likes them as much as me. I'm not as special." Intellectually I know it's not true. I know I'm a great mom, but I can't get rid of all these old messages. I wish I could. And I dread the day when my son weans, because nursing is the only thing I can do for him that *nobody* else can.

Deborah Daly, Wilton, CT

Even when our mothers are no longer with us, nursing can be a powerful reminder of a common, unmistakable bond we share. The next piece comes out of a writing circle I organized earlier in this book's development. The newborn son Elise mentions is now a busy ten-year-old with a six-year-old brother. Her story remains one of my favorites.

☕ A MOTHER'S LEGACY

When my son was a newborn I was trying to learn all that new-mom stuff—how to feed him; when to burp him; how to get him to sleep for several hours at a stretch; and, failing the latter, how to survive. My father, in a valiant effort to help me sort it all out, told me my mother had used a diaper pin on her bra strap to identify which breast to nurse with next.

So I gave it a try. But I was never able to keep straight whether I had put the pin on the side I had most recently used or on the side I should start with *next.* Furthermore, I found that the only way to keep him awake and suckling long enough so he would sleep for more than forty-five minutes was to switch breasts every ten minutes or so—six or eight times at every feeding. So switching a pin around was out of the question. Instead, I began writing it down. In no time, my favorite nursing chair was surrounded by little scraps of paper covered with sleep-deprived scrawls, meandering columns of capital Ls and Rs, with the times listed next to them: L 3:45–3:57, R 3:57–4:15, L 4:15–4:32.

Sometime in those first few months, we visited my dad. In the blanket chest in my old bedroom, I found a smallish box. It was marked, in my mother's handwriting, "for Lise's scrapbook," and it was filled with cards and telegrams congratulating my parents on my birth. Many had little penciled notes, also in my mother's hand: "Pink hat and booties." "White smocked dress." "Silver rattle."

On the back of one card, from our Uncle Zimmie, was a scribbled single column of capital Ls and Rs, with times listed next to them. Suddenly I felt a connection to my mother's early mothering and nursing experience—an imparting of her wisdom I'd assumed I had missed by her death the year before. I could clearly picture my mom, sleepy eyed, smiling in the dim light, nursing, rocking, and writing down cryptic messages only another nursing mother would understand.

Early this morning, my sister gave birth to her first child. When I go to visit her next week, I think I'll bring her the card from Uncle Zimmie and leave the diaper pin at home.

Written by Elise Nelson, Houghton, MI

CHAPTER FIVE

A Balancing Act

STORIES OF READJUSTMENT, IDENTITY, & BOUNDARIES

In breastfeeding one may find . . . the most intense experience of conflict over what the late-twentieth-century American mother is and ought to be.

Linda M. Blum, At the Breast

God, she's beautiful! I lie on the futon nursing my daughter and listen to her breathing become deeper, more rhythmic. I am smitten. Carefully, I guide my finger between her tiny hand and my breast and slide my nipple out of her mouth. Eyes shut, she searches for the lost nipple like a baby robin, eager for its mother to feed him. In a moment she will cry with frustration and wake herself up. I let her mouth return to my breast. She is home.

I gaze at her puckering cheek and possessive embrace of my breast. Her breathing is again deep, her body relaxed. I wait and once more try to reclaim my nipple. Fat chance! Her head follows her mouth toward my receding breast. Clamp! She is back on. Her eyes never opened.

She clings to the breast she believes is hers. I'm getting bored. My neck is stiff. I can't be her pacifier all morning! She sighs and sucks with more determination. This is not the breathing pattern of a baby in deep sleep. I roll my eyes. She sucks.

I've given birth to a leech! I resolve myself to a no-nap/no-work morning and try one last time to separate mouth from breast. She stirs, but her mouth stays shut! Yes! A free woman at last!

I slide my body away and tiptoe hurriedly across the room, eager for a chance to get to my computer. My hand is on the doorknob, and I turn around. My daughter is on her back now, sucking an imaginary breast. I stand there for several minutes staring at her. I am smitten. God, she's beautiful!

I don't remember how old my daughter was when I wrote this piece, probably a year or so, but I clearly remember the battle of my emotions: the overwhelming love I felt for her; the fusion I often felt between her body and mine; and the burning desire to have just a single hour to myself, to feel the satisfaction of having something tangible to show for my time.

The struggle for balance is a central theme of mothering. Not only must we balance the biological needs of our children in our adult-oriented culture, but regardless of how old or numerous our children are, or whether we are parenting solo or with partners, we each perform juggling acts on a daily basis. The stories in this chapter all center around this ongoing quest. (Stories about balancing these needs with the need to make a living appear in the following chapter.)

Finding Time, Finding Self

My experience of nursing my daughter to sleep suggests at least two distinct ways to think about the nursing relationship. On one end of the spectrum, we have mother and child with a physical, almost spiritual connection: the baby cries, the mother's milk lets down, the baby suckles, the mother's uterus contracts. Their boundaries are almost nonexistent. Writer Andrea Boroff Eagan describes this relationship as symbiotic; that is, mother and child have not yet become fully separate beings but are two different yet highly interdependent organisms. On the other end are a mother and child with separate and often competing needs. The baby's need for connection and fusion contrasts sharply with the mother's need for autonomy and self-definition (Eagan 1985).

The day-to-day life of our mothering takes place within the boundaries of these two extremes and constantly evolves and fluctuates. Typically, as our babies mature and begin to acquire separate identities, we in turn look for ways to integrate and balance who *we* are vis-à-vis who *they* are. For many, the issue of balance is inextricably bound up with the issue of identity.

In *The Mask of Motherhood: How Becoming a Mother Changes Everything and Why We Pretend it Doesn't,* author Susan Maushart writes that the transition to motherhood is increasingly associated with a major identity crisis, a "mismatch between expectation and experience, between what we ought to be feeling and how we do feel, between how we ought to be managing and how we do manage" (1999, xi). A friend of mine, a highly educated, professional woman, refers to this as "the oh-my-god-what-have-I-done factor."

Part of the adjustment women experience has to do with the emphasis our culture puts on the need to *accomplish* something, to have something to show at the end of the day. Even though we receive little social recognition for the work of mothering, much of what we do is, in fact, *work*. Although we may know this intellectually, many of us still feel frustrated spending our day doing "nothing" but taking care of a baby.

In her essay "Having a Baby, Finishing a Book," author Mary Gordon reflects on the way having a baby caused her to rearrange her priorities, her very consciousness:

> It is the first hot day of the year. A drugged and meager light sifts through the haze; almost as in a dream I see the chestnut tree through the window, its flowers set within its leaves like little candelabras. I can see the chestnut tree from the bed where I lie with my baby, skin to skin. The pleasure of this is like the pleasure of a drug; it prevents activity. Only I am active. I am feeding. Perfectly still, almost without volition, I nourish. (1991, 220)

This business of nursing, of readjusting our lives to take constant care of another human being, of redefining accomplishment, is a transition some of us undergo easily and others not so easily. The challenge is to find a way to address the biological demands, even pleasures, of being female without falling into what writer Natalie Angier refers to as "the sludge of biological determinism" (1999).

In Their Own Words:
Finding Time, Finding Self

Before becoming a mother, Allegra had an exciting career in New York City and Russia. Forty-one with two daughters, three and a half and one, she reflects on life as a nursing mother vis-à-vis life before motherhood and the surprising way she managed to achieve . . .

A SENSE OF ACCOMPLISHMENT

Who leaves a great job at the United Nations? I had fascinating work, fantastic medical benefits, and three months paid maternity leave. But when I first went back, I missed my baby so much! I asked my sitter to bring her to me at work so I could see her sooner. It was like I was waiting for a date. "Do you think she's left the house yet? Is she on the subway? Do you think she's here yet?"

Before my daughter was born I *knew* I'd go back to work at the end of my maternity leave. But this was a harder decision once I had Kira. Aside from missing her, there was the ridiculously high cost of child care in New York and the inconvenience of pumping at work. So even though I rather smugly think New York is the center of the world, we moved to Texas, where my husband has family. Erik would work, and I would stay home for a while.

This was a huge identity shift for me. I'm goal oriented, and it's hard to feel like I'm accomplishing anything when I just feed the baby, sweep the floor, and play. It feels like work, and it certainly takes up a lot of time, but even *I* don't appreciate it. I have all these things I'm trying to accomplish, things that could bring in a little extra money if I could only complete them, but I don't have the time.

I've had problems adjusting to my new at-home role. It's hard to find a part-time, fascinating, paid position, unless you are already established. I found some volunteer work in an archeological lab, just a few hours a day, once or twice a week, and after a while I started to get some paid work from them. But after I had my second baby I didn't have time anymore. Having watched Kira grow to three and a half, I've seen how quickly babies change to children—it goes by in a blink! And I want to be here to watch every step.

Then I heard about the nearby milk bank and the need for donors.* Here was a way I could be productive without having to leave the house. I've now

* A discussion of milk banks begins on page 82.

been donating for eight months. I try to pump every day or every other day. A few months ago I had a freezer full of milk, but then everyone in the family started getting sick. You can't donate then, because the babies who receive the milk have compromised immune systems.

I still miss putting on nice clothes, looking professional, and talking to grown-ups about anything not related to children. I miss the stimulating environment of the U.N. Donating my milk, though, is a way I can do *something*. When I have a freezer full of milk, I can *see* the bottles and know what I have done. They accumulate, I can count them, and at least I feel I've accomplished something.

Allegra Azulay, Pflugerville, TX

Joyce, forty, has an eight-month-old daughter. Although she had little trouble conceiving, it took her a lot longer to decide whether or not to do so in the first place. Her indecision as she contemplated motherhood gave way to a new kind of ambivalence as she nursed her daughter.

IT'S ALL ABOUT AMBIVALENCE

Sometimes I wish people would be less definitive, less deadly earnest and self-assured in their accounts of breastfeeding. Why not something in between "It's the best thing I've ever done" and "It just didn't work for me"? Why not more ambivalence? Breastfeeding is one of the most gratifying things I've ever done—*and* I wish I were done with it. I'm thrilled at the tidy efficiency of feeding my daughter this way—*and* I want my body back. Below are some random thoughts, events, and memories about these fluctuations.

The Bethlehem, Pennsylvania, La Leche League doesn't seem to fit the stereotype. The leader is a model—sexy, outspoken, and irreverently funny. There's no circa-1970 earth-mother idealism there, but a passion for attachment parenting and biting derision toward formula manufacturers, advocates of early feeding of solid foods, and a lot of pediatricians in the area.

I attended my first meeting a month after I learned I was pregnant. I was afraid I wouldn't know what to do and felt I had to do everything right. And although I had lived here for four or five years, I didn't feel tapped into a community. So, influenced by a few friends, I went to a meeting. And suddenly I was a mother's milk militant. At the end of that first meeting, I was sure: I would breastfeed my baby for two years, maybe longer.

Soon after Anna's birth, a breastfeeding friend who weaned each of her daughters at around age three said to me, "Don't you just love knowing that everything she takes in comes from you and you alone?" I nodded faintly. Inwardly, I panicked. It felt like way too much responsibility.

When Anna was a little over three months old, another friend told me she was beginning to gradually wean her ten-month-old daughter. I was silent—for the briefest of seconds, I'm sure—and she immediately started explaining, justifying, apologizing. I caught myself and started making loud noises of support and understanding. Inwardly, I was surprised, even a little unnerved, at my reaction. There *was* a kind of judgment in my silence, no doubt about it. Where did *that* come from?

Those early La Leche League meetings led me to expect the worst from family members who just wouldn't *get* the breastfeeding thing. At thirty-nine, I hadn't really talked about such things with my mother, but as it turns out, my parents have been two of my most avid supporters. All they seem concerned about was that I might run out of milk. This is a mystery to me. There seemed to be this consensus in my family that at about six months the well would run dry. I think the well runs dry when you start giving bottles in place of the breast. But now I'm hearing that judgmental tone in my own voice again. Enough of that.

I haven't made it to too many more La Leche League meetings, mainly because of conflicts with my work schedule (I went back to part-time teaching this semester). Maybe I imagined it, but at the last meeting I went to, it seemed I got a pretty cool reception when I asked for help or advice for arranging minimal child care (just a few hours a week) when I went back to teach.

I had to stop reading the LLL bible, *The Womanly Art of Breastfeeding*, because it made me feel guilty about going back to work, even part-time.

I guess the main thing I feel about the whole breastfeeding experience is that it's been beautiful and magical (Anna's wide eyes looking up at me when she pauses—there is nothing like that in the world), but it's also been nerve-wracking and exhausting. Still, I wouldn't trade this for anything, and I think I'll be doing it for a while yet.

But I think we should all be a little easier on each other and assume we're all doing the best we can. It's okay to be ambivalent, isn't it?

Written by Joyce Hinnefeld, Easton, PA

Who is a feminist, how one defines feminism, and how our individual understanding of it evolves have long been controversial. In the next story, Roxanne, an actress, writes about how her son's birth caused her to revisit the liberal mantra of gender equality as sameness.

A NEW BRAND OF FEMINISM

I've always considered myself a feminist, even when the mark of a popular girl at my Southern Presbyterian liberal-arts college was to say, "Oh, I'd never call myself, you know, a feminist," as if it were a bad word. I was sure I could have it all, and all at once. I was so adept at combining pregnancy with life that I landed a coveted female lead role in a television pilot when seven and a half months pregnant—playing a decidedly nonpregnant femme fatale lawyer. I was due to give birth in late July, and the producers asked me: "If the show goes, will you be able to report to work on August 1st?" There was not a moment's hesitation before I assured them of my desire not to let motherhood change my life or ambition.

Then God/Nature/the Universe laughed, and I gave birth to a son. Although fully accessorized for my transition to "working mom" with a full-time nanny at the ready, sometime before reality (and milk) settled in, I had decided to nurse my baby. Why? I am a mammal. Mammals nurse their young. Sure, there's formula, but just as I wouldn't amputate a perfectly good limb to trade it in for one of the modern miracles in prostheses, I decided to go with the real thing.

Besides, bottle-feeding just adds work. Buy bottles, nipples, and formula; wash bottles; make formula; warm it up; feed and burp the baby; rinse bottles; start again. An endless lather-rinse-repeat of mothering, and I am way too lazy for that. And I was definitely interested in free milk, a less-often-sick baby, and all the advantages to the mother.

And, truth be known, I know that without nursing I would not have bonded so tightly with this wrinkly little nursing/sleeping/pooping machine we call Cameron. I am an escaper. If a situation gets tense, my preferred coping style is to vacate the premises. And life with a newborn offers many opportunities for tension. With a nanny and no need to be physically in the same room, much less the same state, I might have recuperated from my long and arduous labor at, say, the Golden Door Spa, which does not accept kids.

For several months I couldn't even escape to Bella, my wizard of waxing, for a brow and bikini treatment. I was like Al Pacino in *The Godfather*,

Part III—"Just when I think I'm gonna get out, they pull me back in!" You can't escape the Mafia. And you can't escape a nursing baby. I was tethered, bonded like Crazy Glue due to my milk and Cameron's insatiable hunger for it, which meant hunger for *me*, his mom. So when the show I could have been working on straight from the delivery room wasn't picked up, I breathed a small sigh of relief.

Because I'm nursing, my babysitter has a pretty cool gig. In the first year, it's pretty much the three of us together all the time. I work in the next room or just outside the dressing room and return at the first sign of hunger or need.

They are *my* breasts, and yet, like Häagen-Dazs ice cream, the last cold drink on a hot day, or the blankets in winter, I share them with my family. Sometimes begrudgingly, as when our daughter—cranky, sleepless, and miserable—grabs me and cries, "Nurse, Mommy!" as if her crack high is wearing off and she needs another hit. Sometimes eagerly, like the time our son awoke from general anesthesia, blood crusted on the side of his groggy, swollen face, and I offered the familiar nectar I know will soothe him, the milk that qualifies medically as a "clear liquid." And sometimes I share them with my husband, who, after six years of marriage in which we've had a total of two and a half months during which I wasn't pregnant or nursing, has said, without a trace of irony, "I want my breasts back!"

They are *our* breasts, the Bob and Roxanne Hoge Family breasts, and I laugh when I remember their previous career moves. Propped up in Wonder Bras to sell stupid sitcoms where the female characters always have smooth, round, pushed-up breasts and wear cleavage-enhancing clothing that, in the real world, wouldn't work for a CEO because no man would ever hear a word she said. Breasts on duty, as I like to say. Hey, it paid well.

Now they have a real job, a hard job, and they are slightly the worse for wear. I know it's the weight gain, two pregnancies, gravity, and age that do the most damage, but I hear that breastfeeding gets the rap more often than not. But they work. Knowing that I took this being from chicken-scrawny to a plump and sturdy toddler screams accomplishment and is a great ego booster in a full-time job with no performance reviews.

And so my new brand of feminism finds this lifelong liberal, "we-are-all-the-same" preacher believing that babies need their mommies. Admittedly, being elsewhere is an attractive proposition at three A.M. when I feel like a twenty-four-hour Dairy Queen. But in not escaping my biology or my progeny, I found *myself.* Maybe not a blow-dried, Armani-clad, glossy, multitasking self, but it's me.

And it turns out that nursing is the most radical feminist act I've undertaken recently. I have become an ambassador, educator, and rabble-rouser,

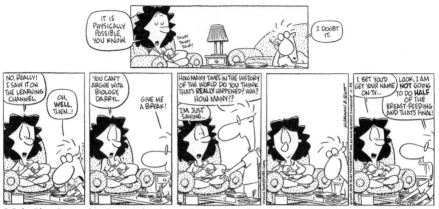

© Baby Blues Partnership. Reprinted with special permission of King Features Syndicate.

defending our right to be out in public with our hungry babies. Instead of viewing my breasts through the distorting prism of Hugh Hefner's bifocals, I now realize that, viewed through the milk-induced drunken smile of my baby, they are the best.

Like many of my friends, I am a fashion-loving, cell-phone-toting chick who likes cabernet with her filet mignon. And who nurses her toddler. The reasons are simple: It's our biology. It's our destiny. It's right for us.

Written by Roxanne Beckford Hoge, Los Angeles, CA

Sam's got two mommies. And I can picture both moms breastfeeding. In fact, the other day at nap time I was saying, "I'll be right up," and before I got there Lisa had put him to sleep by latching him on to her. Sometimes he goes for it, and sometimes he doesn't. It's so sweet when he does. I love seeing Lisa sitting there with Sam in her arms, looking down at him. It's a wonderful opportunity for her to get to experience a little bit of what nursing feels like.

Nina M. Panzer, Ithaca, NY

Diana, thirty-six, makes her home in the "urban and gritty" South of Market Area of San Francisco. Long estranged from her family of origin, she is the only mother in some of her circles of friends. She reflects in the next piece on the fundamental place of nursing in her life and the challenges of single parenthood.

☕ DESCRIBING THE COLOR ORANGE

I am a single mom by choice and have worked hard at maintaining my pre-baby friends and activities. I have never felt shy about nursing in public because I am fairly discreet and know the supreme importance breast milk plays in Jade's physical and emotional development.

As a mom who constantly nurses, I take my daughter with me to many social activities. Jade has attended many hip parties tucked away in her sling. About 99 percent of the people there don't have regular partners, let alone children. We are a bit of an anomaly. But I believe my constant presence and offer of the breast have helped form my daughter into a calm and happy person, and her easy nature has made her popular with my friends and acquaintances.

I get a lot of positive attention as a single, independent woman who doesn't rely on a man for her fulfillment. But since almost everybody in this town is childless, there isn't a lot of understanding about what a little kid wants and needs. Once, for example, my date and I were watching TV with my baby. I had nursed her throughout the evening, but at one point she approached me and suddenly yanked my shirt up. I wasn't ready to nurse her and began to smooth my shirt down. She threw a long tantrum, and the evening was awkward after that. I think if my date had understood that, comparatively speaking, my baby cries about 50 percent less than other babies, he would have been impressed, but since he'd never been around babies before, he didn't know what to think.

I recently ended an engagement because my fiancé and I disagreed about the amount of breastfeeding a child needs for a happy and healthy life. I have always been a "loud and proud" breastfeeder, and my fiancé saw that from the beginning. But along the way he changed his mind and decided he didn't like it. (He said he could never be comfortable with me breastfeeding an infant past the age of six months and that he wouldn't feel comfortable having her sleep in our bed.) He proposed that I change my position on extended breastfeeding and co-sleeping as an effort to get along with him better.

I tried to explain my feelings. But how do you describe the color orange to someone who has no eyes? That's how it is trying to describe parenting to someone who hasn't ever given birth or parented. As a parent, I strive to give my child the best of everything. *Breast milk is the best.* And "Mama Milk" fixes almost everything. When I see how great a difference it makes in her life, there is no way I can take it away with good conscience. And love makes everything easy. Continually being present for my child, being on call for her, is not the trouble it might seem to a non-parent.

I declined the offer of marriage and ended the relationship. Breastfeeding Jade and any other future children is so important to me that I would rather miss out on getting married than compromise on these major tenets in my life. I've felt sad and have missed him since the breakup, but my many pleasurable moments breastfeeding Jade have underlined that I made the right choice.

Diana Greer, San Francisco, CA

. . . And Baby Makes Four (or Five, or Six . . .)

Our culture places a high value on individualism and independence, and the values that underscore dominant child-rearing practices reflect this. Sometimes, however, honoring our children's individuality causes us to recognize their need for connection and dependency. It is *because* they have distinct needs that we don't wean them before they are ready. It is *because* they want to feel our skin and hear our heart beat that we keep them in our beds. Doing our best to meet their needs and honoring their unique developmental time frame, however, takes on a whole new dimension when we have more than one child. This, of course, impacts breastfeeding, regardless of whether we have one nursling or more.

Those of us who can focus solely on the needs of one child may not fully appreciate the issues that arise for women whose attention must be further divided. This next group of stories captures some of the nursing-related issues that arise when nursing mothers have more than one child to take care of.

In Their Own Words:
. . . And Baby Makes Four (or Five, or Six . . .)

The cover of Jane Ribbens's book, *Mothers and Their Children: A Feminist Sociology of Childrearing* (1995), depicts an abstract representation of a mother being pulled in opposite directions by her two young children. All three bodies are faceless, and the mother's feet are turned inward, as if she doesn't know which way to go. Kathy's recollections dramatically personalize this kind of tension.

A TRADE-OFF

My son, Kyle, now twenty-four years old, was the only baby I had ever seen who would nurse and then fuss until I put him down. He didn't want to be held or rocked to sleep. He had to be by himself in the cradle or bassinet, and he had to have his space around him. He's still like that. He's very affectionate, but he needs solitary time, desperately. He gets distracted and is unhappy when there is too much input.

As an infant he was so distractible that for the first month or two he didn't gain any weight. If someone came into the room, he would stop nursing and look around. The pediatrician talked about supplementing, but I wanted him to be totally breastfed.

In order to get Kyle to nurse, I had to take him alone into a darkened room, pull the curtains, and sit with him in a rocking chair. This meant that Ian, my two-year-old, had to stay outside the room while I nursed the baby. I had to say to him, "The baby has to nurse. I'll be out in a little while." I would try to set up some toys or coloring things or sometimes even television, when there was something I thought he could watch. I can still see him standing out there in the hallway as I'm taking the little baby away into the other room, his tiny face looking up at me, pacifier in his mouth, as I'm closing the door. Shit!! It just hurt my heart. I don't know if I've ever cried about that before, but after all these years I'm weepy now thinking about it!

Once Kyle started to gain weight and became more established as a nursing baby, I didn't need to seek out private places. But there were a couple of months when I had to try to be as quiet and private with him as possible. There was that kind of trade-off—to adequately nourish one child, I had to turn away from another.

Kathleen Kramer, Newfield, NY

Much of Kathleen's experience appears on pages 16–20, and she shares her reflections on weaning on pages 278–79.

❍

Because there's been so much activity going on, Larissa has been distracted from day one and hasn't been as good a nurser as Kelsey was. She'll get off my breast to look around just as I'm having a letdown, and breast milk starts shooting out at her! The only times when she latches on and drinks without going on and off the breast a lot, and when I feel like she's actually filled up, have been in the middle of the night or last thing in the day when I'm putting her down to sleep. My doctor said, "You just need to find a quiet, dark place." Yeah, right.

Joan P., Loveland, CO

At the same time that we try to meet the individual needs of our children, our own needs may get lost in the process. Some of us do not view the sacrifices of self as a burden. Others struggle. As much as Gwen adored nursing, her story speaks to the unyielding physical and emotional demands that may accompany intensive parenting, particularly when nursing more than one child.

UNDER WATER

The look on Ava's face broke my heart. It was her birthday, and we were getting a pizza. She was tired, it was hot, and she wanted to nurse. But I had told her that when she turned four she wouldn't have "num num boobie" anymore—her phrase for nursing. I said, "Honey, you're four now, and we're not going to do that anymore." It was a heartbreaking moment, and I just held her in my arms. It was a bad idea to wean her on her birthday, but I hadn't thought about that.

My daughter had loved to nurse, and I had always let her. I would nurse her on the subway, on the PATH train, in the sling. I would put her on a Boppy (a breastfeeding pillow) and would talk on the phone, even read a novel. She just loved to nurse! And so did I. We had a family bed, and when she was about one year old she would wiggle a little bit and I knew it was time to feed her. All I had to do was roll over, and she would find my breast. In the morning my breast was the fullest. I would be gushing, and she could hardly keep up with it. She would be moaning in pleasure and swallowing these big gulps of milk—while sleeping. Those were beautiful moments.

As she got older I realized that nursing was more than nourishment, and I discovered that the most powerful mothering tool was my breast. In fact, in German, the verb "to soothe" is the same as the verb "to nurse."* When Ava would get hurt or feel frustrated all I had to do was open my shirt. She would latch on and go from crying to silence within a second. We called it "the plug."

But as much as nursing was fundamental to my mothering, nursing became painful during my pregnancy and drove me crazy! I began to curb her nursing, cutting her off before she wanted to stop, counting to ten. I didn't want to do this, but it hurt so much!

At the same time, my mother was dying of cancer. She was only fifty-six, and we were very close. I was running back and forth from New Jersey to the

---

* The German word *stillen*, which means to nurse a baby, also means to soothe, to quiet down, to comfort.

Borrowed on 12 Jul 2007

0) Ladder of years
   Due date: 02 Aug 2007
   No.: 33630002580160
1) The breastfeeding cafâe : mothers share
   the joys, challenges, & secrets of
   nursing
   Due date: 02 Aug 2007
   No.: 33630003551335
2) Fast women
   Due date: 02 Aug 2007
   No.: 33630003186439
3) Love actually [videorecording]
   Due date: 16 Jul 2007
   No.: 33630003569535

Item(s) held : 4

> Loan Receipt <

12/07/2007 - 15:54

intensive care unit of a hospital in Michigan. Her death put me in a state of shock for about six months. It sucked the life out of me. I was so angry because she had been a grandmother for only a year, and I was in an emotional tailspin, which is not a good state to be in when mothering.

After Zachary was born and my milk came in, Ava hit the jackpot! Her cheeks blossomed, she filled out like a baby, and her fingers got a little layer of fat on them. She went through infancy on a whole other level again, along with Zachary, who was nursing well. She completely indulged herself in the fountain that had been dried up for about six months. It was a gold rush for her, and she couldn't get enough.

I tandem-nursed for one and three-quarter years, but it was very tough on me. I wanted to, and I believed in it, but I struggled and never found peace. Still, the idea of weaning was too painful for me, and I felt a little nursing was better than nothing.

I can't even describe what a nervous wreck I was that year. My head was under water, and I was spread the thinnest I've ever been. My husband was in his last year of graduate school, on top of a demanding full-time job, and he never saw the children. I was like a single mother. Nobody was getting their needs met, except for Zachary, the baby. As most mothers do, I put myself on the bottom and had no help whatsoever. I didn't know how to balance everything without a housekeeper or an au pair, neither of which we had the money for.

Ava and I suffered, and I always cut her off before she was ready to stop. Because I had let her nurse as long as she wanted to before I was pregnant, this was a big change for her. And even though she hit the jackpot with my new supply of milk, she was heartbroken when Zachary was born because she couldn't be the little baby anymore. To this day I think she still harbors bad feelings and frustrations about not being able to nurse as much as she wanted.

Nursing was a beautiful, incredible experience, and I'm so glad I embraced it. The idea that I could feed a child with my body is an amazing thing. But in retrospect I wish I hadn't had my children so close together. Ava was just not ready to step down from her central position, and four years between my kids would have been much better.

Gwen Shook, Jersey City, NJ

❍

During mid-pregnancy my milk supply was low or nonexistent. Haleigh would nurse only for a second, then roll over and go to sleep. I knew when my colostrum had arrived because she nursed for minute, looked up at me, and said, "Yummy, yummy, yummy." At that point she started asking for "milk please" more often. Once my milk came in after Rebecca was born, Haleigh's "Yummy, yummy, yummy" got even more enthusiastic. Between six and twelve months, Haleigh hummed while nursing, and recently she began humming again. Now I am back to having a difficult time getting my breast back once it is in her mouth.

Peggy Olsen, Elma, WA

Sam's story suggests that tandem-nursing may be an effective way to help reduce an older sibling's jealousy of a new baby. Because the new baby doesn't "replace" the firstborn, the likelihood or intensity of sibling rivalry may be reduced. But Sam didn't just tandem-nurse. She did so while nursing triplets—without relying on formula, ever. A legal assistant until her daughters were born, she talks in the next story about nursing them while also nursing her then two-year-old son.

LIKE PUPPIES IN A BASKET

My husband and I were stunned. We walked around the block about fifty times muttering to each other like an old senile couple.

"What do you mean?" I had asked. "Triplets don't run in our family."

"They do now," the doctor replied.

As soon as the doctor realized I was having triplets (when I was fourteen weeks along), she told me to stop nursing my eighteen-month-old immediately—she was afraid it would bring on premature labor. But I read about breastfeeding while pregnant and couldn't find anything definitive. Since Jordan was already going to have his life significantly turned around, I wasn't about to take nursing away from him. He was an intense nurser, and it was very important to him. At about thirty weeks, though, it was getting harder for me to tell what might be real contractions and what might be Braxton Hicks.* I explained that we needed to stop for a while. "If you still want to nurse after the babies are born," I added, "you can." Jordan seemed to understand.

---

* Braxton Hicks contractions, or pre-labor contractions, do not dilate the cervix as do "real" labor contractions. They tend to be non-rhythmic, unpredictable, and painless. They do, however, help pave the way for later cervical effacement and dilation.

The girls came in healthy, weighing about five pounds each. The day they were born, Jordan crawled into my hospital bed and started nursing. It was something he was a part of—he wasn't shuffled to the back—and it helped him feel less excluded because boy, life sure changed for him overnight! I also feel that having an actively nursing child helped to stimulate a good supply of milk early on.

The girls were gavage (tube) fed for the first several days, so I had to pump as much milk as I could. Then we took nursing slowly. They didn't have a ferocious latch-on, and they were sleepy, but they managed fine. The only problem they had was "bradycardia," a condition where they would stop breathing as they nursed and their heart rates would slow down.* If this happened I would unlatch the baby, give her a minute to catch her breath, and then resume. It was a bit intimidating the first few times, but I got used to it, despite having to deal with

Tandem-Nursing

Tandem-nursing—breastfeeding two (or more) children of different ages at the same time—remains a rather closeted phenomenon. Part of the reason is because it almost always involves nursing a toddler or preschooler, which American culture already views as radical, if not perverse. Beyond that, though, I believe tandem-nursing shatters a sacred and deeply embedded image of one mother, one nursling. "Madonna and children" is not a common cultural image.

Tandem-nursing was something I had never heard about before immersion in the world of mothering and breastfeeding. But during my second pregnancy, had it not felt as if my daughter were using pliers to draw my nipple into her mouth, I could have easily ended up nursing a four-year-old along with my newborn.

Not all women feel discomfort and may indeed choose to nurse through pregnancy. This is generally quite safe, says lactation consultant Kathleen Huggins, author of The Nursing Mother's Companion (1995), even though the amount of milk we make often decreases due to the estrogen secreted by the placenta (personal communication, 2003). In fact, the American Academy of Family Medicine Policy Statement on Breastfeeding expresses strong support for tandem-nursing, noting that a child younger than age two is at increased risk of illness if weaned. (The statement is available at <http://www.aafp.org/x6633.xml>.)

While nursing through pregnancy may overwhelm some women, others find that it helps to maintain our closeness with our children and to reassure them that they will not be replaced by the new baby. And because milk production works on the basis of supply and demand, once the baby is born there is generally plenty of milk for two.

A good book on the subject is Hillary Flower's Adventures in Tandem Nursing (2003), published by La Leche League International.

---

* Nursing does not cause bradycardia, a condition common in preterm babies like Sam's. It is simply a symptom of a preterm infant's general immaturity. In fact, because milk flows more quickly from a bottle than a breast, bottle-feeding is more stressful on premature infants, explains Kathleen Huggins (personal communication), and bottle-fed babies experience bradycardia more frequently than do babies at the breast.

all the monitor wires. Sometimes I felt like I was nursing an octopus, but the nurses reassured me that nothing could come unhooked that couldn't be hooked up again.

Over the next few days we gradually worked toward longer nursing sessions, more frequently. We were all tired and overwhelmed, but the nursing staff was patient, kind, and reassuring.

Everyone assumed I would use formula, though. The hospital sent me home with a little kit, and free, unbidden cases of formula showed up on my porch from Enfamil and some other company. Fortunately I'm pretty ornery, and we didn't use it—I think I ended up giving it to a food bank. Nursing was so much simpler than heating up all those bottles, preparing formula, and getting out of bed in the middle of the night.

For the first two weeks we kind of lived on the couch. I didn't get off the couch much for the first year, actually. Jordan was a self-reliant little guy. He'd bring me diapers and could reach things out of the fridge. Fortunately, the girls were efficient—they got on, they nursed, they got off.

They never nursed on a schedule, but it evened out over time and became less constant. We introduced solids when they seemed ready, between nine and eleven months. They just weren't interested before then, even though we tried.

I was prepared to nurse for as long as I needed to and went into it with a strong commitment. I was already at a significant deficit for individual kid time, and as long as I was nursing I could focus in on that one baby. Each one got at least *that* much of my time, closeness, and attention. That was important. I took it day by day, sometimes hour by hour. When things got trying, I would remind myself that it wouldn't be forever and I was doing the best I could.

Sleep was a precious commodity. If I had it to do all over again, I would throw our mattress on the floor, get a couple of futons, and make one big sleeping room for everybody. Instead, I got used to clinging to my six inches of space at the side of the bed or curling up with my quilt at the foot of it. It felt like a bunch of puppies all rolling around each other in a basket.

All three girls nursed for a long time. I became pretty committed, probably fanatical, truth be told. I was going to do it for as long as they wanted, and that was that. We were going to do it until somebody gave us a reason not to.

Everybody was over four when they weaned, Jordan included. He sat down to nurse one day and said, "I don't think this is working very well anymore," and that was it. He was done. The girls sort of trailed off, stopping within a few weeks of each other.

Now that my kids are teenagers, I joke about how I wish I could go back to a time when every problem in their lives could be solved by sitting down for a cuddle and a nurse. And it made me stop and take five minutes to be with that kid who was having a hard time.

Breastfeeding made me slow down and appreciate where I was, rather than looking to what was coming. And I don't think I realized how connected I could get to another person. I had read ahead of time about the importance of bonding, breastfeeding, and not separating any more than you have to. If I hadn't read all that, I would have been a lot more surprised by the intensity of feelings I had. It was nice to know that someone was saying, "That's okay. That's the way you're supposed to feel."

Sam R., Bothell, WA

When Graham was little enough to fit inside Cameron's lap I would nurse them together in the cradle hold. Graham would come off my breast and Cameron would reach across to him and say, "Nursey, baby brother. Nursey." And he would push Graham's head up to my breast, just like I do, and put the nipple back in his mouth. And Graham would nurse.

Teal Peck, Torrington, CT

Parenting in the Dark

As Sam attests, sometimes balancing our needs and those of our children is less a *day-to-day* struggle than a *night-to-night* struggle. How to *get* children to sleep, *keep* them asleep, and maximize the amount of sleep for everyone in the family becomes the focus of much mental, emotional, and physical work.

One could easily argue that the dominant U.S. culture is obsessed with babies' sleep habits. What new parent has not been asked, "Is she sleeping through the night yet?" as if the answer is a reflection of one's skill as a parent and the maturity of one's baby. Given the cultural emphasis on fostering independence and self-reliance, the notion that the parental bed is sacred, and an emphasis on privacy, it should come as little surprise to know that the United States today is the *only* society in which babies most often sleep in their own bed, in their own room. Anthropologist Meredith Small points out that 90 percent of babies around the world sleep with an adult and that for almost all of human history babies have slept next to their mothers. This model of nighttime parenting, though, is lost in the rush to fix the nursery, find the right crib, and buy a baby monitor.

It should also come as little surprise to know that Western expectations of babies' sleep are based on infants fed formula. Such babies are able to sleep longer and more deeply because formula is more slowly absorbed and metabolized. Moreover, babies who sleep alone have more difficulty rousing themselves from deep sleep—a factor that may contribute to SIDS (sudden infant death syndrome). Nursing babies, on the other hand, tend to wake more often because they digest their food quickly and easily. And co-sleeping babies tend to follow the sleep patterns of their mothers, whose mere presence helps them develop more mature sleeping and breathing patterns.

Unfortunately, co-sleeping is not well understood by most American pediatricians, the very people to whom most American parents turn for advice. And because medical science is typically deified in this country, doctors' opinions are often accepted without question. Small reports that a survey of American pediatricians found that 88 percent advocated for babies to sleep in a crib outside the parents' room and 65 percent suggested that babies receive no parental body contact during the night at all! (1998, 118–19).

Anthropologist James McKenna challenges these beliefs. Director of the Center for Behavioral Studies of Mother-Infant Sleep at the University of Notre Dame, he asserts that many of the nighttime struggles we experience are based on our own unrealistic expectations rather than on anything pathological with our babies.

Well-known for his pioneering studies comparing the physiology and behavior of babies who sleep alone with those who sleep with their mothers, McKenna offers solid evidence in support of co-sleeping. Babies breastfeed more often, cry less frequently, and spend less time awake. And because breastfeeding is related to reducing the risk of death from SIDS, co-sleeping, which facilitates breastfeeding, may help to prevent it. In Japan, McKenna notes, where co-sleeping is the norm, the SIDS rate is among the lowest in the world (McKenna, Mosko, and Richard 1997; McKenna, 1995).

Dr. William Sears, author of *Nighttime Parenting: How to Get Your Baby and Child to Sleep* (1999), offers another compassionate voice in support of shared sleep and, along with many of today's midwives, has helped women feel they have "permission" to go against the cultural grain. Moreover, babies are not the only ones who benefit. Co-sleeping and nighttime nursing reduce breast engorgement in women and help to prevent breast infections. And mothers who co-sleep with their babies can simply roll over, offer a breast, and get on with their own sleep. Nursing mothers who don't sleep with their babies are apt to find nighttime more challenging—a prime example of the tension required to keep those two adjacent magnets from snapping together.*

Despite a deeply ingrained bias, more parents today are recognizing, even if subconsciously, this clash between a baby's biological need for physical contact and our culture's denial of it. This is not always easy. Our society is based on schedules and routine, in which women need a good night's sleep to function the next day, not only as a parent but also as part of the paid labor force. But co-sleeping is far more compassionate—and often yields more sleep—than listening to the desolate sobs of one's baby, who seeks nothing more than human contact.

There are, of course, alternatives beyond the two extremes of letting your child scream itself into a bereft and abandoned sleep and keeping your child "in arms" twenty-four/seven. My own family, for example, often played musical beds. For a while my husband slept downstairs on a futon and my daughter and I shared the queen-sized bed upstairs. When she became mobile and we worried about her rolling off the bed, we brought a futon mattress into our room, she slept there, my husband slept on the bed, and I shuttled back and forth between the two. Eventually we moved the futon to her own room, and sleeping with her there was the easiest thing to do. When she got her "big-girl bed" on her third birthday, I returned, once and for all, to my own bed and my husband—at least until daughter number two was born! The second time around was much easier. I basically bid my husband adieu and spent the better part of most nights cuddled with my baby. My husband didn't care—he just wanted to sleep!

---

* Just as cribs must be designed for safety, co-sleeping must take safety into consideration as well. Parents who smoke in bed or abuse drugs and alcohol create risky environments for co-sleeping. Likewise, water beds, soft couches, or beds with gaps or ledges that could trap a baby should also be avoided. For most of us, though, sleeping with our babies is quite safe.

What worked for my family, however, wouldn't work for everyone, and each family has to find its own solution. These next several stories address the relationship between nursing and sleep.

In Their Own Words:
Parenting in the Dark

Nighttime parenting constantly evolves. Trina illustrates some of the challenges we face in the early days.

☕ RISING IN LOVE

Once my son got home from the hospital, he nursed every two hours. Nobody ever told me about that! What the hell had I signed up for? Why should I even go to sleep when I would just have to get up and change his diaper? After a while, though, I got used to not sleeping. I was like a zombie. Eventually, he started to sleep for four hours, an improvement, but then came the nights when he couldn't *fall* asleep or get *back* to sleep. Even breastfeeding wouldn't do it. He would cry until midnight! I'd have to keep moving with him, walking him in the living room, even putting him in a stroller and strolling him through the house. It was also very hot, the air conditioner didn't work, and the fans weren't doing it. So I'd go outside and bounce him around. *I* was falling asleep, but *he'd* still be awake.

By about ten months it started to get easier. He'd wake up, I'd nurse him, and he'd be okay. By about a year he started sleeping through the night. Now at two and a half, he still sleeps in bed with us. I'll nurse him for about fifteen minutes, and he sleeps through the night. It's a breeze.

Trina Odetta Sandress, Sacramento, CA

○

Now that I am breastfeeding and pumping, if I have a bad night's sleep, my milk production is half what it is when I have a good night's sleep. I can't believe how closely related it is. I can say, "Look, I'm not getting much milk. I have to get a really good night's sleep tonight, and I have to eat really well today." My husband is very supportive of that—I can sleep until noon if I want to.

Laura P. Burke, Syracuse, NY

The next two stories illuminate some of the ambivalence we may feel as our babies-turned-toddlers continue to sleep with us. Nursing in the middle of the night may get old after a while, but that doesn't necessarily mean that we want to quit. At least not yet. At least not all at once. At least not when they're so cuddly . . .

TAKING IT ONE NIGHT AT A TIME

People think I'm insane that I would not mind waking up two or three times a night when my child is two years old. But even though it's been really hard, I've never questioned doing anything else. I'm raising my child as I see fit, not as others tell me I should.

Part of the problem is that Allison has always awakened a zillion times a night. At about eight months she began to sleep for two or three hours at a stretch. But she still has waking peaks that are exhausting for me. The other night she woke up about ten times. In her entire life, she's only had one night when she woke up once and fewer than ten nights when she woke up twice.

Before we were even married, my husband and I talked about how much we like to sleep together, and we agreed it was weird to put children in a separate room, by themselves, when they're infants. It's just nice to sleep with someone, to be close. We felt strongly about that, even though we knew nothing about attachment parenting or having kids.

We have queen-sized and double mattresses next to each other on the floor, and it's nice sleeping next to Allison, in the way that it's nice sleeping next to my husband. It's an intimate, connected feeling. And to be able to nourish her in the middle of the night is very nurturing, very loving.

I do wonder, though, if this is contributing to her being awake all the time. If I'm in the other bed, she'll sleep longer, but if I'm next to her and turn over or move, she wakes up and wants to nurse.

I was really irritated a few weeks back and decided, "That's it. I'm going to wean her." I called my favorite La Leche League leader, who had a lot of helpful things to say. But as the day went on I felt my anxiety level increasing. And by the time evening came, I realized I wasn't ready. That was kind of a revelation and helped me mellow out a little. Because it's been so hard, I often end up talking about the negative. And yet, when I actually considered stopping, I realized I hadn't been paying very much attention to the pleasurable part of it. And because she doesn't eat that much and is such a little peanut, I worry that she's actually hungry. But I go back and forth. I'm getting to the point where I feel like the positive aspects are starting to diminish. If I'm yelling at her in the middle of the night, I'm not doing either of us a favor.

I *would* like to night-wean Allison, I just don't know when. As she becomes more verbal and we can talk about it, I expect to impose more limits. Already she's able to take some of my feelings into consideration. I can say, for example, "My nipples are sore and you have to be gentle," and she'll come right off.

I have always thought that I was not lost in Allison's needs, that I would know when I had to make a change for *me*. And I believe when that point comes she will be able to do it, and we will be able to move forward into the place we need to be as a mother and child.

Nancy Paranka, Denver, CO

Leslie is a single mother who works in TV broadcasting. Her story dispels the assumption that women who engage in extended breastfeeding and co-sleeping are full-time, stay-at-home mothers.

DAVID'S LIEDOWNMILK

My son, David, calls nursing liedownmilk. All one word. We liedownmilk in the chair, when he stands on the toilet seat while I'm getting out of the shower, when I'm getting dressed in the morning. Now it's become a game where everything wants liedownmilk. Sometimes its his guitar. Or Pooh. He'll hold Pooh to my nipple for a minute and then say, "Okay, Pooh, you've had enough. It's my turn." Sometimes David even wants to liedownmilk with Grammy. She says, "There's no milk in there, David. Sorry. It's a dry well."

In David's mind everybody liesdownmilk and sleeps with their mommy. That's how the world is. I didn't plan it this way—it just evolved. I was so exhausted when he was a couple of days old, and it was so much easier to nurse and have him fall asleep on top of me. He's been sleeping with me ever since. I did get a crib when he was about five months old and would lay him down when he was already asleep, but he'd wake up as soon as I'd put him down. That crib has been through three families now, and not one of the kids has slept in it!

Now David has a toddler bed that he knows is *his*. I had thought he would decide it was fun to have his own bed, that he would like it when my mother came up for the summer and his little bed would be in the same room as hers. But he doesn't. He'll take a nap in his bed or fall asleep on the couch, but at night we go to sleep together. When he was little, he would nurse, fall asleep, wake up, nurse, and keep nursing. I'd always have to pry his mouth off. Now I sort of say, "Um, Mama has to go to the bathroom. Could you roll over?" and he'll roll over and go back to sleep. Sometimes there are nights when I'm so tired and he wakes me up totally. But nighttime doesn't seem like a good time to fight about where he sleeps. And I love it when he wakes up and is happy and cuddly.

Nursing is a touchstone, our little cocoon, a time when I tell him how much I love him and it's just us together. I made up a little song with his name, weight, and date of birth, and I've sung it to him since the day he was born. Sometimes I'll tell him stories. Occasionally he'll open his mouth and pipe in to make a comment, but usually it's like he's saying, "I'm here, *you* talk."

Sometimes if he's really thirsty he'll ask for a cup of milk first, but he tells me, "Mommy's milk is the best." I'll ask him what flavor it is, and sometimes he says, "Banana." Yesterday he was hot, and he wanted me to put my breasts in the refrigerator!

David is so happy nursing and smiles with my nipple in his mouth. He has a sweet habit when he wants to nurse on the run or is just looking for a little close comfort. He'll nurse on my right breast until it's almost empty and then go on the left breast for about five seconds. It's almost like a kiss to let it know that it's not being left out. He tells me he has to kiss both breasts each time he nurses.

It's also his way of making total contact with me after I've been at work all day. I think this is part of the reason we still nurse. Many times when I come home from work David's eyes just light up. He looks right at my chest. It's like he's saying, "You're home! The breasts are home!" Now he tells me, "Mommy, I was missing you when you go to work. Please don't go. Please stay with me." It tears me up. It's really hard to be away from him ten hours a day. When I ask him where *he* lives he'll say, "Natick, Massachusetts," but when I ask him where *I* live, he says, "You live at Channel 7 News and Weather in Boston."

"No, David, I live with you," I'll say.

"No, Mommy. You live at Channel 7."

I know nursing won't last forever. In a couple of years he's not going to want to be held, cuddled, and kissed all the time. So even though it would be nice if he would sleep through the night in his own bed, I don't actively say that I have to stop next month, that this has to end. And I like to think I'm raising a sensual male who someday will appreciate a woman's body, who will love to stroke her arm and put cream on her shoulders. Everyone says that children's memories really start at three, so he'll remember lyingdownmilk. And he'll remember the closeness and sensitivity and be a strong, loving man when he grows up.

Leslie Shocket, Natick, MA

Permeable Boundaries

Some women love being pregnant. I was not one of them. Apart from excitement in hearing the heartbeat and delight in feeling the baby move, there was little about pregnancy I enjoyed. By my seventh month, I couldn't wait to have my body back. Bodily autonomy—how I missed it! In fact, this was at the root of the only parenting argument my husband and I had during my entire pregnancy. I was in my fifth month, and we were on vacation visiting friends. We were dining in an Italian restaurant, and I longed for half a glass of wine to enjoy with my meal. I hadn't had any alcohol since being pregnant and figured since the French and Italians don't impose the same standards as Americans, what was the harm in a little bit, just once? My husband disagreed. Vehemently.* My feminist self interpreted this as an example of men trying to control women's bodies, of taking away our rights and responsibilities to make informed choices. On the other hand, I could (sort of) understand that this growing baby belonged to him, too, and when it came right down to it, he *was* rather powerless in what happened to this dependent creature.

Women like myself thus anticipate childbirth as the end of this period when our bodies are ours—but not totally; when we are autonomous—but not really. We soon discover, though, that our child's dependency on our bodies does not end with childbirth. As long as we are nursing, whatever *we* take in, our children do, too. This doesn't mean we must stick with a 100 percent organic diet, that we can't eat Cheetos, have a beer now and then, or take a Tylenol. But it does mean we may have to consider the pros and cons of consuming certain substances, medications, and foods.

---

* I am not trying to present a cavalier approach about drinking during pregnancy! It is well-known that abusing alcohol can cause physical and mental birth defects, and the March of Dimes does indeed recommend that pregnant women completely avoid alcohol. They add that even though drinking at any stage of pregnancy can affect fetal development, birth defects are more likely to result from drinking in the first trimester, while growth problems are more likely to result from drinking during the third trimester. Visit their Web site at <http://www.modimes.org>.

This should not be the responsibility of mothers alone, however. In her fascinating and provocative book *Having Faith: An Ecologist's Journey to Motherhood* (2001), biologist Sandra Steingraber illustrates the obligation we have, as a society, to provide a nontoxic environment for pregnant women and breastfeeding mothers. The food chain we all studied in high school is incomplete, she argues. It is not "man" who constitutes the final link, but the baby who suckles at its mother's breast. Steingraber presents a frightening assessment of the degree to which traces of pesticides and toxic chemicals are found in the breast milk of women all over the planet. Since these dangerous substances become increasingly concentrated as they move up the food chain, the world's nursing babies become the ultimate repositories for toxic wastes.

Having nursed her own daughter for two years, Steingraber is a strong proponent of breastfeeding. Breast milk, she rightfully argues, is still healthier than formula. Her point is not to prevent women from nursing, but to bring the problem into the public eye. Keeping it hidden, she argues, is not a good public health strategy and prevents us from having an informed discussion about a serious problem.

Throughout the day-to-day minutiae of motherhood, we are often too exhausted and preoccupied to do anything about the impact of industrial waste, potentially thousands of miles away. But we are still confronted with more immediate decisions concerning the quality of our breast milk. Based on our distinctly female bodily experiences, the stories in this next section challenge the deeply entrenched American myth of individualism and independence. And they illustrate another way of thinking about the kind of balancing that women must undertake.

In Their Own Words:
Permeable Boundaries

 BREASTFEEDING AND THE PILL

For about two weeks after I started the Pill, my three-month-old daughter was miserable. Unfortunately we didn't make the connection until I tried pumping and noticed I was practically dry! I had asked my obstetrician about birth control, and he said that while the Pill does affect some women's milk supply, he didn't see any problem with me going back on it. Besides, I had tons of milk and leaked all the time.*

Dena was tiny, and I wanted her back on breast milk. so I stopped the Pill immediately. We started her on formula, and after a few days she enjoyed it. I was relieved that we had figured out the problem, but even though only a few days had passed, Dena had lost interest in the breast. I was disappointed but felt it was more important for her to get the nourishment, even if it *was* formula. This is probably taboo to admit, but I was getting a break and it was a little bit freeing. It was a relief that she wasn't just pulling on my nipple and crying.

A few weeks later in the bath I offered Dena my breast—she used to love nursing in the tub—and she completely ignored it! Clearly that was the end.

Hopefully, our next baby will be calmer and will enjoy eating more. And I'll do things differently and won't go back on the Pill. I'm still a believer, and I really want breastfeeding to work.

Laura Rosenthal, Ann Arbor, MI

The majority of breastfeeding mothers don't have to eliminate dairy or other foods in our diet because most babies do not have adverse reactions to them. Some do, however. L'dia, in the next story, shares her experience. For another aspect of L'dia's experience, see pages 68–69.

 DIETARY DILEMMAS

It took me a while to figure that out that my daughter's allergies were caused by what *I* ate or drank. When *I* stopped drinking milk, *my daughter's* body cleared up! That's how I learned that a lot of things I ate affected her. Dairy. Citrus. Tomatoes. Nuts. Looking at what I was eating and working through all that was very challenging!

Because of what I learned with her, my other children didn't eat solid foods until they were a year old. My second daughter wasn't allergic to any-

---

* According to Kathleen Huggins, IBCLC, nursing babies are not harmed by their mothers taking birth control pills, but pills that contain estrogen, even in low doses, may indeed reduce one's milk supply. However, some birth control pills (known as the Mini-Pill) contain only progestin, and these are less likely to adversely impact milk production. Nor are progestin-only injections or Norplant, two birth control methods that Huggins asserts are safe during breastfeeding (personal communication, 2003).

thing. But my third and fourth children were also allergic to dairy. I would eat ice cream, for example, and within an hour or two they would start scratching their ears and get ear infections. When I gave up eating ice cream, they wouldn't have them.

L'dia S. K. M. Muhammad, Berkeley, CA

There was never any question in Liz's mind that once she became pregnant she would breastfeed. At thirty-seven, she felt quite healthy, and she and her husband were preparing for a natural childbirth at the local birth center. A nurse in upstate New York, her main worries were about changes in her body image, losing her youthful body, and getting stretch marks. This all changed when, in her ninth month of pregnancy, she felt a lump in her breast.

BORN UNDER THE SIGN OF CANCER

It was Thursday, June 29, and it was becoming harder to get myself out of bed and out of the house on time. When I woke up, for no special reason I rubbed my chest and felt a lump on the upper part of my right breast. My midwife had checked my breasts at the beginning of the pregnancy and had not felt anything. What was this lump? It was hard. Harder than a cyst.

I went to work, and the gynecologist I work with agreed to check it and, if necessary, send the tissue to a pathologist, who could tell if it was normal or not. We waited a week, and the results came back with less explanation than a Pap smear. It just said "No abnormal cells." Period.

Meanwhile, I was feeling this lump every morning, and it seemed harder and bigger. I was scared. After mulling it over for several days, I went to a surgeon I know. "Could you please get a second opinion on this pathology report?" I asked. He called me a couple of days later, saying the specimen was in poor condition, but abnormal cells were definitely present. The surgeon thought I should have an excisional biopsy. "Do it now," I said.

Two days later, on Friday, July 14, two weeks before my due date, he called me at work. I was in the middle of seeing a patient. "Liz, I have some bad news," he said. "It's cancer."

I couldn't believe it. I was about to have a baby! My father was the one with cancer. He had been diagnosed in January with lymphoma and was undergoing chemotherapy. The surgeon told me to come right over. I left, and that was it. I never went back to work for fourteen months, not even to pick up my plants.

My husband and I met at the doctor's office, and he went over all our options. "You're going to need more surgery," he said, "and a lactating breast is hard to operate on. You'll need radiation if you don't have a mastectomy, and we don't know whether or not the cancer has gone deeper. And you certainly can't breastfeed during chemo."

"This is impossible," I said. "You can't tell me I can't breastfeed. I'm having a baby!"

I had never considered bottle-feeding. From the time I was eighteen I always thought of breasts not only aesthetically but as functional organs. My training in nutrition and nursing only strengthened my feelings. There was no question in my mind that I would breastfeed.

That weekend we went to the local Breast Cancer Alliance, borrowed several books, and had a crash course in cancer. On Monday I was on the phone *all* day, getting information and making appointments. We were looking for a doctor with whom we felt we could work and get what we wanted. The doctors all seemed concerned with conserving the breast from an aesthetic and sexual perspective. "What about function?" I asked. "I'm about to become a mother!"

Two of them told me I could nurse, and two of them told me I couldn't. One of them wanted to hit me with the big guns right away. He told me I should have an induced labor or Cesarean and go right from the delivery room into the operating room, have a full mastectomy, and start chemotherapy right away. He said, "We don't know that much about pregnancy with breast cancer, and your hormonal state could really increase the speed at which it's growing and spreading. It's best not waiting, and breastfeeding is out of the question." No one else was that radical. They said there was no evidence I had to have a mastectomy; a lumpectomy and radiation statistically were just as good. They told me I could have the baby naturally, give myself two weeks to recover, have a lumpectomy and axillary dissection, and breastfeed until chemotherapy began.

I couldn't endure what the one doctor recommended. I didn't want my birth experience stolen from me, as well as my breast. I would not be giving my daughter what I wanted—an all-natural, no anesthesia, nonmedicated birth. I wanted her to come into the world clean and clearheaded, and I wanted to make my birth experience as separate from my cancer as was medically and emotionally possible. That was clear. So we decided to have the baby naturally.

We saw our oncologist on Friday and remembered we had weekend passes to a local music festival, already under way. A strategy became apparent: (1) enjoy the festival; (2) get the baby out, and start breastfeeding;

(3) decide on a surgeon; (4) have the lumpectomy and axillary dissection; (5) take it from there.

We knew that dancing and making love could induce labor, so we went to the festival and danced for about five hours. All our friends were there dancing around us under a starry summer sky. It was like coming home, being purified, cleansed, and taken care of. I prayed for the health of our baby and for me to live to see her grown with children of her own. We danced until we were exhausted, then went home and made love, thinking, "If we start now, maybe by the end of the weekend . . ."

We went to sleep about two thirty A.M., and I woke up two hours later, in labor. Hannah was born completely naturally and beautiful at three o'clock the next afternoon at the birth center. Her daddy caught her. She was born under the astrological sign of Cancer, literally a week after I was diagnosed.

Hannah seemed to know that if she were not a good nurser from the start I was not going to be able to deal with it. But she took to my breast immediately. Because I was able to have her at the birth center and was able to breastfeed, at least initially, I felt like her birth was a separate thing, a little cocoon of time between the diagnosis, her birth, and my second surgery.

I gave myself two weeks to make a plan. Two doctors said they were willing to operate on a lactating breast, but the others said it was too messy and would slow the healing process.

"If I'm willing to deal with the long healing period," I said, "and you're willing to deal with the mess, I'm going to do it while I'm lactating. Now what about the anesthesia?" It turned out the anesthesia wasn't going to be in my blood for more than twenty-four hours, so I would just have to keep my milk supply up.

Of the two doctors who said I could do it, I chose the one with experience operating on lactating breasts. As it turns out, he never told me that he *didn't* have experience doing an axillary dissection on a lactating woman, a procedure where they remove the lymph nodes from the armpit to see if the cancer has spread. In retrospect I'd say he really didn't know what to expect.

We went to New York City and stayed with my parents for a week. August 6 was my dad's birthday and my parents' wedding anniversary. We found out his cancer was in his liver. My surgery was the next morning, and the result was no lymph node involvement!

They put a drain in me, underneath my armpit, to drain the serous fluid that inevitably accumulates around a deep wound. It was like an IV tube sticking out, attached to this little thing you squeezed, like a bulb syringe. It would slowly suck fluid out, and I would have to empty it every day and measure the amount of fluid. It was gross. Most people have this in for three or four days. I had it in for a month. I was draining milk.*

We had some breast milk in the freezer. Another woman's baby was premature, and she was pumping copious amounts of milk with a baby only drinking a couple of tablespoons a day. The midwives at the birthing center connected us, and she ended up giving me a month's supply.

Hannah was *so* good. She was only fussy when she needed something. Most of the time she would let anyone hold her and be happy, wherever she was. She was the baby I needed her to be, this little angel.

By the end of six weeks I was starting to feel fairly normal but incredibly detached from Hannah. I was pretty numb. I did what I had to do, but I felt like I was going through the motions of mothering.

I did feel strongly about her nutrition, though, and I did not want her to get formula. I felt like it was heresy, poison. When I had to start looking at formula because I was going to start chemotherapy, I did all this reading, trying to figure out if I could make my own out of nut butters, soy milk, and goat's milk, and then I just said, "No. I can't do this. I have to choose my battles."

They were pushing me to start chemotherapy six weeks after my surgery. Hannah would have been eight weeks old. But I wasn't sure I wanted it. I wanted to spend as much time as possible with my father, and I was having such a hard time giving up breastfeeding.

My surgeon said, "You're losing sight. You've got to raise your daughter and be around for her to graduate from high school. You've got the wrong idea if you think you're not going to do chemotherapy."

My oncologist said, "You will not have a 70 percent or 80 percent survival without recurrence. For you as an individual, it is 0 percent or 100 percent."

I read a lot of studies about breast cancer survival rates and the different kinds of treatments and wasn't sure what to do. "I *know* I'm going to do the radiation," I said, "so why can't I do the radiation first and the chemotherapy later?" Nobody could tell me I was going to kill myself by delaying it for six weeks.

Even though I used my own health as an argument, I really wanted to breastfeed for another six weeks. I decided to live with my parents and get

---

* Not all surgeons insist on the use of drains. See, for example, *Dr. Susan Love's Breast Book* (2000), written by the founder and director of the National Breast Cancer Coalition.

my daily radiation there. I'd get to spend time with my dad, he'd get to spend time with Hannah, and I wouldn't be sick with chemotherapy.

Hannah and I moved in with my parents, and Dave commuted for long weekends. My radiation oncologist thought I was crazy but didn't tell me I couldn't nurse through radiation. She did convince me, though, that I should not feed Hannah on the side getting radiation because radiation irritates the skin. She didn't want me breastfeeding over that and risking an infection in my nipples, because then I would have to stop radiation, take antibiotics, let it rest, and she wanted to make sure I got through the treatment. So I let the milk in my right breast dry up, and I only fed Hannah on the left side.

I had my first dose of radiation on our second wedding anniversary. The next day my father asked to have his treatment stopped and be discharged from the hospital. He died in the living room two days later, with me and my mother there. The funeral was on my mother's seventieth birthday.

I didn't know exactly when I would nurse Hannah for the last time, as the last day kept getting pushed back. I thought it was going to be six weeks after my surgery, and then I realized we were going to have six more weeks. When I was done with my radiation, I called my oncologist, thinking he would want me to start chemotherapy right away. He said, "We've got to give you a couple of weeks to heal from the radiation first," so I got another two weeks. Ultimately, I nursed her until she was four months old.

That was very painful for me. I pumped as much breast milk out of my one functioning breast as I could to freeze and give to Hannah after she was weaned. The midwives also helped me find other nursing mothers who were willing to donate breast milk. In the meantime, I had to train her to take a bottle when she really wanted my breast. I felt like I was torturing her. I was taking away something she really loved. Out of all of this, weaning was the hardest thing. I felt like Hannah was being ripped from me, like my ability to mother my child was ending. I had this feeling that the chemotherapy was going to make me so sick, weak, and listless that I wasn't going to be able to take care of her. And I was so tired as it was. My mother, David, and my friends were taking care of her, and I felt like my only connection with her was through breastfeeding. I was afraid that when I stopped I would be just like anyone else to her.

My first dose of chemo was the Monday after Thanksgiving, and my last dose was in April. I had decided that chemo wasn't the enemy—cancer was. And I had to do everything possible to ensure that I would be here to mother the child I had just given birth to. I had acupuncture, took herbs, went to yoga classes when I had the energy, went to physical therapy to get my arm moving and loosen up the scars that had adhered to my chest wall, and more.

Now, a year later, I feel like I'm Hannah's mommy. David and Hannah have a more special relationship than they would have had if I hadn't had cancer. I would have wanted to have everything my way, and I had to let go. It's much easier for me to do that now. And it's also allowed me to better appreciate David's enthusiasm, perspective, and willingness to be flexible and helpful. This could have been a disaster, and it wasn't—our love has grown.

For information on breastfeeding and cancer, a selected bibliography can be found on the La Leche League International Web site. The link is <http://www.laleche league.org/cbi/bibcancer.html>.

Medicine is not an exact science. And because what I learned *was* conflicting, it made me realize that it was my choice. No one else really knew, so I had to make it up. So far, I'm lucky. My period is back, and I'm considering another pregnancy. I'm back to work part-time and have joined a breast cancer support group. I'm trying to live so that every day counts and I will have no regrets. And Hannah is an exceptional child.

Liz, Ithaca, NY

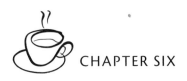 CHAPTER SIX

Doing It All

STORIES OF
MOTHERHOOD & LIVELIHOOD

*There are three major cultural themes in this country: patriarchy,
commercialism and technology. And breastfeeding doesn't fit any
one of those. It's not valued. Breastfeeding is a female thing. Those
three cultural themes are male things. Women don't get rewarded
for breastfeeding. They get rewarded for going to work and earning a paycheck.*

Marsha Walker

Motherhood is full of contradictions. When breastfeeding rates
in the United States were at their all-time low, the majority
of women stayed home with their children full-time. Our job was
motherhood, but not on our own terms. We were taught to ignore
our instincts, trust our doctors, and put our faith in scientifically superior formula. Ironically, breastfeeding rates began to climb at the
same time more women than ever before were saying good-bye to
full-time, stay-at-home motherhood in exchange for a paid position
in the job market. As recently as 1975, not quite one-third of married women with children under a year old were in the labor force,
but by 2000, this figure had shot up to well over two-thirds (Statistical Abstract of the United States 2001, table 578).

At the same time that we hear "breast is best," an unprecedented
number of new mothers are now in the workforce. Breastfeeding

thus reveals a main paradox of women's lives: how can we provide our children with what could be considered their nutritional birthright without impairing our ability to earn a decent living? How can we take advantage of the pleasurable and potentially empowering aspects of motherhood without reinforcing financial dependence on men or public assistance and without sacrificing the part of our identity that we derive from our jobs?

Despite the fact that the majority of mothers are in the workforce, many of us work in positions in which our time and activities are externally controlled, often monitored, and almost always based on the assumption that our bodies are our own and unencumbered. But when we carry babies within us, when they depend on us for sustenance, and when our breasts become engorged and must be emptied, we shatter the illusion of bodily autonomy.

A number of countries around the world recognize this, far more than the U.S. government. The International Labour Organization (ILO) has created standards involving maternity leave and time to breastfeed or express milk during work hours. The standards are:

- Twelve weeks maternity leave, with extension if necessary,
- Cash benefits during leave of at least 66 percent of previous earnings,
- Breastfeeding breaks totaling at least one hour per day,
- Prohibition of dismissal during maternity leave.

Over three-fourths of the world's countries conform to these standards, but the United States does not (Maloney 2002). In fact, we remain the only industrialized country in the world that does not offer women paid maternity leave. Even the Family and Medical Leave Act, enacted in 1993, offers only twelve weeks of *unpaid* leave, and a relatively small percentage of women either qualify for it or can afford it.

Studies document that maternal employment does not seem to affect our decision to *begin* breastfeeding, but it has a huge influence on whether or not we stick with it (Visness and Kennedy 1997). Both the number of hours we spend at our job during the week and how quickly we return to the workforce after our babies are born impact how long we nurse. This is true regardless of age, ethnicity, or educational level. The workplace environment and the kind of work we do also influence our decision to continue nursing. Women in manufacturing occupations and who work on assembly lines, for example, are less likely to be nursing, in part because they are not likely to have a private, clean place to pump their milk. Race also comes into play. African American women, for example, are not only more likely to return to work sooner (at eight weeks post-partum) but often return to jobs that do not enable them to succeed at breastfeeding (Bronner et al. 1996).

Part of the problem has to do with how our society defines work. "Work," as commonly understood, refers to the activities we do in exchange for money, the economic value we "produce" as members of society. Much of the real work women do, however, is excluded from this definition—namely the work we do to maintain our families, which is known in academic and activist circles as "reproductive work." This does not have to be the case. In Norway, for example, the production of breast milk is counted in national food statistics. Unfortunately, the United States has a long way to go before the economic value of breast milk is calculated and included in the gross domestic product (GDP). The practice of including the value of manufactured baby foods but *not* the value of breast milk illustrates one of many ways in which our society devalues breast milk and the women who produce it.

If we truly lived in a breastfeeding culture, we would value the reproductive work mothers do, along with our productive work, and we would support nursing mothers to do both. Focusing on reproductive work, however, emphasizes the *differences* between men and women, whereas the mainstream women's movement in this country has mobilized within a framework of equality and *sameness*. Women have had to prove (and still do!) that we can perform in a man's world and behave like men. Pregnancy, childbirth, and lactation, of course, do nothing to support this claim of sameness, and many women's groups have been opposed to maternity protection or "mommy track" options fearing that they would perpetuate discrimination in the workplace (Baumslag and Michels 1995, 200).

So how do women do it? How do we manage to combine paid work with breastfeeding? The stories in this chapter center around this pivotal question. Perhaps more than any other set of stories in the book, this group tends to reflect a middle- to upper-middle-class bias. Simply put, it was hard for me to find women in entry-level, blue-collar, and unskilled positions who were able to keep their job and nurse. Many women with these kinds of jobs use formula. Others simply leave the workforce.

We do not yet live in a world in which what makes women *different* from men is imbued with the same cultural value as what makes us *similar*. It is within this cultural context of devaluing and disempowering what is uniquely female that we each have to figure out how best to meet the needs of our babies within the unique conditions of our lives.

Plugged In

An ability to express one's milk is crucial in allowing women to continue breastfeeding. Before a chance encounter in my mid-twenties, I'd never heard of such a thing. I'll never forget entering the bathroom across the hall from my office at an international aid organization to see a colleague sitting there with a strange-looking contraption attached to her breast. I was fascinated! Not only didn't I know that women could express milk, but I didn't know it could actually shoot out in streams! Fortunately my curiosity didn't faze her, and she patiently explained what she was doing.

Expressing milk on a regular basis presents an interesting issue. While it clearly enables babies to receive the nutritional and immunological benefits of breast milk, Lydia Furman, a part-time practicing pediatrician, argues that there is a distinction between nursing and lactation. Lactation is to produce and secrete milk from a mammary gland, while nursing is "to give milk from the breast to an infant" (1993, 2). Having a substitute caregiver give a baby pumped milk in a bottle, she asserts, is not enough: "The closeness, warmth and gratification of the nursing relationship are built upon the synchronization of baby's hunger and mother's letdown, a bodily relationship that a pump or bottle can only intrude upon, not simulate" (Furman 1993, 2).

This points to an interesting paradox: at the same time that most medical discussions of breastfeeding focus on the *product* of nursing and not the *process*, some breastfeeding advocates do just the opposite. This is complicated. If we place too much emphasis on the milk itself rather than on the nursing *relationship*, we risk devaluing the mother (see, e.g., Emma's story on pages 110–12); if, however, we focus too much on the embodied interaction between mother and baby, we risk reducing women to their biological functions (Blum 1993, 301).

The ways in which our society accommodates the needs of nursing mothers further support this distinction between product and process. Sociologist Linda Blum, for example, suggests that employers with large, low-paid, female-dominated workforces will be more likely to provide electric breast pumps to their employees rather than offer on-site nurseries, job flexibility, and paid leaves (1993, 303). Thus they choose to focus on the *product*, rather than on the relationship on which it is based. In other words, they are more supportive of *lactation* than they are of nursing.

The average mother probably has little time for this kind of theoretical conundrum, however. More important is how to make breastfeeding a viable option for the vast majority of us, not simply a luxury for those who can manage it. We need the security that we don't have to choose between work and family.

This first group of stories is a window into the private (and sometimes not so private) world of pumping our milk. It should be of no great surprise that most of these stories come from professional women who had advantages that the majority of employed mothers lack, particularly a clean, private place to pump; a place to store the milk; some degree of control over their schedules; and access to a good-quality, affordable pump. The experiences of Niesha and Lauren, two young mothers who lacked these workplace advantages, provide a striking contrast. (See their stories on pages 170 and 175–76.)

In Their Own Words:
Plugged In

Dawn, an environmental data analyst for a consulting firm, talks about how she handled pumping in an office of male coworkers.

☕ DEMANDING PRIVACY

I was able to stay home with my daughter, Claire, for her first three months, and that last month, our first month when breastfeeding wasn't painful, was heaven. So when I started back to work, I wasn't about to drop breastfeeding.

My first day back I began a twice-daily ritual of asking my sweet and supportive office mate, George, to vacate the room; posting on the door my "Do Not Disturb" sign with the hand-drawn portrait of Elsie the Cow; and settling in for a pumping session.

Months went by, no one said a word, and I became pretty complacent. I got to the point where I could balance the bottle on the computer table and pump while typing my reports. I even stopped posting Elsie on the door, figuring everyone knew what the closed door meant. Wrong.

The first break-in was when our office nemesis, a marketing guy with the ego development of your average fourteen-year-old boy, burst in on me. I covered myself up as best I could and dove under the computer table. He figured the scene out and retreated, mumbling, "Oops, sorry, didn't know . . ."

The next time, another coworker, childless and clueless, opened the door and peered in, even though Elsie was clearly posted. "I just need to get something off George's desk," he said.

"Get out, please," I said.

"I just need to get that memo."

"Get *out*, please."

"Is this a problem?" he said, clearly annoyed.

I matched irritated glance for irritated glance and spat out, "I'm PUMPING MILK. GET OUT NOW!" Finally, recognition dawned, and the guy quickly shut the door and left.

It was clear that I needed to make a statement, and while still pumping I wrote and e-mailed the following:

Author: Dawn Wendt

Subject: Elsie

Message Contents: Okay, no more subtlety. I thought that most people had figured out why the door is closed to my office so often (and why George leaves). I thought my cleverly drawn picture of Elsie the Cow was a pretty good clue. But having been broken in on once again, it is clear that subtlety has no place here. So here's the deal:

I had a baby. Babies drink milk. I make milk. I am broke and therefore I work. I pump milk at work. If the door is closed to my office, STAY OUT, or I will stand up and squirt you in the eye.

Thank you.

Other than a couple of inquiries as to the accuracy of my aim, the issue never came up again. Overall I'm proud I stuck with it. Claire weaned herself at one year. And I like to think I made it a little easier for the next woman who needs to pump for her baby and gets stuck with those guys in a work setting. One by one, we change the world.

Written by Dawn Wendt, Caledonia, NY

Since the late 1980s, hundreds of companies have invested in corporate lactation programs to make their workplace more "nursing-mother-friendly." In fact, 81 percent of corporations listed in the 1998 *100 Best Companies for Working Mothers* offer this benefit to their employees.* Congresswoman Carolyn B. Maloney, a breastfeeding advocate, reports that in its first year, Aetna, Inc., saved an estimated $1,435 in medical claims and three days of sick leave per breastfed baby—a total annual savings of $108,737 (Maloney 2001, xvii). Joan, whose story also appears on pages 97–98, talks about how a supportive company and boss eased her life as a nursing mother.

THE MOTHER'S ROOM

As a project manager at Hewlett-Packard, I was lucky enough to be in a position where I could schedule meetings around times when I needed to pump. I also have an excellent young boss, very supportive of me doing whatever I needed to do.

I went back to work part-time when Kelsey was four months old. My husband would drop her off at a home day care around eight or eight thirty with a frozen bag of milk. The day-care provider would put the milk in her freezer, thaw it out later, and give it to Kelsey. Initially I got off work around noon, so Kelsey was there for a total of twenty to twenty-four hours a week. Then, because I got additional benefits if I went back to work for thirty-two hours, I stepped it up. I didn't go back full-time until she was just shy of a year old.

The company has a special place called the Mother's Room for nursing moms to pump. You would sign up on the reservation sheet, and there was a sign that would say "In Use." It had dim lighting, soft couches, and some magazines. It was off one of the bathrooms but had a door you could lock

---

* For the statistics, see the Medela Web site at <http://www.medela.com/New-Files/corplactprgm.html>.

for privacy. I would go in there midmorning. After I pumped, I would freeze the milk (there are freezers all over) and later put it in my freezer at home.

I had one of those great Medela pumps, so I could sit down and in twenty minutes pump out eight to ten ounces. I took it back and forth every night because sometimes I would pump at home in the morning. I pumped for a little longer than eight months, and it wasn't a big deal.

Joan P., Loveland, CO

I was a flight attendant for Northwest Airlines. After a nine-month maternity leave, I returned to work, flying domestic trips only. I didn't want to be away from home for long, and I wanted to continue nursing.

I pumped my milk to stay comfortable, using a hand pump because the electric one would have been too big to haul around. I pumped in hotels, airport bathrooms, bathrooms of employee lounges, and, on longer flights, in airplane bathrooms. The latter was actually more comfortable than in more public places because the engine noise was loud enough so no one could hear me. I just threw the milk out, though I did fly with friends who saved theirs and carried a cooler. It felt a little strange, throwing it all away, after the time and work I put into getting it out, but I did what I had to do.

Pam Bryce, Willseyville, NY

In the fall of her senior year of high school, Daniel found out she was four months pregnant. She had gone in for a pre-qualification test to join the Army, which, to her surprise, included a pregnancy test. Stunned because her period had always been irregular, she wasn't showing, and she didn't have any symptoms, she planned to abort. But while she waited for another paycheck so she would have enough money, her ethics class started talking about abortion. She decided to keep the baby.

NOT JUST ANOTHER STATISTIC

When I was about six months pregnant I left the family I'd been living with since running away from home, and I moved in with my boyfriend's family. (My mom had been beating me for things like getting Bs on my report card instead of As.) Joan, my boyfriend's mother, started telling me about breastfeeding and showed me a couple of books. It seemed weird to me because, like everyone else in my family, I was bottle-fed, and my mom thought nursing was disgusting.

Then about a week before my son was born, some friends asked me if I was going to breastfeed. "Try it. You might actually like it," they said. "Besides, it's the cheapest way you can go. But you're probably going to have to pump or stay home with your kid until he gets old enough to start eating regular food before you can go back to school."

Well, I had too many friends who dropped out because they'd gotten pregnant, and I didn't want to end up like that. I wanted to be able to do something, to get a job and help raise my child successfully.

Daniel was born the next week and was making little sucking noises when the doctor gave him to me. It felt like he knew there was something waiting for him when he got out, and that kind of pushed me over the edge to nurse him.

It's kind of a cliché, but it was like this little bonding thing as soon as he started nursing. I felt like this was what was going to separate me from every other woman in the world. He was going to know I was his mom because of this one thing that I did.

I was expecting it to hurt, but it didn't. He'd nurse for two minutes, then let up, and my milk would spray all over his face and he'd get mad. I felt I was doing something wrong. Joan was like, "Don't worry about it. It happens. They suck and then let go, but the suction is still going."

Daniel's birth had been easy, and I didn't really feel uncomfortable after the first couple of days. I had kept pretty active while I was pregnant, healed fast, and was back to school full-time a week later. I would leave at seven and be home around three. Joan stayed with the baby. Before I left I nursed him to the point where I felt empty, and then I pumped two or three times a day in the nurse's office. At first I had a pump that I squeezed, but I wanted something quicker, so eventually I got an electric pump that I carried in a little diaper bag.

It was hard because I would have to take twenty minutes out of a fifty-minute class to pump, and I wanted to make sure I was making the grades in all my classes. So I might do it second period one day and in fourth period the next. Fortunately I had understanding teachers, and the school nurse thought it was great! Sometimes it was kind of embarrassing, though. I'd be walking to class, and someone would say, "There's something on your shirt," and I'd run down to the nurse's office, pump for a while, and change my shirt. I kept a spare shirt in my locker for that reason.

In my ethics class, we kept journals and had discussions about articles we read. In a newspaper editorial someone wrote about her disgust at women nursing in public. People in my class asked, "Why do people look at lower-class women who are nursing and go, 'Ugh,' but when they look at upper-class people nursing, they say, 'Oh, that's so beautiful'?" It was kind of weird, since I was actually living what we were talking about, but I was able to put in a lot of my own two cents.

In June of 1996 I graduated from the biggest high school in St. Louis. Most people just walk across the stage and graduate, but I felt I actually had *done* something. Not only did I graduate, but I had this baby. For a while I felt like I was just another statistic, another one of those teenagers who was nutty and got pregnant. But now I feel that I'm special because I've got this little boy who's really great.

Daniel René Luna-Workman, St. Louis, MO

Pumping can be productive and successful—or a disaster. It all depends on choosing the right kind of pump. In jobs involving travel, an effective and reliable pump is key. Melanie writes about the trials and tribulations of providing for her daughter, even when on the opposite side of the country.

PUMPING, PLANNING, AND PROVIDING

Like most women who choose to combine career and family, I have constant and simultaneous worries that I am neither spending sufficient time with my child nor working sufficiently hard at my job. When I returned to work after my daughter was born, I was fraught with worry about my capabilities as a mother. I was insecure and unsure of everything except one thing: exclusive breastfeeding. It's just one of those things, like getting a Ph.D. years earlier, that I just knew I would do. I never worried that I might not be able to produce or supply enough milk, and physiologically and philosophically I had few troubles. Instead my concerns were all about logistics. Specifically, the logistics of pumping: where and when to pump, and how much to tell to whom.

I count myself lucky. I have a marvelously competent husband who stays home to raise our daughter. My coworkers support, in principle at least, my choices and my need to balance family with career. I have my own office, and I was able to purchase a high-quality breast pump to make relatively quick work of pumping. So you'd think it should be easy for me. And sometimes it is.

But the little things add up. Traveling for work, for example, takes on concerns of epic proportion. When my baby was young, my breasts filled up so fast that even a five-hour flight seemed like eternity. If my plane was delayed or airport security delayed me with questions about what "electrical device" I was carrying, I thought I would burst! More than once I had to crank the pump up to max to unplug a plugged duct or two and push at the sore nodules, until all the milk came out. And unlike a male colleague with a new baby who revels in a few good nights' sleep when he's away, I must get up in the middle of the night, as if my child had awakened me (since she's still a big night nurser) and pump. But instead of her warm snuggly body and soft, expert lips, I'm greeted with a chair and my pump.

Planning has never been one of my strong suits, and preparing for a trip now means trying to calculate how much milk my daughter will need and, even more difficult, pumping that much extra before I go! I always bring some home from trips (imagine explaining that stuff to airport security), but there's never enough stored away, so I've always got to pump more. It's not like I can just sit down one Saturday and crank out 150 ounces of milk for the five days I'll be gone! So, painstakingly, for months, I add another pumping session and collect and collect and hope that I've guessed the right amount to leave.

I don't always guess right. The all-time low for me in the "I-can-do-it-all" super-mom business came during a cross-country trip to Seattle. It had been a difficult few months for me, and despite pumping three times a day for up to thirty minutes a session, I was barely keeping up with my daughter's growing needs, let alone putting any extra away in the freezer. I hoped she would need less than she had the last time I had traveled, since she was now eating solids. I called my husband during the lunch break of the second day of a four-day trip. We did a quick calculation and realized our daughter had consumed nearly half the milk I'd left; she'd never make it until I got home. I hung up the pay phone and fell apart. I walked back to my hotel, fighting back tears: my daughter would go hungry *and* I was missing an important meeting. I was a complete failure as a mother and a scientist. I tried to change my flight. But the earliest flight would still get me home hours after she'd consumed the last of the milk, and, of course, I'd miss nearly the entire meeting I'd come so far to attend. In desperation I called the hotel business office and asked if they could send a package of a "perishable" nature for me. After inquiring about the contents, the young woman said, in a tone tinged with disgust, "We don't send that sort of thing." But she did put me in touch with a local mailboxes store.

I'll never forget that wonderful man. I called, nearly crying, and asked if he could send my package. I explained what it was. He was not the least bit taken aback. He could send the package, but I would need to get ice packs. He gave me directions to the fish market, where I could purchase ice packs, and back to his shop, assuring me we could do it all before the five o'clock P.M. UPS overnight deadline. I counted my packages of milk I'd stored in the hotel refrigerator: twenty-four ounces. My daughter would need at least thirty! I looked at the clock: three thirty. I rapidly pumped out eight ounces, yelling at my breasts to empty out faster, and cooled it on ice while I packed the other bags. I then wrapped the box in a sweater and took off at a near run up and down the steep hills of downtown Seattle. Fortunately the man's directions were precise. I purchased ice packs at the fish market and made it to his shop by four forty-five.

All Pumps Are Not Created Equal

Apart from Medela and Ameda by Hollister Products, the two leading manufacturers of pumps, many of the semi-automatic and double breast pumps sold at chain stores provide too little stimulation to release the milk and may cause discomfort or pain. This includes pumps made by formula manufacturers and bottle manufacturers (e.g., Gerber and Evenflo). For more information on breast pumps, an excellent Web site is <http://www.artofbreastfeeding.com>. Also contact Medela at 800-TELL YOU or at <http://www.medela.com> or Ameda by Hollister at 800-323-4060 or <http://www.Ameda.com>. Both Web sites also offer lists of rental locations.

He was waiting. My package made it to my husband's anxious hands by nine A.M. the following morning, after a long night spent tracking it on the UPS Web site.

My child is now over a year, and my other pumping friends have quit. It *is* difficult, and I *do* dream of the day when I can leave town or even leave home without my constant companion, the Medela Pump In Style. So why do I carry on? Maybe it's my training as an evolutionary biologist, or maybe it's all my travels into the "less-developed" world that led to my conviction that breastfeeding was meant to go on for years, rather than weeks or months. Maybe it's because I sometimes feel it's my only real contribution to her day-to-day well-being. Maybe I'm just stubborn. Or maybe it's the look of sheer gusto on my daughter's face when she lifts up my shirt and pounces with great satisfaction onto "her" boobies when I return home from work each day. I don't know. But for me, for now, it's still just the right thing to do. So off I go on another business trip, Palm Pilot in one hand, breast pump in the other.

Written by Melanie, East Coast

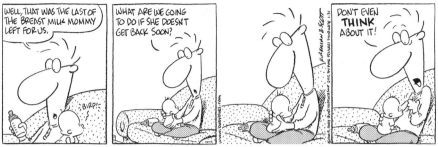

© Baby Blues Partnership. Reprinted with special permission of King Features Syndicate.

OF (FIRE)HOUSE AND HOME

As a firefighter for the city of Chicago, I work a total of eight twenty-four-hour days per month. I was planning on going back to work at three and a half months, and my initial intentions were to only nurse for this time.

But I attended La Leche League meetings while pregnant and learned about pumping. I had never heard of this before! I rented a Medela Lactina pump for two months and then bought my own, using it for ten months with my son and fifteen months with my daughter. Pumping was like exercise—it was just a matter of getting used to it, and within two weeks I was comfortable and it became part of my routine.

Depending on which firehouse I was at, I pumped in the community locker room, the bathroom, an officers' room, a spare room, and the female quarters. I've also been walked in on and teased (good-naturedly) about the guys using my pumped milk for cream in their coffee. But I did a good job of educating them and have actually found them to be more accepting of breastfeeding than women have been. In my experience, women who bottle-feed tend to be very defensive, and I don't wish to fight with them.

At times I have had to leave everything on the table because we got a call. I heard that breast milk stays good at room temperature for ten hours, so I would keep it and make sure to use it the next day.* The only time I ever threw milk away was after I went to a fire. Then I pumped and dumped, just in case the toxins from the fire passed into my milk.

I live close to the firehouse, and often when I would go out shopping for firehouse groceries, I would stop at home for a quick nursing before heading back. Sometimes on weekends my husband would come by with the baby every three hours for me to nurse her.

---

* According to studies, freshly expressed breast milk can be left at room temperature for between six to ten hours, depending on the room temperature.

On the days I was home, I nursed on demand. My son didn't nurse much at night, which is maybe why he weaned so early, but my daughter nursed once or twice a night until she was a little over two years. Overall, the best times were when I came home from work and my babies had big smiles for me and wanted milkies! I loved when they would just nurse and keep looking up at me and smiling—I guess to make sure I was really there—and then fall asleep with that milk-drunk look.

I've become a breastfeeding peer counselor, with the local La Leche League leaders referring mothers to me. They wanted me to become a leader, but the organization turned me down because I was separated from the baby for too long and had to use artificial nipples. But my success rate has been pretty good. I've helped quite a few women, and most of them have nursed for almost a year. I plan to find out if there are other moms in my community interested in going back to work and wanting to nurse. It's nice to have someone to talk to about breastfeeding because it seems that everywhere you look someone has a bottle. Here in Chicago, you can feel very alone.

Cindy Fagiano, Chicago, IL

When my son was three weeks old, I went to work at a telemarketing job. I'm no executive, I didn't have my own office, and I couldn't pump my milk at a place like that. And who else was going to hire me? I'm seventeen. After a week I said, "Forget it." I decided I couldn't be away from my baby for that long. I didn't want them cussing me out, I missed my baby the whole time, and my breasts were so engorged when I got home. I decided to be home with him until he's of an age where I don't have to worry about pumping when I'm gone.

Niesha Vann, Glendale, AZ

Beyond the Pump

All of the lip service to motherhood still floats in the air, as insubstantial as clouds of angel dust. On the ground, where mothers live, the lack of respect and tangible recognition is still part of every mother's experience. Most people, like infants in a crib, take female caregiving utterly for granted.

Ann Crittenden, The Price of Motherhood

While expressing milk makes it possible for many employed mothers to continue nursing, it is only part of the solution. Even though meas-

ures enacted to support breastfeeding employees actually sav
nesses money, workplace environments must become more "
feeding-friendly." That means greater availability of on-sit
care, longer maternity leaves, more flexibility in work schedu..__,
helping employers better understand why supporting breastfeeding is
a win-win situation. As Marsha Walker, an international board-certified lactation consultant and nationally known breastfeeding advocate, asserts, "It's hard to encourage women to breastfeed when children and breastfeeding are looked at like a hobby, as something you
do in your spare time so you can get back to the stuff that's really important, which is your job" (personal communication, 1996).

Some of us may decide that we can't do it all. Arlene Rossen Cardozo, author of *Sequencing: Having it All but Not All at Once . . .
A New Solution for Women Who Want Marriage, Career, and Family* (1986), writes about the process of going from full-time career to
full-time mothering, and finally to a stage of life in which these two
aspects of life become creatively integrated. This "sequencing" approach, she argues, evolved as a response to the "superwoman"
myth of the 1960s and 1970s, a myth, she claims, invented by women
who did not have children.

Sequencing, however, is not an option for everyone. Apart from
the long-term financial consequences vividly described in Ann Crittenden's best-selling book *The Price of Motherhood,* Cardozo's
strategy is irrelevant to any woman who is not married and middle-
class. Not all women can choose to leave the workforce, nor do all
women want to. As writer Mary Kay Blakely asserts, "Being asked
to decide between your passion for work and your passion for your
children was like being asked by your doctor whether you preferred
him to remove your brain or your heart" (1994, 199).

Of course, millions of women do find ways to integrate their private, unpaid work of mothering with their public and paid work in
the labor force, but the struggle for balance continues. This next
group of stories sheds more light on what this means within the context of women's daily lives.

In Their Own Words:
Beyond the Pump

According to the National Coalition for Campus Children's Centers, over eighteen hundred child-care centers are available on col-

lege campuses. Not all of them, however, offer infant care. As inspiring as this next story is, the availability of on-campus child care would have made a huge difference in this mother's life.

☕ BREAKING THE RULES

When I was a graduate student, the director of women's studies talked about bringing her babies to her office with her in the 1960s and putting them under her desk while she was doing her doctoral work. She was nursing twins, and there was no available child care. This image has always stayed with me—a woman who did what she felt she had to do for her children, while still meeting her professional responsibilities. I think of it as a kind of legacy.

In 1992, while working on my dissertation, I, too, had a baby. I supported myself by working part-time as assistant to the dean of my school. His wife had recently had a baby, so he was very sensitive to the issues. He gave me enormous support and said, "Of course, Elaine, when you have the baby, you'll bring it to work."

I worked until the day before I went into labor, had the baby, and returned two weeks later. I had an ongoing commitment to give my son the healthiest start I could, and that included nursing. I wouldn't let anything come between me and achieving that aim. Benjamin was with me all the time, and I basically did everything I did before. Nursing satisfied him, so when he stirred, I just nursed him, and he was not disruptive. I nursed him a lot. Most of the time I don't think people even knew. They had so little experience with babies that they didn't know that when a woman is holding a baby across her chest, there's a chance it may be nursing. Benjamin stayed with me in my office until he was six months old, when he suddenly became noisy and more challenging.

During this time I had great support from my extended family. I wasn't married, and my mother, who was retiring about the time he was born, came to help me. She actually stayed for a year, until I finished my dissertation. Eventually, I quit my job to finish writing it. I moved to my mother's house, left my baby with her, and went to my brother's house during the day where there were no people around.

When my son was fifteen months old, I was still working on my dissertation and was exhausted from the dual responsibility. By then he was only nursing in the morning and at night, and my mother really pressed me to wean him. She told me I needed to be able to go away overnight, finish my dissertation, and meet with my advisor. I weaned him very gradually. I remember putting him to bed and nursing him for the last time, not knowing if I would ever have another baby or nurse again. It was a very poignant moment.

Eventually I finished my dissertation, earned my Ph.D., and worked a series of one-year jobs at different universities. I married and became pregnant in December of 1994, which meant I would give birth at the end of the following summer. In academia you start looking for a job in the fall preceding the year you need one. I was looking for a permanent job, and the market was very bad. My husband had lost his job and was starting to develop a business, so he could not support us. I went to a colleague and said, "I'm pregnant, I'm on the job market, and I'm going to have this baby. What do I need to tell people when I'm interviewing?"

"If you are not going to take a leave," she said, "you don't have an obligation to make this an issue in your interviewing process."

So I didn't. I wore a big jacket, and when people met me, they didn't know if I was heavy or what. The subject never came up. Eventually I was given a one-year contract at a university forty-five miles from my home. When I began the job and was given the contract, I explained that I was expecting in early September, intended to take one week off, and then I would be back. My colleagues told me they would cover my classes for the one week.

I taught my first class on Monday, August 28, and William was born the next day. It was a wonderful birth—five hours of labor—and everything was fine.

I returned to work the following Wednesday, having been in the department for only ten days, with William in the car-seat carrier. My mother also came with me to be sure I would be okay and not pass out. No one expected my baby to be there with me. At the first faculty meeting of the semester, where new faculty are introduced, the president was making his speech and looked up from his notes when he saw me in the middle of the room with the baby. He sort of gasped, which I interpreted to mean, "Oh, my God! This baby's going to cry in the middle of my speech!" It seemed to be a terrifying moment for him. But when the dean called my name and I stood up in the middle of the crowd—holding this baby no one knew was there because he was so quiet—the dean just gasped! She said, "This is just the way things should be!"

On my second day of teaching, I took the baby in the carrier to my classes and put him under my desk because, not knowing his schedule yet, I didn't know when he would want to nurse. Upon leaving that day, one of the office administrators said to me, "So how long are we going to have to put up with this?" I just smiled and got in the elevator with my mother and baby and went home.

I understood that the people around me had no experience with a faculty member bringing in a baby, and I realized I would have to help them find ways to articulate the experience and ultimately support me. So I did the diplomatic work of helping them to understand what I was doing at each stage of the baby's development.

The first stage of diplomacy was to educate the students in my classes. I explained that I had just given birth and was nursing. As a commuting mother with no campus child-care facilities, I needed to keep the baby with me. Since it was legal to nurse in public, if the baby stirred I would step out of the room, attach him, and then come back into the room and continue to teach. About two times in both classes I did have to nurse during class.

This arrangement lasted for six weeks. By that time some of the students had told me that if I ever needed child care during the day, they could help. So I found students who stayed with the baby in my office while I taught. (I continued to have him with me during my office hours, though.) I informed both my department chair and my division director of the change, so they would have a response to anyone who would ask them about it.

William was a very contented baby who fit the circumstances and lived up to my best hopes. He became known as "that baby you don't know is there." He was charming and sweet-natured, and everyone in the building adored him.

Ultimately, those same people who asked me how long this would be going on came to be my greatest supporters. And I learned that if you are going to ask people to help you do something, you need to help them understand it, especially if it's the first time they are going through the process.

Toward the end of the semester, William started to get noisier and needing to play. I met a woman who lived off campus and was returning from maternity leave. I would bring the baby to my office, and a student would get him, get the car seat, get my car, drive down the hill to the professor's house, and stay with her baby and mine through the day. I would use the professor's car to drive down at noon to nurse, come back, and then at the end of the day, the father of her child would return home. The student would get in my car, drive back to campus, and bring William to me. Eventually he didn't need to nurse at lunch time, and I didn't need to do all that.

When my class evaluations came through, two students commented, "It was totally inappropriate to nurse a baby in a class." Two others said, "This is the most incredible thing I've ever seen—a baby nursed in a class!" What was interesting to me is that the chair included the two negative statements, but *not* the two positive ones, in the annual letter that summarizes one's course evaluations. I don't know why, but the chair felt some obligation to make a note of this.

Still, my contract was renewed for a second year. I experienced no long-term negative professional consequences, and I believe that because I made it work, the sum total of this experience has been extremely positive. I teach sociology of medicine and women's health issues, and those kinds of experiences strongly inform my teaching. And I was thrilled that I could be working because at forty-four it was part of me that defined most of my life.

Overall, I was able to achieve my goals and do two things I really loved. And it gave me real comfort to meet my son's needs and attend to him in a way that was meaningful and made sense. At the same time, though, I understood from the beginning that there was a very critical social-class issue. My professor who had brought her babies with her in the 1960s had explained that the people who resisted the most were the women who had not been able to bring their children because they were in positions that didn't support it.

Interestingly, at the end of the semester, after all had gone well, the division director came to me and asked, "So how's it going, Elaine? How's it going with the baby?"

I said, "It's been great. Everybody's been very supportive."

And he said, "You know, it's against university regulations to have a baby in your office." It was an equity issue, he explained. Because secretaries don't have a private space to keep their babies, university regulations stipulate that no one is allowed to have a child with them on campus. Then he added, "But the rules are never enforced unless someone complains."

Since nobody told me I couldn't do it, I assume it was because I had done the diplomatic work.

While I did what I felt was important for me, I also have a commitment to make it possible for all women with children to do what I did. What we need are facilities to enable women to do what they feel is best for them and their children. We need the array of options so women can decide for themselves.

Elaine R. Cleeton, Western New York

Lauren's story is representative of women who have no power or control while on the job. Despite her experience, Lauren, seventeen when her daughter was born, has been working hard to get on her feet. See her inspiring story on pages 69–71.

NO BABIES ALLOWED

When Taea was two months old I started a job as a reservation agent at a cab company. I worked eight hours a day, from six A.M. until three P.M. My dad worked at the same place on a three o'clock to eleven o'clock shift, so he watched the baby while I worked and brought her to me as I was leaving. I would nurse her on the subway ride home.

During this time, Taea refused to take a bottle and would be hungry all day and scream. It didn't even enter my mind to have a pump, and by the end of the day, I would be painfully full.

Taea spent 90 percent of the time crying, unless she was asleep. I felt so bad for her, but my job was so strict. I would ask, "Can I bring my daughter in? She won't eat, and she's crying."

And they said, "You've got a problem, then."

I quit after a couple of weeks. It wasn't fair to Taea.

Lauren Leigh Humphrey, Kensington, MD

Melissa is a senior policy analyst who works full-time for the Women, Infants, and Children program (WIC), a federally funded supplemental nutrition program that operates out of state health departments and local clinics. Among the services WIC offers is the provision of supplemental foods to pregnant and nursing women, other newly postpartum women, and children under the age of five years. Still, the program combats an image of being nothing more than government assistance that gives out free formula and food vouchers. In recent years, the U.S. Department of Agriculture (USDA) and state WIC agencies have spent an increasing amount of money on public education and breastfeeding promotion.

Melissa is nursing her twenty-one-month-old son, Ian, and previously nursed her daughter Lucy, now five. Forty years old and four months pregnant when we spoke, she tells a story that reveals the contradictions between workplace policies and lived experience.

RHETORIC VERSUS REALITY

While the WIC clinics and health departments I visit have been very friendly and supportive of breastfeeding, my agency has been slow to come around to giving anything more than lip service to "supporting nursing mothers in the workplace," as touted in a 1998 employee memorandum.

After my daughter Lucy was born, I took three months off. I found a day care near my office so I could nurse her at lunch. Seeing her made it easier to get through the day, not only physically but emotionally. I could visit her, eat lunch with the other breastfeeding moms, nurse her to sleep, sit and rock her, and put her down for her nap.

Still, I pumped at work until she was a year. My boss was philosophically supportive but hadn't breastfed her own children and had no practical concept of the time it would take, the need for privacy, and the importance of feeling relaxed.

According to agency policy, the staff was given two paid fifteen-minute breaks per day and an unpaid lunch break of thirty minutes. If someone went over that unpaid period, they had to count it as annual or sick leave. My boss didn't charge me leave for the few extra minutes it took me to pump, but there were a lot of people in the office, including the personnel officer, who said that she should. I had to explain that it usually takes longer than fifteen minutes to pump, especially since I didn't have a room where I could leave my supplies. And I pumped in a conference room where I had to put sheets of butcher paper on the windows so people couldn't see inside. Even so, if someone had gotten on a chair, they could have peered right in. And they could *hear* everything from their cubicles. Because of the constant pressure I felt to be at my desk, I wasn't able to pump enough during the workday to keep up with my baby. Instead, I pumped extra in the evenings and on weekends.

In exchange for being on "limited travel" for the first six months, I agreed to do all the backup and office support for the people who *were* traveling. Despite this, I had to take my first business trip when Lucy was about six months old. Luckily, my sister offered to travel with me, welcoming the chance to bond with her new niece.

Whenever possible I had her meet me so I could breastfeed Lucy at lunchtime. A coworker actually raised a stink that my baby was on the trip with me. To place this in context, it is common and accepted for nursing babies to accompany their moms to WIC program conferences at the state and local levels, even during meeting times. The babies are peaceful and secure. Instead, my coworker raised suspicions: Was a person from the state taking care of her? Was I using my position to my advantage?

There is supposed to be an agency policy against having your child at work with you, and the president of the local union felt it was important to make an example of me. At this multi-agency meeting, I was literally standing on the threshold of the conference room during a break because people wanted to see my baby, and this person reported that I'd had the baby in the meeting room. That was my first of five or six trips over the next year.

One day, when Lucy was about twelve or thirteen months old, my boss asked me if I was still pumping.

"No," I replied. "I stopped."

"Then you can get back on travel again," she said, thinking that because I didn't pump anymore, my breastfeeding relationship was over. I explained that I still went to my daughter's day care to breastfeed at lunch time and I still nursed in the evenings, overnight, and first thing in the morning. It was a wonderful and intense part of our relationship, and I knew she still needed me.

"I can't justify it anymore," she said. "You're not taking on your part of this business travel."

It pulled the rug out from under me, but I went back on travel. My sister came along for a while. But when she was no longer able to do that I decided to wean because travel commitments reached a peak and I no longer had anyone to come with me. My daughter was just about two and not yet ready to wean. It took several weeks to wean her, and the last couple of them were tormenting because she really didn't like being cut back that far. I'd give her a cup before bedtime, and she would just sit in my lap sobbing. She didn't want a *cup*—she wanted to *nurse* until she fell asleep.

Lucy was almost two and a half when I became pregnant. After my son Ian was born, I really didn't want to go back to work, but I have tenure in this job, and my husband doesn't have the fringe benefits I do. I also have financial security and the independence my job brings. I extended my maternity leave, used all of my accrued sick and annual leave, and took additional leave without pay.

According to the Family and Medical Leave Act, the organization had to protect my job for me while I was gone. I talked with my new supervisor, as well as my longtime boss, both of whom said if I didn't come back before six months, the front office could not guarantee I would have the same job, and I might be put somewhere else in the agency. They were also afraid that if I didn't come back, they would lose the position on the organizational chart because of cutbacks.

So after taking off five and a half months, I went back. I put Ian in the same day care in which I had put my daughter and hoped for the same support as before. Unfortunately, I discovered that management support had completely shriveled up. My boss gave me what seemed like a prepared speech, explaining that the new union contract was constraining what she could do. She declared, a little stridently, that she was proud of what "we" had done to "allow me" to continue breastfeeding before but added that we had "done some things wrong." This time I was going to have to take leave for every minute I was out over the thirty-minute lunch period and the fifteen-minute breaks. I couldn't believe she had changed her tune so much. Despite all her previous support, I was now on my own.

It was really stressful. Two of my close coworkers had left the agency, and I was surrounded by people who thought that any minute I was away from my desk was giving them extra work. I felt like they were nickel-and-diming me to death over each little thing.

During the next six months I had to travel out of town three times for about a week each. Like before, I brought Ian with me, this time lining up day care in each town I was traveling to. Suddenly, though, it became a big deal. When I had traveled with my daughter, we could all travel in a governmental rental car, but with Ian I had to rent a separate car, at my own expense, because they said I couldn't transport my child in a governmental car unless he were on official business.

The agency made it clear that I was responsible for all of Ian's travel-related expenses. To me, this was so obvious it had never been an issue before. I had always made it clear that any food, child care, or travel expenses were personal and *not* claimed for reimbursement by the government. Upon my return, I had to demonstrate that *I* was paying day care and wasn't somehow finding a way to charge the government.

When Ian was about nine months old, I started working at home two days a week. This was the result of national union negotiations. I was skeptical about even attempting to exercise that option because the policies are very stringent and not family-friendly. They specifically forbid you from providing child care while you're working at home, and that includes sick children. You could have someone else in the house, but you would have to show that they, not you, were taking care of the child.

One time my son was home with my husband and was crying when the phone rang. It was a coworker from my office. We talked, carrying on business, and immediately afterward I received an e-mail from my supervisor: "It is my understanding that you have your baby at home with you. If this is the case, you will need to take sick or annual leave instead of claiming to be on duty." I called immediately and explained that the baby was at home, but my husband was watching him.

The greatest irony is that I work for WIC. And yet, as a nursing mother, I was given the least amount of support in terms of time and place to pump, ever-decreasing flexibility regarding traveling, limits on work schedule, and people presuming I was doing wrong. I wish I could say that the government is great to work for, especially in a program supposedly focused on maternal and child health, but my agency is constrained by union contracts and management stagnation. Union involvement in setting and enforcing employee policies is dependent on the self-interest of the top cronies. For example, smoking on duty time is not only condoned but sheltered in a safe, open-air patio for employees to enjoy at any time without having to turn in any request for leave. No one asks for apologies to coworkers when they "take up the slack" while the *smoker* spends an unlimited amount of time away from the office.

One might think that the government is in a prime position to set policy standards for corporate America by piloting and modeling family-friendly policies to retain the workforce. After all, government salaries certainly don't have the competitive edge. Instead, downsizing makes utilizing the remaining workforce a very sensitive issue. Even people who want to be considered family-friendly feel it's a luxury they cannot afford.

My story is not done. I'm still nursing Ian at twenty-one months, and I'm four months pregnant. Again, I'm at this crossroads. Do I quit or take a longer absence?

In the meantime, there was a woman in another work unit here who was assigned heavy travel during the first year of her baby's life. She objected but didn't get any relief and traveled almost every week for days at a time. More than one coworker has told me that her case was a great example of why there is no need to make exceptions for anyone, certainly not for new mothers. However, I know that she began supplementing with formula by the time her baby was seven months old, feeling terrible about it. "At least," she said, "it didn't affect his growth rate." She told me she had to throw away the milk she pumped while on the road because there was no practical way to save it until she returned home. Perhaps not surprisingly, she is no longer with this federal agency.

I can guarantee that I will not let this kind of forcible separation happen to my next baby and me. But the pressure is on. One close coworker already outlined a full travel schedule for me once I come back from maternity leave. Thus, the stakes are always getting higher, and the expectations never ease up, no matter what.

I guess if I were to buck up the courage I could quit, but it would not be a wise move. I have a career of over fifteen years. I'm forty years old, and this economy is pretty scary. For all this job's inflexibilities and illogical policies, I am still able to take leave, I can work flexible hours, and I occasionally work in my home office. I have a secure financial future for my growing family. And there are certain aspects about the job that are satisfying. My kids are only going to be little for a short time, and I hate to miss out on that during so many hours of the day. But at the same time, I still need to provide for them. I'm getting older, so I've got to do all I can.

Melissa

I am a senior U.S. Army officer and currently work for a man who has four children. His support alone has allowed me to continue nursing my child. First, he granted me three months of absence right after Chyanne was born. Then he reduced my work hours to accommodate my nursing schedule. I was also given a private office so I could pump, which I stopped doing when Chyanne was fifteen months old. I am still allowed to work reduced hours so that I can spend more time with my child, and I strongly believe that if all women received the type of support I have, the percentage of breastfeeding mothers would increase by at least 50 percent!

Brooke S. Oestreich, Woodbridge, VA

Thirty weeks into her pregnancy, Lee went in for a routine check-up. After discovering that her blood pressure was dangerously high, she was admitted to the hospital for testing. When the doctors discovered that her liver, kidneys, and other vital organs were on the verge of shutting down, they insisted she deliver her baby right away. Her daughter, Caroline, now six years old, was born via C-section, weighing only two pounds, fifteen ounces. Lee pumped her milk, and the nurses fed Carolyn via a feeding tube and, later, bottles. Lee talks about the challenges she faced in getting her premature daughter to nurse and how this experience was shaped by her obligations at work.

 ## FROM BOTTLE TO BREAST TO BOTTLE

Two weeks after my daughter, Caroline, was born, when she was still in the hospital, I went back to work part-time. I would get up in the morning and pump; go to the hospital, visit Caroline, and pump; leave for the office, spend three or four hours there, go back to the hospital, see Caroline, and pump again. After an hour or two I would go home, and my husband and I would visit again that night. My coworkers were very supportive, and a lot of them felt sorry for me. But given that having a baby in the hospital was the only scenario I'd ever known, I didn't have an overwhelming sense of loss that she was not at home.

If I had to do it over again, I would have spent more time at the hospital, but I wanted to save my maternity leave for when she was home. For several weeks I couldn't even hold her, except at feeding time. Her skin was ultra-sensitive, and even the air could irritate it. So there was no point in being there when I couldn't even pick her up. I had left with my computer still on and a lot of things unfinished, so I was able to go back, hand off projects, and get some closure.

When Caroline was six weeks old she left the hospital, still four weeks be-fore her due date, and I started my maternity leave. Because I'd had constant support at the hospital, with a nurse looking over my shoulder when I changed Caroline's diaper, took her temperature, or gave her a bottle, by the time we came home, I felt like I'd mastered the basics of baby care. My *moth-ering style*, on the other hand, was something that evolved as Caroline and I got to know each other.

I continued pumping and trying to get her to latch on, enduring many tearful moments. I kept thinking, any day, any day, any day . . . Finally, within a week of her due date, she was able to open her mouth wide enough! It was pretty miraculous given how long she'd been given a bottle. I couldn't be-lieve it! *This* was what it was all about!

At first, she slept in a cradle next to my bed, and I nursed her in a bed-room chair. Eventually I stopped getting up and took her into bed with me. I would lie down because I was so tired and then wake up in a panic, won-dering, "Where am I? Where is she? Did I lay on her?" But about this time I began reading Dr. Sears and the ideas of attachment parenting. It all made sense, and I realized how much better we slept when we were together.

It was at this point that I really began to relax and enjoy being a mom. She was healthy, home, and exclusively nursing. It was also at this point that I realized it wasn't going to last forever. I had worked so hard to get her to nurse and to nurture our relationship, and now I had to start planning for a different routine for both of us.

Ironically, I had a hard time getting her to go back onto the bottle when I returned to work. We tried different nipples ahead of time, and she pitched a fit! By the time I went back, when she was four months old, she was still having trouble.

I went back part-time and gradually increased my hours so I was full-time when she was six months old. I didn't want to, but I had to—quitting would have cut our income in half. I had used up my maternity leave, and they had even let me have extra time off from using days in what's called a sick-leave pool.

Leaving her felt as if someone in my family had died. I cried a lot. She was in day care, not too far away, and I would go nurse her at lunch. I also pumped—two times a day at first and then three times after my supply dropped.

I worked full-time for eight months, during which time I kept pumping. I nursed her before dinner, at bedtime, and at least twice during the night. Many nights I would pump again before going to bed to have enough milk for the next day. Weekends were the best—no pumping, no bottles, just nursing. It was great for my milk supply. Monday was always a big production day.

I really wanted to stay home. Even before she was born, I knew that juggling motherhood and work was not for me. But I conceived the first time we tried, and I hadn't thought I would get pregnant so quickly. I figured out that by selling my car (which was paid for) and going without one, I could stay home. Ultimately I quit when Caroline was fourteen months old. Our other car did not get repossessed, we ate three meals a day, and we paid our mortgage. Somehow it worked out.

It was about this time that Caroline kind of weaned herself. She just stopped asking for it, and I kind of stopped offering. I think I was glad to have my body back, but in retrospect, now that I'm nursing my almost two-year-old son, I wish I had nursed her longer. I can sit down with my son, cuddle him, and give him the comfort of mother's milk. It soothes him, especially when he's frustrated, and it's just a balm for his soul.

I don't think weaning her at fifteen months affected our closeness or my ability to parent her. But I do wish we could have continued the benefits of nursing, given how hard we both worked to establish it. Only after my son was born, and I was able to nurse without the worries of prematurity and switching from bottle to breast to bottle, did I realize how lucky I am that we made it as long as we did.

Lee Harris, Austin, TX

Lori's story fits within the discussion of the *process* of nursing versus the *product* of breast milk. For Lori, it was the process that was more important. To read more about her determination to nurse, a fierceness that caused her to redefine the meaning of *feminine*, see her story on pages 108–9.

☕ IN AND OUT OF THE WORKFORCE

I've never been successful pumping and storing my milk. Somehow, I just couldn't see the value in the milk if it wasn't coming directly out of me. This means I've had to be available all the time for the first year of my children's lives and that I have entered and exited the workforce several times.

I have four kids—eight and a half, seven, three, and five months. I nursed Bishop, my oldest, for ten months. It was me and the boy, and we were the world. For nine months, I didn't even look up. I was completely immersed in him. I did not anticipate the intensity of the relationship, and I don't know if I'll ever be that close to another person again. But I stopped nursing because my nipples started to hurt all the time. I didn't know it right away, but it was because I was pregnant.

My second son, Mitchell, was born during a difficult period in our lives. My husband's mother had cancer and was dying, and my father had just had heart surgery. I'm amazed we made it through. I nursed exclusively for about four months, but by that point, I was burned out. I had been pregnant for nine months, nursing for ten months, pregnant for nine more months, and then nursing again. I think if I'd had the skills I have now to go out and create relationships with other mothers and find the things I enjoy about being home, it would have been a different experience. But at the time, I was running for the hills. I really needed to be out of the house, and financially, we needed me to work.

I got a job making good money, more than my husband, with health benefits and all the things we didn't have at the time. Brad stayed home with Mitchell. I nursed when I was home, and Brad gave him a bottle of formula when I wasn't. I didn't do any pumping. I felt like the benefits from breastfeeding were not from the milk itself, but because I was there.

Brad and Mitchell developed a bond similar to the one Bishop and I formed, and it lasts to this day. Brad really feels like Mitchell was *his* baby. And going back to work was great for my self-esteem. I needed to be out of the house and successful in my own right. I didn't regret my decision—it was the best thing to do at the time—but I realized I missed out on breastfeeding and the baby relationship with Mitchell.

So my third child I absolutely had on purpose. Because Charlie was going to be the last one, I savored every moment and stayed home with him. But it's difficult for me to be at home, and I'm not incredibly good at it. So when he was ten months old I went back to work full-time. My husband and I did whatever we had to do to keep the kids out of day care. Brad worked nights at the time, so we sort of had split shifts. He would bring Charlie to me at lunch, and I would feed him. It was difficult for me to mentally shift from being at work to feeding the baby, and I had to wear clothes I could nurse in without getting completely naked. I needed him to nurse quickly so I could get back to work, and it was hard to find a place where he wouldn't be distracted. I didn't love the arrangement, but it only lasted for about a month or two, and then I just fed him at night and in the morning.

By the time Charlie was thirteen or fourteen months old, I was good and ready to be done nursing. I wanted a little more freedom, and I wanted my body back. I was ready to stop, but I thought, "Why torture the child? He'll give it up." And he did at about sixteen months.

Our lives then fell into an acceptable, comfortable pattern. I found a different position that I enjoyed very much. My husband and I were able to arrange our work schedules to minimize the time the kids were in child care, and we had a great provider for Charlie. It was the first time since we began having children that we were both working during the day and could spend time together in the evenings and on weekends.

And then our birth control failed. I was devastated. I was on my knees in the bathroom sobbing in disbelief. I didn't tell anyone except Brad for over a month. I was so pissed off! But when I had a sonogram at sixteen weeks and saw that, after three boys, I was having a girl, that turned the whole thing around.

Somehow the circumstances of my life fell together. I got laid off on Wednesday, and Olivia was born on Monday. I got a huge severance package, the best maternity leave I've ever had, and I feel like it was meant to be.

My parents have not understood why I just can't leave my kids. But I just cannot imagine taking my six-week-old child and giving him to someone else for the day. That, to me, is horrific, and not necessarily because the baby would be uncomfortable or upset but because I couldn't stand to be away from him. I'm responding to an instinct that I cannot overcome, regardless of financial ruin or whatever circumstances might come my way. The circumstances would have to be completely dire before I would do it. The only reason I was able to leave Mitchell was because he was with Brad.

Breastfeeding, for the most part, has kept me home with my babies. I really don't think of the decision to breastfeed as a nutritional one. I'm glad breast milk is good for babies, but the actual milk itself has never been my motivation to nurse. My motivation has always been the intense relationship, the incredible feeling I have doing it. I was lucky enough to share that with three of my children for an extended period of time. I love my husband, and we are very compatible, but it doesn't come close to what I've felt with my babies.

I provide 50 percent of the income, and it's a big deal for me not to be working, but I'm going to see how it goes. Olivia is now five months old. I want to be with her at least until she's a year, and we're going to stretch the money until it dries up. Right now we are stuffed into a townhouse. Olivia sleeps with us and doesn't take up any space—I can't imagine if we had a crib since there's no place for it! But I'm just going to see how it goes and take it day by day.

Lori Bishop, Jacksonville, FL

BREAST MILK: WORTH ITS WEIGHT IN GOLD

When Christopher was about a month old, a friend's mother was at a dinner where she met a doctor who told her Monsanto was doing a breast milk study. "We're paying women 250 dollars a liter for their milk," he said.

She gave the doctor my phone number, and he contacted me. I guess they were putting it under a microscope to study the immunological qualities, proteins, and stuff like that.

It would take me two days to pump thirty ounces. I would nurse the baby, then pump milk and freeze it. Chris ate every one and half hours, so for two days I was either nursing or pumping. He'd be asleep, and I'd watch TV and pump. Sometimes he would nurse on one breast while I would pump the other.

I pumped a total of three liters and made about 750 dollars from the study. We got hit at the last minute with quite a large hospital bill to pay. My milk paid it. I teased my husband that this was the epitome of working at home.

Susan A. Keen, St. Louis, MO

 CHAPTER SEVEN

An Embodied Relationship

STORIES OF CONTRADICTION, SEXUALITY, & INTIMACY

Who wants to dwell on the thought that breasts can look like ud-
ders, that breasts are udders, full, swollen, dripping with milk,
squeezed, sucked on, raw, tender, in pain—and ultimately used up
and withered. No, we're Marilyn Monroe in her calendar pose.
We're Friday-night entries in a college town wet-T-shirt contest.
We float down the avenue in a Maidenform bra and the nipples
don't show.

Susan Brownmiller, Femininity

One of the great cultural paradoxes to confront women in the
United States is the seeming incompatibility between sexual-
ity and motherhood (Rodriguez-Garcia and Frazier 1995). Marilyn
Yalom, author of *A History of the Breast,* sums up the matter nicely:
"The mandate to nurse and the mandate to titillate are competing
claims that continue to shape women's fate" (1997, 5).

Clearly, the biological purpose of breasts is for nursing children.
But it is impossible to understand the cultural context of breastfeeding in the United States without recognizing the unmistakable
assumption that breasts are primarily to "turn on" a man, not to
latch on a baby. This assumption is decidedly culture bound. Apart
from the fact that humans are the only species in which mammary

glands play a role in sexual behavior, this role is not culturally universal. In some cultures in Africa and the South Pacific, women rarely cover their breasts, and no one gives this a second thought. Katherine Dettwyler, a biocultural anthropologist, points out that women in the African country of Mali, for example, were either "bemused" or "horrified" upon hearing of American attitudes toward breasts, particularly their role in sexual foreplay. They regard adult mouth-to-breast contact as unnatural, perverted behavior (1995a, 171–72).

However interesting it may be to know how women in Mali view the breast, it is of little practical relevance in a culture as breast obsessed and misinformed as ours, where the breast is arguably the most scrutinized, eroticized, objectified, manipulated, commercialized, and worshipped part of women's bodies. Women in the United States nurse in a culture in which our breasts are used to sell everything from cars to beer; in which deep cleavage dominates the checkout aisle; in which a nationally franchised "family" restaurant markets "hooters" more aggressively than hamburgers; and in which the number of women who artificially enlarge their breasts has increased 593 percent from 1992 to 2002.* The American Society of Plastic and Reconstructive Surgeons, the group of surgeons (almost exclusively male) who profit from breast augmentation surgery, do little to remind women of our breasts' primary biological function and have even diagnosed small breasts as "deformities" and a disfiguring "disease"—"micromastia"! (Barbara Ehrenreich, quoted in Dettwyler 1995a, 176).

Despite the message that "bigger is better," even well-endowed women can't always win. A friend of mine, for example, who bottle-fed during the mid-1970s, admits it was because of her emotional and psychological discomfort with her double-E breasts that she did not nurse her two children. Twenty-five years later, she still regrets her decision. Is it any wonder, then, that we often feel self-conscious and ambivalent about our breasts? As Susan Brownmiller, the author of *Femininity*, suggests, "Breasts are a source of female pride and sexual identification, but they are also a source of competition, confusion, insecurity and shame" (1984, 40).

---

* See the Web site of the American Society of Plastic Surgeons at <http://www.plastic surgery.org/>.

The stories in this chapter center around what it means to breast-feed in a society in which breasts are so sexually charged. How does our sexuality affect breastfeeding, and how does breastfeeding affect our sexuality? How do we meet our children's needs when we're out in public? How do women both accommodate and resist the cultural assumption that our breasts serve a sexual purpose more than a functional one?

The "Official Breast"

In our money-can-fix-anything culture, where we are still judged more for how we look than for who we are, what we do, or how we think, it comes as little surprise that more and more women are choosing to alter our bodies to meet the cultural standard du jour. If Goldilocks were to grow up today, she would want her breasts to be neither too small, nor too big, but just right. Laurie Nommsen-Rivers, IBCLC, points out that our understanding of "normal" is becoming increasingly narrower, creating a society "where performing surgery to the breast, despite a fairly high rate of complications, is becoming more 'normal' than having an A or DD cup size" (2003, 7).

This ever-narrowing standard has resulted in the "Official Breast," one that negates all others, asserts feminist author Naomi Wolf. "Looking at breasts in culture," she writes, "one would have little idea that breasts come in as many shapes and variations as there are women. Since most women rarely if ever see or touch other women's breasts," she continues, "they have no idea what they feel like, or the way they move and shift with the body, or of how they really look during lovemaking" (1991, 247). This lack of access to a full range of real breasts makes it easy for us to feel that our own pair is inadequate or imperfect.

In most cases, nobody "forces" us to alter our bodies. It is an individual choice, based on myriad psychological factors and the degree to which we have internalized the messages we receive about our bodies. We often make these life-altering decisions, however, long before we consider the impact they will have on our ability to feed and nurture our children.

One of the main controversies centers around the ability to maintain an adequate milk supply. Lactation consultant Nommsen-Rivers contends that many plastic surgeons interpret being able to nurse as the ability to produce milk, regardless of whether a woman will have to supplement. This is quite different from the ability to breastfeed exclusively with an ample supply (Nommsen-Rivers 2003, 7).

While some of us who have altered our breasts go on to successfully breastfeed, studies and anecdotal evidence suggest that both breast reductions and augmentations *can* adversely impact our milk supply and reduce how long we nurse (e.g., Souto et al. 2003; Neifert et al. 1990). And, contrary to what plastic surgeons may believe, it has nothing to do with breast size, since size is determined by the amount of fatty tissue we have, *not* the glandular tissue that produces milk. There is thus no relationship between cup size and volume of milk (Nancy Hurst, personal communication, 2003).

In the case of implants, both silicone and saline, whether or not they reduce our milk supply may depend, in part, on whether the implants are placed on top of or beneath the chest muscles. No studies, however, have critically examined how this may affect milk production (Scott L. Spear, personal communication, 2003). Nor are there statistics concerning *trends* in the kind of implant surgeries women receive. The American Society of Plastic Surgeons, the largest plastic surgery organization in the world, does not track this.

The ability to nurse may also be related to how the surgeon inserts the implants. Nancy Hurst, director of the Lactation Program at Texas Children's Hospital, found that women who have an incision around the nipple (known as a periareolar incision) may be more likely to experience nursing difficulties than women who have incisions under the breast or near the armpit; cutting the areola is more likely to sever the milk ducts, meaning that although women may *produce* milk, the milk can't flow well to the nipple (Hurst 1996). Her conclusions, though, are based on small sample sizes, and, as with the placement of implants, no well-designed studies address how the different types of implant incisions may affect nursing (Spear, personal communication, 2003). Consequently, plastic surgeons are left to rely on their own assumptions.

"We don't have a lot of information about how breast implants influence a woman's ability or motivation to lactate," says Scott L. Spear, professor and chief of plastic surgery at Georgetown University and spokesperson for the American Society of Plastic Surgeons. "Someone would have to spend the time and money to do it. Not all women want to breastfeed and not everyone can.

Where breast implants fit into this, I don't know" (personal communication, 2003).

In a culture that uses scientific evidence as the basis for recommending all sorts of health behaviors, it is shocking that so little research exists concerning the possible relationships between breast implants (not to mention other breast surgeries) and the ability to lactate. The fact that the medical community has given so little thought to how surgical procedures could potentially obstruct our ability to nurture our children illustrates one more way in which nursing is devalued and the well-being of women and children is minimized.

A second issue concerns the *safety* of breastfeeding with implants, particularly for women whose implants are filled with silicone gel.* Although the Food and Drug Administration took silicone implants off the open market in 1992, no indisputable link between implants and harm to babies has ever been established. Moreover, a 1998 study found that the silicone level in cows' milk was ten times higher than in breast milk, and even higher in infant formula (Semple et al. 1998).

On the other hand, Susan M. Zimmerman, author of *Silicone Survivors: Women's Experiences with Breast Implants,* mentions a woman from Long Island who found over fifty cases of children afflicted with strange symptoms after they were breastfed. All their mothers had received implants prior to pregnancy (Zimmerman 1998, 40).

It is within this quagmire of studies and statistics, claims and counterclaims, that those of us who have altered our breasts—or who are considering it—confront the need and desire to nourish our babies. As outraged as I feel that so many of us are made to feel inadequate or uncomfortable about our bodies, and as much as I want to push for a culture that embraces and celebrates the beautiful diversity of our breasts, I want neither to blame nor to judge any woman for the choices she makes. What I do want is to show how these profound, embodied contradictions arising from the overarching sexual role of the breast can affect our nursing relationship. The stories in this next section are a beginning.

---

* After the Food and Drug Administration (FDA) in 1992 restricted silicone breast implants to women participating in clinical trials, saline implants became the only option for cosmetically driven breast enlargement.

In Their Own Words:
The "Official Breast"

Lisa has breastfed two children, and in most ways, her experience is like that of many other nursing mothers. Six years before giving birth, however, Lisa had breast implants. Given the ambiguities concerning the possibility of leaking silicone, her story could have easily fit within the "Permeable Boundaries" section of chapter 5. It appears here, though, because the underlying issue centers around the cultural aesthetics of women's breasts.

☕ OUR CROWNING GLORY

I was a "late bloomer," teased in school because my friends were developing breasts while I was not. I was still a size 32AA when I got married. Four years later I decided to have implants. I was twenty-three and away from home for the first time. I was working, newly married, and having a great life, but clothes never fit me quite right. I was, and still am, a little heavy at the bottom and felt out of proportion.

I had no immediate plans for children. My husband and I knew how hard it was to raise them and decided to wait until we had grown up a bit. Still, I remember consulting with the physician and specifically asking if I would be able to nurse afterward.

At the time there were only two types of surgery: under the breast, where a one-inch incision is made and the implants are pushed in through the cut; and the other, where the areola is removed and the implants are put in through the opening. I chose the "under the breast" cut since removing the areola damages more tissue and nerves associated with milk production, making nursing less likely.

After the implants, wow! I felt taller, more in balance, even stronger. My husband had never said anything about the size of my breasts, but after the implants I found out how he really felt. He himself hadn't known how much he would like the results afterward.

Six years later, I got pregnant. I never had morning sickness, ate well, and continued to do aerobics until I was eight and a half months pregnant. It was about this time that everyone was getting concerned about silicone's effects. I believed the information I read stating that the number of women who claim to have autoimmune diseases brought on by silicone implants is the same as the percentage of women in the general population who would have contracted those diseases anyway.

Nursing went well, and my husband was my biggest supporter. I was concerned about "normal bleeding," however—small amounts of silicone that would leak into my breast milk as the shell broke down. But through my own research and earlier involvement with the Coalition of Silicone Survivors, a group that informs women of their legal rights, I concluded there was no scientific evidence of harm through nursing. My participation in a study by Children Affected by Toxic Substances (CATS), which examines the children of women who have silicone breast implants to see if there are any adverse effects via pregnancy or nursing, also helped me to reach this conclusion.

At the request of CATS, I sent them a sample of my breast milk when Taylor was six months old. The study is not yet complete, and to this day I have no official information about the results.

When Taylor was seven months old, I became pregnant again and nursed through the first four months. My milk supply dwindled, and she was down to nursing twice a day. I would place her at my breast when I came home from work, and one day I didn't offer it to her and she never asked for it. She was weaned.

I quit work three months before my daughter was due, so I could have some time with Taylor. I felt great most of the time, and Mackenzie was born after a shorter and easier six-hour labor.

We had a few problems at first, but after about three weeks we clicked, and she nursed for about ten minutes every one and a half to two hours. When Mackenzie was several months old, though, she began to have a lot of ear infections, fussiness, and rashes. I got scared and began to wonder if my implants were the problem. A friend of mine, posing as me (since I was sleep deprived and so distraught by this time that I couldn't do it myself), called CATS. They told her there *was* silicone present in my breast milk but no more than in women who did *not* have silicone implants.

I believed them, felt relieved, and started thinking about possible food allergies. Another friend, a La Leche League leader, commented on Mackenzie's red cheeks. I had thought it was the cold weather, but she suggested a sensitivity to citric acid. I removed everything she was eating that had citric acid, and in about two to four days her red cheeks disappeared. I'd also heard that excessive spitting up might be linked to wheat sensitivity. I removed wheat from her diet, and she stopped spitting up!

By the time Mackenzie was fourteen months old, she was still getting sick fairly often. I wondered if she was sensitive to anything *I* was eating and thought it might be easier to initiate weaning than to alter my diet. I stopped offering her my breast, and when she started asking by pulling at my breast, I would offer her juice or a snack. It was as easy as that.

Taylor is now four years old, Mackenzie is three, and they appear to be as healthy as the next kid. While there is not a lot of information available about the safety of nursing with silicone implants, there *is* a lot of information about the benefits of nursing. I have no idea what the future holds, but I have no regrets about my decision to nurse. Nor do I regret having had implants. I still enjoy them, and if I had to do it over again, even with the information I have today, I would.

For more information on breastfeeding and implants, the La Leche League International Web site has a selected bibliography. The link is <http://www.lalecheleague.org/cbi/bibimplant.html>.

Now that I'm older, health is more important than anything, and breast size is not as important to me as it was eleven years ago. But I wouldn't say it's completely unimportant. I am a woman, and there is symbolism associated with our breasts. They are, so to speak, our crowning glory.

Lisa Chamberland, Morrow, GA

Where Lisa felt her breasts were too small, Jennifer thought hers were too big. Her story looks at how breast *reduction* surgery can impact nursing and the tendency of some physicians to minimize the impact on breastfeeding and prevent women from making fully informed decisions.

☕ SHADES OF GRAY

They came when I was twelve—with abandon. I stood alongside my best friend before the mirror, both of us topless. "Yours are so big," she said with awe. "You're lucky." I didn't feel lucky—I felt annoyed. How dare they come so early and so large?! I wanted to get rid of them.

I bounced through high school and jiggled through college. I ran on the cross-country team and ached in the chest after every race even though I wore a normal bra, a sports bra, and a leotard under a big extra-large t-shirt. I squeezed myself into 36DDs and popped out of them on every occasion, not knowing that bras came in bigger sizes. I was a freak.

By the end of college, I had gained the freshman ten, plus another ten. It all seemed to go to my chest. After I graduated, if I sat cross-legged on the floor with poor posture, the ends of my breasts would tickle my belly button. They were huge, floppy things. They disgusted me.

My boyfriend—who became my husband—sweetly said, "I love them because I love everything about you," but I didn't believe him. Four months after our marriage, I looked up plastic surgeons in the phone book. One of the ads said, "Hundreds of breast reductions performed!" This was my man! I sped to his office immediately. "Chop them off," I said. "I hate them." He understood . . . he'd seen it before. "Does your back ache sometimes?" he asked sympathetically. "Yes." I said. "Do you feel uncomfortable wearing clothes that fit you?" he asked. "Yes!" I exclaimed. "Do you think you could live a more normal life as, say, a 36B–C?" he asked. "Yes, yes!" I shouted. This was going to be great!

I filled out the paperwork. The surgeon sent pictures to the insurance company of me topless, slouching, and looking like my miserable self. They immediately faxed their approval, confirming what I had always believed— there was indeed something wrong with me. I needed medical attention, after all.

"Oh, and one more thing," said the surgeon, right as I was about to sign on the dotted line. "If you decide to have children, you probably won't be able to breastfeed."

This gave me pause, but only a small one. I knew one day I would have children and want to breastfeed. But heck, he'd only said *probably*. I was all for the power of positive thinking, so I shrugged and said, "Oh, that's okay," and signed my name with a flourish, smugly thinking I would breastfeed my children, no matter what he said my odds were.

What I didn't understand at the time was that it isn't black or white, all or nothing, you breastfeed or you don't. With breastfeeding and breast reductions it's all about shades of gray. I didn't learn that until I was pregnant with my second child, over ten years later.

When I was pregnant with my first child, the OB waved his hands in the air when I told him I wanted to breastfeed and was worried about the breast reduction. "Pshaw!" he muttered. "I've been in the business of birthing babies since before you were born, my girl, and I have never heard of breast reductions causing problems with breastfeeding. Anyway," he added, "if there *are* problems, you can always use formula." He then continued rambling about how silly the medical establishment is: how one year they recommend formula and the next they want you to breastfeed and it's really all the same and doesn't mean anything after all.

So, after a long and grueling labor, fraught with interventions and the threat of a C-section, I gave birth vaginally to an eight-pound, four-ounce baby boy. I brought him to the breast, and he latched on like a pro. Things were going great until we realized it's probably not normal for a new baby not to pee or poop for four days. And what was with all of the screaming? Was something truly wrong here? Could it be possible he wasn't getting milk?

We took the baby to the pediatrician, and he was down to six pounds, fourteen ounces. I burst into tears as the nurse read the scale. The doctor walked in and saw the tears streaking my face. "It's all right," she said soothingly. "We can fix this. Here is a can of formula."

It was, of course, the beginning of the end, though I pumped and nursed around the clock. When I couldn't cover the bottom of a tiny bottle, everyone around me took it as proof that I was wasting my time. "Honey," said my mother, "why are you doing this? You're exhausted. There's no harm in just bottle-feeding him now. After all, look at how smart and beautiful you are, and you were bottle-fed!"

But I persevered, even though their comments escalated. "What's the point?" said my husband. "He's not getting any milk from you anyway." And my mother said, "You're being selfish. This baby needs to eat, and you're frustrating him by forcing him to nurse at your breast. Look at how he's crying, the poor thing."

They were right. I was wasting my time. What was the point of all this effort and frustration?

So I quit.

One and a half years later I found myself happily pregnant again and as determined about breastfeeding as I had been before. I found an on-line site about breastfeeding after breast reductions and gleaned two new and exciting pieces of information: (1) if you've breastfed before, you will probably make more milk the next time; and (2) there is a drug you can take to help boost your supply.

I also learned that even though I had very little milk for my first son, I could have continued breastfeeding. There are many benefits, and not all of them have to do with providing 100 percent breast milk. Now that I knew this, nobody was going to stop me, no matter how much milk I did or didn't make.

So there I was, nine months pregnant and armed with everything I could think of: fenugreek, blessed thistle, Mother's Milk tea, alfalfa tincture, fennel, nettles, More Milk tincture, a nursing pillow, a brand-new top-of-the-line breast pump, my La Leche League leader's phone number, two supplemental nursing systems, a year's supply of oatmeal, feeding syringes, the miracle prolactin-inducing drug Domperidone, a rocking chair, and a cursed can of formula. I secretly and fervently hoped and prayed I would need none of this stuff besides the rocking chair and the nursing pillow, but having been through this once before, I was damned well going to be prepared.

The birth was even more long and arduous than the first one. My nine-pound baby boy was born screaming in chorus with me. We bonded right away, and he latched on like a pro, just as my first baby had. Things looked good.

But by day three, I realized my dream of nursing exclusively was not to be. My son had already lost nearly a pound, was not peeing or pooping, and looked dehydrated. I started a strict regimen of drugs, pumping, and herbs to try to up my supply, and I fed him formula using a supplemental nursing system.

I did not give up. Since my family offered no support, I looked elsewhere— La Leche League and an on-line mailing list of women who had breast reductions and were breastfeeding. These groups gave me the information, support, and motivation to keep going.

Today, my son is twenty months old and still nursing. He eats plenty of solids and doesn't need the supplemental nursing system anymore. I figure I was able to produce 60 to 70 percent of his needs with breast milk, and since he is still nursing as a toddler, he has received more mother's milk than the majority of North American babies. For that, I am extremely proud. As I look down into his peaceful face while he nurses, dozing off at the breast, relaxed and calm, there is no doubt in my mind that despite all the crap I had to deal with, it has definitely been worth it.

But how do I feel about the breast reduction now? Well, I'm

If You've Had Breast Reduction Surgery

BFAR, Breastfeeding after Reduction, is an organization that provides information and support to women who wish to nurse after having had breast reduction surgery. It also helps to educate health care providers on the subject so they can be better informed to help their patients. BFAR is on the Web at <http://www.bfar.org/index.shtml>.

There is also a comprehensive book on the subject: Defining Your Own Success: Breastfeeding after Breast Reduction Surgery, *by Diana West, published by La Leche League International (2001).*

---

ambivalent. Yes, I am thrilled that even after having two children, I can no longer truthfully sing that song that goes: "Do your boobs hang low? Do they wobble to and fro? Can you tie them in a knot? Can you tie them in a bow? Can you throw them over your shoulder like a continental soldier? Do your boooobs haaaang loooow?" But I also mourn the fact that I will never be able to have a "normal" breastfeeding relationship with my children. For me, breastfeeding is intricately linked with images of pumps, herbs, drugs, scales, and constant worry. This takes something from the experience, some small piece of my womanhood. The surgeon's knife removed something more than fatty flesh, and for this loss, I will always mourn.

Written by Jennifer Haymore, Valencia, CA

Opal is a professor of literature and creative writing, a poet and performer with a passion and exuberance for life. Her experience growing up in Jamaica greatly influenced her perceptions of nursing. Her cultural observations create a perfect segue into the next section.

BREASTS ARE FOR MILKING

I came up in a culture where it was just assumed I would breastfeed. It never occurred to me that I would have to be so discreet. But American society, it seems, is hostile toward breastfeeding. I always felt I had to cover my breast or put myself in a corner, car, or restroom so people wouldn't be offended. "Am I doing something wrong?" I wondered. "And what is this about?"

When my oldest was about fifteen months old, I fed her just before I went to teach my morning class and at lunch when I went to her day care. I had done that for several weeks, nursing in the rocking chair, when the director came up to me one afternoon and told me other parents were concerned that their children (no older than four) were seeing my breast. I thought, "Oh! This is ridiculous! What kind of parents would be concerned that my breastfeeding would ruin their kids or give them wrong attitudes about breasts? What kind of absurdness is this?" I took her out of that day care as soon as I could.

There were other smaller incidents that made me wonder what kind of society thinks there is something offensive or sexually violating about a woman breastfeeding her child. I remember going to Mexico when Shola was a baby and sitting on the side of the road, nursing. I didn't cover my breast, and nobody said anything. I was in Jamaica and St. Croix, and no one said anything there, either. I remember being in Africa years later. Women would just take out their breast in the marketplace and pop it in their baby's mouth, without the idea that they had to put a cloth over themselves, smothering their baby's head.

Prior to being pregnant and feeling my breasts fill up with milk, I saw my breasts in terms of sexuality, in terms of the sensations I got with a lover and, later, with my husband. That changed when I had a kid. It's not that they didn't produce sensation, but the *functionality* of them really took precedence over their sexuality.

I teach my kids that breasts are for breastfeeding. They can also be desirable, and both desire and functionality can collapse and become one, but plain and simple, a woman's breasts are for milking.

We live in a patriarchal society that tries to divorce women from their bodies and their basic processes, a society where a woman's body is supposed to be for a man's pleasure. It's almost like women who choose to breastfeed their children are committing a crime—not only are they denying their husbands, but they are supposedly diminishing their own beauty. I think women who breastfeed in this culture are brave. I feel a sense of honor and pride that I breastfed my kids.

Being pregnant, carrying a child, and breastfeeding gives me a totally different appreciation for my body and how awesome and complete it is that my body could sustain a life. This is an incredible miracle, and I'm so grateful. My body's not ninety-five pounds anymore, but after three kids I'm enormously appreciative of it.

Opal Palmer Adisa, Oakland, CA

In the Public Eye

One of the most obvious ways in which our nursing experience is affected by the oversexualization of our breasts concerns our ability to nurse in public. I think back to an experience in 1972 when the staff of my Midwestern elementary school was all abuzz. According to my mother, a teacher there, a woman brought her baby to a parent-teacher conference and nursed *right in the middle of the conference!* She hadn't even the sense to be embarrassed. She just attached her baby to her breast with the same nonchalance as if she were taking a sip of coffee.

Influenced by the adults I respected, I was similarly horrified. This is my first memory of breastfeeding. I was ten years old, and breastfeeding rates in the United States were at their all-time historic low. The shock was only partly because this woman had nursed her baby in a public, professional setting; it was also because she was breastfeeding, period. The teacher who had been so embarrassed had never seen a woman breastfeed before. She was young, twenty-two, and came from an upper-middle-class family. The parent was older, quite poor, and had little formal education.

What I find significant today is not simply that this event took place but that I clearly remember it thirty-plus years later. It speaks to the degree to which breastfeeding had ceased to be the cultural norm, the extent to which it had not only disappeared from the public eye but was derided and scorned.

Fortunately, much has changed since the early 1970s, and women have the legal right to nurse in all fifty states. Still, over twenty states

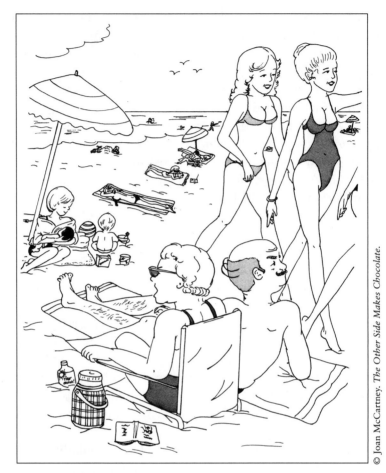

*I think that woman over there is breastfeeding
her baby. How any woman can expose herself
like that in public is beyond me!*

have enacted breastfeeding legislation to prevent women from being
charged with indecent exposure, lewd behavior, or obscenity. In fact,
much of the current breastfeeding legislation has been designed to
amend the laws surrounding indecent exposure and lewd behavior
to make it clear that they don't apply to breastfeeding women. Additionally, some state laws provide mothers with legal recourse if
they are told to stop breastfeeding, explained the late attorney Elizabeth N. Baldwin, who was a national authority on breastfeeding
legislation (<http://www.lalecheleague.org/Law/Bills4.html>).

The fact that lawmakers have passed such laws sends an important message. But as Opal's story illustrates, women who nurse in public continue to do so under an often judgmental eye. Consequently, women typically try to be as discreet as possible, resulting in the strange paradox that the less visible we become, the more approval we earn. We sling blankets over our shoulders, purchase special nursing tops, turn our backs to others in a crowd, and ultimately try to disguise our behavior. Sociologist Cindy Stearns (1999) points out that given how much time new mothers spend with a baby at the breast, we end up hiding much of the early work of mothering. And instead of directing our focus to our babies' needs and our own, we find ourselves worrying about how others will perceive us. Even when we receive no direct disapproval, many of us assume a hostile environment and feel vulnerable and nervous. Stearns adds that we also use "code words" to refer to nursing (e.g., "nummies," "eeshies," "nu-nu," "bow-bows," and my all-time favorite, "buddies") as a way to disguise what we are really doing, thereby helping us to resist the cultural norms of what's considered appropriate.

A woman's nursing experience is influenced not only by the setting but by how comfortable, confident, and secure she feels. While some of the women in this chapter felt self-conscious and awkward, others emphasize how surprised they were to find themselves feeling comfortable. Among one woman's favorite memories is the time she met a friend at a bagel shop and they sat in the back, nursing their daughters. She describes it as "cool." This is significant not because she felt comfortable nursing in public but because she felt moved to mention it at all. We wouldn't make it a point to mention how wonderful it felt to eat a muffin with someone or walk our babies together. Nursing our babies should be no different.

At stake is more than our comfort level. Until our society becomes more comfortable for and accepting of nursing mothers, we compromise the health and well-being of our children. This is particularly problematic for women who can least afford formula and the higher medical bills that formula-fed babies commonly accrue. For example, one reason why breastfeeding rates are so low in communities of low-income Hispanic women, explains Judy Hopkinson, IBCLC and assistant professor at Baylor College of Medicine in Houston, Texas, is that some illegal immigrants are afraid to nurse in public for fear of drawing attention to themselves and being deported (personal communication, 2003).

I've long believed that to nurse in public does more than meet the needs of a child; it does a public service—indeed, we are committing a political act. For despite the ways in which the cultural milieu makes our nursing experiences more complicated, one feeding at a time, one woman at a time, we change the world.

In Their Own Words:
In the Public Eye

A common theme running through women's stories is how we become more confident, even defiant, over time and with subsequent children. But this increase in self-confidence is put to the test as our babies grow older and discretion becomes more difficult. Even women who assert their right to nurse in public still admit to feeling susceptible to how others view them. The next few stories address this.

☕ MAKING IT NORMAL

When Katie was around six weeks old, I wanted to go places and do things but was so nervous that someone might get a glimpse of my bra as I opened it or, God forbid, a flash of skin. I practiced nursing discreetly, in front of mirrors and in front of my husband. After a few weeks my attitude changed, and I got resentful and angry. I hated that I couldn't focus on my daughter's needs but on whether somebody might be seeing more than they should.

After about two or three months I began to feel like, "I can feed my baby wherever you can feed yours." I would actually seek out places that might ruffle a few feathers. I learned quickly that I could nurse in the dressing room at Penney's, but I might just do it on the bench in the mall. I was recently shopping at Nordstrom's, and they had a room next to the ladies' room called the "mothers' room." My friend and I were thrilled to find a nicely decorated room with a changing table and sink, a sofa, and two chairs. At the same time, I see the possible trend of all women being expected to retreat to the "mothers' room." Perhaps that's why I also fed Katie that day on the couch in front of the register at Limited Too.

I'm big on breastfeeding in public, both for my convenience and to ensure that the practice is seen. But despite my defiance, there are still times when I worry. For example, Katie was about seven months old when I flew to see my parents. It was over Thanksgiving, and I got a middle seat. On one side of me was the grandmother of a nursing toddler, and on the other was a stocky, older guy who I thought for sure was not going to be able to deal with Katie flailing at him. I felt a little guilty about being relieved to learn he was blind! In fact it took a few minutes of her gulping for him to actually ask me, "Are you traveling alone?"

Katie is ten months old now and sometimes gets distracted, so I may need that quiet place in the dressing room. But if I don't think that's necessary, then I seek out a place where teenage girls might see me, so they'll have the benefit of seeing someone nurse in public. I just hope that the more people see it, the more normal breastfeeding will become.

Stephanie Weishaar, Camp Hill, PA

As a first-time mother, Cheli rarely nursed in public and spent much of her first nine months feeling isolated at home. (See her story on page 45–46.) Her life was considerably different six years later when she discovered she was pregnant again.

☕ BLENDING IN

When my first child, Brandon, was a baby, my whole world revolved around him—the prince. But when I had my second child, that prince was a six-year-old with numerous activities outside the home. My new baby would have to be schlepped from here to there.

I had gained a lot of experience and knew that nursing would be a big part of my parenting style for a good two to three years. I decided to buy a nursing wardrobe with enough clothes to sustain me for two weeks. I received a few catalogs for nursing mothers, and to my surprise, the clothes had greatly improved since 1993, when Brandon was born. There were fewer prints and florals, more solids and sleeker designs. And by searching the Internet I was able to find even more nursing fashions. To my delight, I found I could put together a nursing wardrobe that would make me feel confident and able to nurse discreetly.

While fashion was somewhat important, it wasn't primary. It was more important that I had clothes in which I could nurse discreetly. We were in a fairly conservative, Christian homeschooling group that met weekly, and some of the mothers didn't want their children exposed to another woman's breasts. We needed to stay with that group for social reasons, so even though I didn't agree with their attitude, I needed nursing clothes with flaps that covered everything and where it wouldn't be apparent that I was nursing.

To the extent that I have needed to blend in to society at large, I've had to adapt my behavior. This is not simply out of respect for other people's feelings but also to protect my children and myself from possible ridicule. For example, I had been taking my daughter with me to my hairdresser's for her entire life. Nursing her in the shop was fine at three months, four months, even twelve months. But when she was a bit older, we were waiting a long time when she got restless and wanted to nurse. We'd hear, "You're a big girl nursing like that. You don't need that anymore!" I didn't want my daughter to hear these messages, and I stopped nursing her there.

Even though I used to nurse her everywhere, I guess I'm bowing to societal pressure. She is tall enough to be mistaken for a three-year-old and is quite verbal. Rather than having to deal with strangers saying, "What are you doing nursing that big ol' kid?" I'm now selective in the situations in which I allow her to nurse. It's not as automatic as it used to be.

Cheli English-Figaro, Bowie, MD

❁

Today, at four and a half, Taylor continues to nurse about three times a day, though we have become "closet nursers" except for the friends and few family members who know we are still doing so. I abhorred stepping inside the closet and resent society for keeping me in there. I hated having to explain to Taylor that we couldn't nurse in public because "some people think that nursing is only okay for babies, but not for children." Nursing has meant everything to Taylor. It has been such a natural, normal experience for her—how could anyone think that was wrong?

Michelle L. Miller, Kirkland, WA

Gwyn's experience, following, one of my personal favorites, shows the importance of maintaining a sense of humor!

ON ACCOUNT OF A PLATTER

I used to attend an extremely conservative church where no one else breast-fed and everyone was mortally uncomfortable with the whole topic. At the time, I was nursing a four-year-old (eeek! no one there knew that!) and a newborn. This church had such a "thing" about public nursing that men and older children of both genders weren't allowed in the nursery on the off chance that a mom might be breastfeeding and they actually might *see* something.

One day, I had finished feeding the baby in the nursery, was in a big hurry, and just pulled the flap of my nursing bra up but didn't clasp it. I was then called into the kitchen by an older woman. She slid an empty platter across the table and asked if I would deliver it to its owner on my way home. Her eyes were fixed on my chest. I immediately looked down and saw the tip of my nipple poking out of the nursing slit in my dress. Just then, a rush of folks poured out of the sanctuary. I grabbed the platter and clutched it to my chest. As I shifted it, I could feel the coldness of the dish against my bare skin. "Holding it so tightly must have opened up the nursing slit even more," I thought. "Thank God for this dish." The feel of the platter was reassuring— as long as it was in contact with my skin, I wasn't exposed.

I relaxed a little. I made my way out of the church in no particular hurry, chitchatting here and there, smiling warmly, graciously greeting newcomers. People were looking at the platter a lot, though, which I couldn't figure out. "Must be something odd on it," I thought. "I hope it's nothing offensive." I was curious but didn't want to draw any more attention to the platter than necessary. After all, I couldn't put it down anyway. I held it tighter and felt the coolness against an even larger area of skin. A usually dignified gentleman engaged me in an animated discussion. "Wow!" I thought. "I never knew he enjoyed my company so much!"

At last we were in the parking lot, and I was free to look down. Clutched tightly to my chest was a large *clear* glass platter! Smack dab in the middle, skwooshed against the glass but rosy pink and clearly identifiable, was my right nipple—a milky rivulet meandered downward to the rim, where one white droplet hung, swaying gracefully with each breath. I gasped and sprinted to my car.

No one at the church ever mentioned the incident. Ever.

Gwyn, New York

Nursing outside of the home yields a wide range of situations, responses, and reactions. Here is just a sampling.

A SUPPORTIVE STRANGER

I was at Kmart in Bay City, Michigan, with Ava, about one and a half years old at the time. I had been shopping, was tired, and needed to nurse. I sat on a little bench by the exit. This woman was sitting next to me, polyester from head to toe, perfect makeup, and so much hair spray supporting her perfect beehive that she probably could have taken a shower and her hair would have stayed put—a perfect throwback to the fifties. I was gearing up for a minor confrontation, and I was ready to spout off about my civil liberties. That's the kind of mood I was in.

The woman and I made no contact whatsoever. She didn't look at me or talk to me. All of a sudden she got up and, still without looking at me, said out of the corner of her mouth, "You should be proud for doing that," and walked out the door, heels clicking. It was a great moment.

Gwen Shook, Jersey City, NJ

BREASTFEEDING WITHOUT APOLOGY

◐

When my mom took me out to lunch at a local restaurant, I tucked Emma under my shirt to nurse, and our waiter avoided eye contact with me and asked my mother, instead of me, for my lunch order!

Amy C. Condra-Peters, NH

◐

I got a call from an old friend today. She has been breastfeeding for many years and is not particularly discreet or easily intimidated. She was eating in a nice restaurant while nursing her twenty-month-old, when her young waiter advised that she was not allowed to nurse in the restaurant. She replied, "Oh, honey, he's not nursing. He's just licking my nipple while he falls asleep."

The young man was flabbergasted and did not return to their table for the rest of the evening. She had a nice meal while the baby slept peacefully.

Cathy Liles, TX

◐

When I first had Sam I met another nursing mother. We were walking one day when she asked me, "When did you first start breastfeeding in public?"

"The first time I went out of the house," I said.

She replied, "Oh, I haven't yet. And I never did with my first."

That was unbelievable to me! I love nursing in public and don't put a ton of effort into hiding it. I don't carry a cloth to cover up but just use my shirt and his head and don't worry about what's showing or not. I'm not saying that breastfeeding should be about shock value, but I feel strongly about nursing and being proud of it. I don't look down, don't feel embarrassed, and look people right in the eye.

Nina M. Panzer, Ithaca, NY

POOR ACCOMMODATIONS

There were a few times when I actually sat in the stall and nursed the baby while sitting on the toilet. I'd just put down a lot of toilet seat covers—a lot of them!—and sit there and nurse with my clothes on.

Patti Murray, San Francisco, CA

When Alvin was about three weeks old, I went to Wal-Mart or Target. I was nursing him in the baby section, and one of the managers came up to me and, trying to be as nice as he could, said, "Excuse me, ma'am, could you go to the bathroom?" He said there were male customers in the baby section shopping with their wives. I felt offended but went out to my car. Now I wouldn't do that. I'll stay right where I am. There are people who walk around stores half naked, and me feeding my baby is nothing different. If they don't like it, tough. I'm sorry. My baby's hungry.

Niesha Vann, Glendale, AZ

JUDGMENTAL EYES

The most challenging part of breastfeeding was when I didn't have a place to nurse my son. I was comfortable about nursing in public, but my husband had issues about it. Every five minutes he would be like, "Make sure you cover up! Make sure you cover up! You got perverts watching!" He didn't want people to get a free peek.

Vonjerita Trevon Boyd, Tulsa, OK

I was sitting in a mall, nursing my fourteen-month-old son. It was the end of a long day, and my breasts were extremely full. I was twenty-six, going to college, and had been away from him for four hours while I was in class. Nursing felt sooo good. And he was glad to see me, too.

Out of nowhere this older woman came up to us, with her fists balled up, and said, "You look like you're enjoying yourself!"

"Well, yes," I replied. "If we both didn't enjoy it, I wouldn't do it."

"You should nurse the baby, at least in the beginning," she said, "but for the baby's health! People like you should be turned in for child abuse—you're using your baby to gratify yourself!" Then she walked off as though she'd won an argument.

Julie B., Adirondacks, NY

Not only is the percentage of women who nurse their babies unevenly distributed across the landscape (e.g., the South has the smallest percentage of women who nurse, while the far West has the largest), but there are also variations within ethnic communities. The next two stories illustrate regional and cultural variations of what it means to nurse in the public eye.

AN ANOMALY IN ALABAMA

I come from a family where we were breastfed until we were three and a half or four years old. When you come from a family like this, breastfeeding is just normal. My mom had such a big impact on me that I considered breastfeeding to be my only option.

Here in Alabama, though, everybody asks you at your baby shower, "Which formula are you going to use, Isomil or Similac?" When I took a Lamaze class in Alaska, where my first baby was born, the nurses recommended breastfeeding and positive thinking so you didn't have to get an epidural. The Lamaze class here? They tell you when you'll get your epidural and that after your baby is born they'll give you a bottle of formula.

I'm definitely abnormal compared to most of the women around me. Here in the South, women tend to be quiet, they don't cause a lot of ruckus, and they certainly don't breastfeed in public. People really look down on you for that! Instead, women go into a bathroom or something.

I remember my mom seeing women breastfeeding in public and going up to them and saying, "Good for you!" It was embarrassing when I was sixteen, but now I understand it.

Danielle Haven, Bessemer, AL

Laos is a small, landlocked country in southeast Asia, sandwiched among Thailand, Cambodia, Vietnam, China, and Burma. An agrarian people of highland Laos, the Hmong fought for the United States during the Vietnam war. Beginning in the 1970s, thousands of Hmong fled Laos, escaping civil war, persecution, and genocide. After they had spent years in Thai refugee camps, 1975 marked the beginning of an exodus of Hmong into the United States, where most of them encountered an industrial, urban society for the first time (Lao Human Rights Council and the United Hmong International 2001). As of 2001, it was estimated that there are about three hundred thousand Hmong living in the United Sates. This next story offers a fascinating glimpse into how breastfeeding practices are influenced by our cultural origins.

☕ FROM REFUGEE TO ACTIVIST

I was married at seventeen years of age in Laos. Our first child, born when I was eighteen, died in childbirth. Within two years I had Mee. I breastfed, like all mothers did, but I was very shy and covered my breasts and Mee's head. My mother-in-law told me there was no need to do that. She said everyone fed their babies in public and let their breasts show. I took her advice and stopped covering my breasts or Mee. If I had to go to the garden to work, my mother-in-law would take care of her. If Mee got hungry before I returned, my breastfeeding friend would help feed her. If my friend had to be away, I would breastfeed her child. We helped each other.

When I was pregnant again, war came to our city. Our extended family was forced to go to the jungle when Mee was one year old. I breastfed her until my third baby was born. Toua was born in the jungle. We lived there for three years with only the clothes on our backs. If the Viet Cong got close to us, our men dug a deep hole for each breastfeeding woman to lie in and feed her baby quietly. I was very skinny. We ate only rice and jungle potatoes, which we dug with a stick. I had to feed Toua often because I didn't have much breast milk. When he was six months old, I also started to chew cooked rice, jungle potatoes, and green leaves (black nightshade) and spit them into his mouth. This kept him satisfied so he wouldn't cry and the Viet Cong wouldn't find us.

After three years in the jungle, it still was not safe, and we had little food. We decided to move to Thailand. We walked for four nights, because it was unsafe to travel during the day, and then for twelve days to get to the Mekong River Delta. As we traveled, I carried Toua at my breast and breast-fed him whenever he cried. We got across the river safely and entered Thailand. We lived in the refugee camp for about nine months. During the time we lived there, I had Leng. While in the camp I was fed well and had plenty of breast milk to feed him. Even though the camp was very crowded and I didn't know many of the people living there, I still breastfed openly and did not cover my breasts. All the women did the same.

On October 12, 1980, my family came to the United States. Mary Ann was born in a hospital, one week later. I was very shy. I had all my other children by myself with no one else there but my husband. It was scary having so many people around me who I didn't know. They seemed mean because they wouldn't leave me alone. I couldn't speak English, so I couldn't tell them I wanted them to leave so I could push.

The translator came after Mary was born. The doctors told me very little. The translator told me that now I live in the United States and everyone needs to go to school. When you go to school, you need to wear nice clothes and your breasts will leak, so it's best to bottle-feed. So that is what I did.

When I bottle-fed Mary, I felt sorry for myself. I was not close to my baby. She was sick all the time. When I breastfed my babies in the past, they were healthy. I was close to them because as I breastfed them, we looked each other in the eye. To pay for the formula, I got WIC. I also had to use some of the family's food-stamp allotment to pay for it. It was difficult. Every time I wanted to go someplace, I had to bring bottles, formula, hot water, and a cooler for the uneaten formula.

I had Pang four years after Mary was born, and I breastfed him. Neither my doctor nor WIC talked about or encouraged breastfeeding at that time, but I decided bottle-feeding was not good. By this time, I knew it was okay to breastfeed in the United States but that I should cover myself. I went to Family Literacy School, but only for three hours, and I realized I could go to school and still breastfeed. Inside, I knew my child would be closer to me and healthier. I was right. Pang was a very healthy guy. I felt very close to him, too. I was happy. I could go anywhere. All I had to take was Pang, diapers, and a blanket. No cooler!

When I was thirty-two, Nou was born. I had to have a C-section and was in a lot of pain. My husband, Ting, was worried about me and told me not to breastfeed, to just get better. In our traditional culture we must listen to and do what our husbands say. Even if you don't agree, you listen to your husband. If you don't, he will not be happy, and you will have problems. So I bottle-fed Nou. When she was three months old, she got very sick. Ting said, "I should have listened to you and let you breastfeed Nou, too."

This was my experience with breast- and bottle-feeding. I encouraged my cousin, my friends, and every other mother I know to breastfeed, even if they couldn't do it for a long time. I heard about a job opening to encourage Hmong women to breastfeed. (Only about 10 percent of Hmong mothers were breastfeeding.) I was excited to get the job. I taught a lot of Hmong women to breastfeed. If the husband did not want the woman to do it, I told the couple about my experience. I worked with the project for three years and was successful! The percentage who breastfed over three months tripled from the first to the second year and was almost five times greater in the third year, compared to the first. I wish I still had that job, but the funding ran out.

Doua X. Thao, as told to and written down by Nancy Coffrey,
UW Extension Wisconsin Nutrition Education Coordinator, WI

The last three stories address the importance of speaking out and taking a stand.

EFFECTING CHANGE

A couple of years ago a woman was breastfeeding in our local mall, and a salesclerk from one of the department stores went up to her and said something like, "Can I show you to the bathroom?" The woman said, "No, I'm perfectly comfortable right here."

The salesclerk left, and a security guard came back, saying, "I'm sorry, but you cannot breastfeed in the mall."

The woman was upset and left. I don't know where she found them, but she came back the next day with about twenty breastfeeding mothers. They all sat down in the middle of the mall and started nursing! It was very successful. The management spoke with the women, and they put in a nice room to change diapers with a big stainless steel sink, as well as a nice La-Z-Boy recliner to breastfeed. There's practically a waiting line to use it. And I'm sure if you were to go and breastfeed in the mall now you would have no problem.

Laura P. Burke, Syracuse, NY

☕ STANDING UP

I was asked not to nurse at a hoochie-coochie bar for the under-twenty-one crowd. I was with my precocious teenage nieces, they needed to eat, so why don't we eat there, they joked—after all, it *was* a family restaurant. I decided I was up for it. My son was about two and asleep on my back when we went in. We were still waiting for food when he woke up and wanted to be fed.

I scootched wa-a-a-y back in the booth, with one leg on the floor and the other on the seat, my head just clearing the top of the table. We were sort of sitting under the table, as if in a recliner. I was trying to be discreet, but that wasn't good enough for the manager, who offered us free food but told me I would have to eat mine in the bathroom. Given that we were about the only women there, besides the servers, in this highly charged sexual atmosphere, there was no way I was about to leave my nieces unattended!

Well, after her suggestion, I decided it would be a good idea to stand up while continuing to nurse Nicholas. A hush fell over the entire restaurant, and my nieces were flashing me a thumbs-up sign. The manager, turning more and more red by the minute, said she would give us a discount coupon for a meal later—if we would leave. Here she was, braless, wearing a tiny tank top that hardly covered anything—the required attire for female employees. You could see a lot of their breasts, but you couldn't see any of mine. Clearly, to actually *use* my "hooters" was a no-no!

We kept on haggling, and I kept on nursing, with the whole place watching. We ended up walking out hungry, but with three vouchers for free meals—when we didn't bring the baby! I never went back, though, and gave the vouchers to someone else.

Julie B., Adirondacks, NY

☕ THANK YOU FOR NURSING YOUR BABY IN PUBLIC

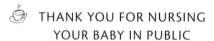

I was in a shopping mall watching a grungy-looking mother of a filthy three-or four-year-old and a tiny infant, less than three months, trying to give the baby a bottle, with her mother and mother-in-law over her shoulder, giving her unwanted advice. Finally she got up and left them. She returned from the restroom with the baby on her breast and tossed the bottle into the trash. The mothers were mortified that she would do this in public, and she did a wonderful job of shutting them up.

I wanted to "connect" with this woman, to show her some support beyond the usual smile and nod. I went home and couldn't stop thinking about this incident. I wished I could go back in time, sit down next to her, and offer my support. Instead, I wrote her a note. I made five hundred copies of it, cut it into quarter-page sizes, and now I distribute them in shopping malls, restaurants, museums, bowling alleys, parks, buses, airports, everywhere I see women nursing in public. I put an address on the bottom for people who are interested in distributing them.

Here is what the note says:

> Thank you for nursing your baby in public. You are not only nourishing your child, but the hearts and minds of everyone here. When nursing in America is more common and understood, the credit will go to women like you. I thank you on behalf of my grandmother, who had never heard of breastfeeding. I thank you on behalf of my mother, who hadn't a single soul to support her nurturing instinct. I thank you on behalf of my daughters and granddaughters, may they never think twice when their children thirst. May they never search for a "secluded corner," a dressing room, or a restroom. I thank you on behalf of every woman who ever was or ever will be. Have a beautiful day.
>
> Copyright 1999, Lisa Russell
>
> For more information, e-mail Lisa at lisa@nursingnotes.org.

I usually just hand it to the woman and walk away without saying a word. Sometimes I'll hide around the corner and watch them read it. They usually cry and look around for the mysterious "stranger" who gave them the note. I imagine it's posted on people's refrigerators. Hopefully, though, they keep it in their wallets and pass it on again. You never know!

Lisa Russell, Yakima, WA

Update: Because a version of this note appeared on the Internet, it has been distributed in all fifty states and has been reworded for use in Canada, England, New Zealand, and Australia.

Sexuality, Sensuality, and Intimacy

Not only does our culture falsely compartmentalize the dual functions breasts serve, but it falsely compartmentalizes women's sexuality. Take a seemingly trivial example. When I wanted to buy a sexy black nursing bra in the mid-1990s I couldn't find one anywhere. In our consumer-oriented culture, where we can buy edible underwear and vibrating tampons (yes, they really exist!), it shouldn't be difficult to find sexy nursing attire.* The message, of course, is that we are supposed to be maternal or sexual, but not at the same time—and certainly not if we are nursing! In fact, it wasn't until the year 2000 that researchers even undertook a study to focus specifically on sexuality and breastfeeding (Avery, Duckett, and Frantzich 2000).+

Much of what has been written about our sexuality in the postpartum period is designed to help us be better lovers for our partners: how to please them when our vaginas are still off-limits and all we want to do is sleep, how to make intercourse more comfortable. Personally, I can't think of anything more counterproductive to sex than the birth of a baby. Most of us are exhausted, sore, and perhaps recovering from an episiotomy or C-section. Our hormones are raging wildly, and our bodies don't look the slightest bit familiar. Sex? At least for me—and for many women I spoke with during this time in my life—it was pretty nonexistent. Now add nursing to the nonerotic pajama party. Most men don't want to hear that this can further dampen our already challenged libido, particularly if they are waiting at home with a bottle of champagne after our six-week postpartum checkup.

But when we lactate, our bodies produce more prolactin and less estrogen, a combination that can not only diminish desire but can also affect our bodies' ability to lubricate. Combined with the fact that we have been intimately involved with another little body, sometimes all day long, the last thing many of us think about is sex.

But our sexuality changes and evolves (as do our hormones), particularly past the first couple of months. Some of us find that lac-

---

* The rising popularity of the Internet suggests that the consumer landscape for this may be changing. When I entered "black nursing bras" into the search engine Google, I easily found a number of sites that market them. (I noticed on one site that they even offer a leopard-print design!)

+ In a 2000 study that looked at the sexuality of first-time mothers who were breastfeeding, the authors thought one of their most interesting findings was the wide variety of responses they received to their questions, indicating (*not* to my surprise) that women experience their sexuality in vastly different ways.

tation enhances our sex lives with our partners or at least adds a little spice to it. Given that there are pornographic magazines, videos, and Web sites specializing in depictions of lactating breasts, it should be of little surprise that some of us discover our partners are turned on by our bodies' ability to produce milk. Unfortunately, honest discussions of such topics are hard to come by.

Equally silenced are discussions surrounding the pleasures of nursing. In fact, writer Lynda Marin refers to this "erotic bond" as one of the best-kept secrets of motherhood. "We like to make a clear distinction between motherly affection and female passion," she writes. "If there were not a clear distinction, what would stop mothers from engulfing their children forever in their own hedonistic designs? We may say our children are cute and extol their individual virtues," she explains, "but we seldom acknowledge our erotic feelings toward those most desirable of objects, our children" (1994, 13).

Thus, in a culture that believes in the selfless, desexualized mother, it is not easy for some women to admit that nursing is pleasurable. Nursing our babies is supposed be a selfless act we engage in because it is *healthy*, not because we enjoy it. It shouldn't *hurt* us, we are told, but, as Julie was reminded, it shouldn't feel *too* good. Indeed, sociologist Linda Blum asserts that, given the strict parameters within which we are supposed to use our bodies, to enjoy nursing is almost subversive (1999, 182).

But life is rarely orderly and distinct. For when our bodies are constantly accessible to our children, when we lie together skin-to-skin, it can be profoundly sensual. When my youngest daughter was four years old, for example, she relished a morning snuggle. Without failure, she came into my room, took off her pajamas, and cuddled up next to me, proudly and completely naked. She would rest her head on my shoulder and place my arm around her, my hand falling naturally on her tush. Although she had stopped nursing a year earlier, she still liked to rest her cheek on my naked breast, cup my "eeshies" in her little hands, and shower them with kisses. This is how we began our days. It was absolutely delicious, and if that isn't sensual pleasure, I don't know what is.

While many feminists, myself included, have decried the quick attribution of women's behavior to hormones, they can't be ignored when it comes to breastfeeding, and they play a key role in understanding the biological basis for the pleasures associated with nursing. In fact, prolactin and oxytocin, the two main hormones involved in breastfeeding, have earned the warm and fuzzy nicknames of the "mothering hormone" (prolactin) and the "love hormone" (oxytocin). Prolactin, the hormone that drives milk production, often creates a feeling of well-being and relaxation. Oxytocin, responsible for the milk "letdown" reflex and the same hormone released during labor contractions, lovemaking, and orgasm, triggers feelings of nurturance and affection.

It is perhaps not surprising that we may occasionally feel aroused while nursing or that we sometimes feel our milk let down during sex. This, of course, does not mean we want to have sex with our children; rather, it means that Western society distorts a woman's honest and full sensuality.

While not all anthropologists would agree (Dettwyler 1995a), anthropologist Sarah Blaffer Hrdy examines this issue from an evolutionary perspective, arguing that the "eros of suckling" evolutionarily predates the erotic sensations of our experiences with lovers and conditioned our ancestors in ways that kept their babies alive (1999, 139, 537). In other words, the pleasure inherent in breastfeeding was an incentive for them to continue the very behavior necessary for our species to survive. Hrdy adds, "It would be more nearly correct, then, to refer to the *afterglow* from climax as an ancient *maternal* rather than sexual response" (1999, 139).

In *The Eros of Parenthood,* author Noelle Oxenhandler asserts that there is an unease that makes it hard for us to speak of the sheer pleasure we take in our children's bodies and they take in ours. Even putting the words *eros* and *parenthood* in the same sentence, she writes, is to step into forbidden territory. But the pleasure exists, drawing parent and child to each other like a kind of gravity. In its intense physicality it is deeply akin to the love between lovers. But unlike the eros of adult sexuality, the eros of parenthood is a sheltering and protective love. "Its predominant rhythm is serene and relaxed," Oxenhandler explains, "quite different from the climactic movement of adult sexuality" (2001, 3–4). To be sure, given that sexual abuse was kept hidden for so long, it is understandable that people are fearful to speak of the physical dimensions of the love we share with our children. But Oxenhandler cautions that in an atmosphere filled with such tension and anxiety, it is difficult for parents and children to enjoy intimate moments with each other. Eve Ensler, author of the bold and acclaimed play *The Vagina Monologues*, adds, "What we don't say becomes a secret, and secrets often create shame and fear and myths" (1998, xx).

Failure to understand the physiology and intimacy of nursing can have devastating consequences, as in the infamous case of a woman who, while nursing her two-year-old, was concerned about feelings of sexual arousal. She called a crisis line for insight, but instead of helping her understand what was happening, the Department of Social Services ended up taking her child away from her for more than one year. In the process, the legal system turned her into a "bad mother" who posed a danger to her child. Lauri Umansky, who has written about this horrifying situation (1997), emphasizes that the case shows the dangerous result of decompartmentalizing "selfless maternity" and "female sexuality." To mention breastfeeding and sexual arousal in the same breath is taboo.

Those of us who experienced child sexual abuse ourselves may not be comfortable with the kind of intimacy breastfeeding entails. Andi, for example, a mother in Pennsylvania, recalls: "I had been taught that breasts were a sexual organ, not a way to feed and nourish new life. To use a sexual organ on or with a baby was abuse."

Research shows that as many as one out of every five women was sexually abused as a child (Kendall-Tackett 1998). Such experience can affect nursing in different ways, explains Kathleen Kendall-Tackett, a researcher with the University of New Hampshire. The close skin-to-skin contact can trigger flashbacks of the abuse, as can the physical sensation of milk on one's breasts or hands. Similarly, so can seeing milk squirt out of one's breast. Some women may find it difficult to nurse at night if that is when their abuse took place, while others may become particularly anxious and confused if they start to experience nursing as sensual or pleasurable. Responses and reactions vary. While some survivors cannot stand the thought of breastfeeding, others find it to be healing (Kendall-Tackett 1998).

The stories in this last section attempt to remove the mystique surrounding nursing and intimacy. They address some of the ways breastfeeding can affect our relationships with our partners, and they speak to the need for a decompartmentalized, more inclusive understanding of women's sexuality.

In Their Own Words:
Sexuality, Sensuality, and Intimacy

When Ellen and I spoke, she had two children, but she and her husband have since added two more to their brood. A knitting enthusiast and a member of her church choir, she tells a story that proves you should never judge by appearances. Her story is one of several similar ones I heard.

LETTING LOOSE THE WILD SIDE

Initially I was somewhat disturbed that my husband was turned on by the fact that I was lactating. I had a hand pump, and he would get an erection from watching the milk drip out. "This is too weird," I said. "Just go away. Don't watch me do this."

I used to like having my breasts touched before I had kids. But I leaked a lot early on and didn't want my breasts touched because they would just make more milk. I told my husband they were off-limits and I'd let him know if I changed my mind. We had a long, long dry spell, first because I was recovering from the delivery and then because I lacked the time or inclination.

I'm trying to think about what changed. We were on vacation together, and he was slightly drunk and just 'fessed up that he still thought it was a huge turn-on that I was lactating. So I let him play with my breasts. And it was fun. I was able to shift gears. There was milk all over the place. It was really wild. It wasn't so much that he wanted to taste it, though he wanted to do that too, but he just wanted to have the milk dripping out. I thought, "Whatever. He's made enough accommodations to me over the years—this is one I can make for him." And he'd done a lot of stuff for me first, so I figured, "What the hell. He's earned it." It was strange because I had thought that compared to an infant's mouth, a toddler's mouth is so much bigger. Now I was thinking, "Wow, this is a *really* big mouth. And he doesn't know how to suck well, either," though he *was* able to get some milk out.

It's not a regular part of our sex play now, but it certainly comes into it. And now that I'm pregnant again, he has started saying, "Oh, it's going to be so nice when the milk comes back!"

The thing with breasts and sex is that it's not the kind of thing that comes up in conversation. Even in Nancy Friday's books on sexual fantasies, there's no lactating section. There is some stuff about people pretending to be babies and pretending to nurse, but there's nothing about people really getting milk. I wonder if some of this whole breast thing for men is that they were denied appropriate access as children and are trying to make up for it as adults.

I don't know how often we had sex before I got pregnant—two or three times in a good week. Now it's like two or three times in a good month, and there are many months when it's not that often. But it seemed like once we had that experience with the milk, it just cut loose this totally wild, creative side of myself. Somehow I'm a lot more open and creative. We tell each other stories now, and I think we've gotten into that because of the hormonal changes with breastfeeding. It takes me a lot longer to respond—vaginal dryness and all that. And with the distractions of the two kids, sometimes it just doesn't seem worth the effort. We have to work a little harder at it.

Ellen, western NC

SEXUAL SNAPSHOTS

❍

I would get a letdown during sex, especially after an orgasm. It would just come out—everywhere! I guess it was my hormones. Occasionally my husband would get drenched, and of course it would be all over me, too. He thought it was funny that occasionally he would get covered in milk when we were making love. But it's only milk. If he felt really sticky, he'd get in the shower, and that was the end of it. It never bothered us very much, and eventually the leaking stopped being much of a problem.

Vicki Duncan, Columbia, MO

❍

It doesn't matter whether I'm nursing or not—I like it when my husband stimulates my breasts during sex. It's a big part of sex for me, but it feels completely different from nursing. I've heard that some women have orgasms when they nurse. I wish! I'd nurse my babies way, way longer if that were true! I would just shut up, wouldn't tell anyone about it, and just enjoy it! But that's never happened. Nursing is pleasurable and feels good, but not in a sexual way.

Lauren, northern FL

Debby makes a conscious effort to help her children feel at home in their own skin. Her story emphasizes the false separation of sexuality from motherhood and depicts the kind of comfortable intimacy that can become a natural part of family life.

AN OPEN RELATIONSHIP

There would be times when I would be nursing and look at my husband and think, "Oh man, I want to have sex." I'd read that this was a possibility and at the time thought, "That's disgusting." But now, knowing how hormones work, I understand it. It wasn't about holding my baby at my breast and feeling sexual toward that child. It was just a passing moment. It may, however, have brought my husband and me closer to having sex on that particular evening.

For the first four or five months after having a baby, though, I'm not really interested in sex. I'm more interested in mothering my child. Later, when my husband and I kind of get back into the groove of our sexual relationship, I don't want him to *touch* my breasts. "Stay away from them. That's not what they're for!"

Now we have to plan sex because both kids sleep with us. Sometimes I nurse Kayla to sleep, get up, we begin to have sex, Kayla wakes up, and I have to go nurse her. That throws me. It's hard to go from nursing to sex, back to nursing, then back to sex.

But breastfeeding has probably enhanced our sexual relationship because my husband would love to nurse as much as Kayla does. He *loves* breast milk! He says it tastes like very skimmed milk with lots of sugar. It's more of a nurturing part of our relationship than a sexual part.

We're very open. We'll wake up in the morning, and Kayla insists on sharing with her daddy. "This one's Kayla's," she'll say, "and this one's daddy's." It's really cute. And he'll nurse for a minute. Any time of the day when she'll start to nurse she might say, "Daddy!" He'll come in, and she'll say, "Nurse, Daddy. Nurse."

I want my kids to be comfortable with their bodies and how beautiful they are. My husband's family was always open about taking showers with each other and things like that. My family never was. And Billy's much more comfortable with himself than I am. I've had to get over initially feeling uncomfortable about myself, especially after gaining weight and getting stretch marks from having babies. Nor have I ever liked my breasts because they didn't look like they were supposed to in the magazines—first I never had enough, and then I got too much. I can't say that I really like them now. But I'm more comfortable with them, and it's okay if they don't look like the ones in magazines. They don't have to.

Debby, Charlotte, NC

We never planned it, but a handful of times we were in the middle of lovemaking when our daughter woke up and needed to nurse. I nursed her, and we continued to make love, not as intensely, but we didn't stop. I've done that a handful of times over the years. I have rather big breasts, so I can lie on my back with my arm under my head and my breast will flop to the side enough for her to nurse. Or I can be on my side nursing her, and my husband can be behind me, in a spooning position. It was always very natural, and I thought it was fabulous.

Erica, NJ

The intimacy that can develop between a nursing mother and child is a strong magnetic force. For Kate, it was all-consuming. Her story speaks to the emotional fragilities of family life. Nursing did not *cause* the challenges she and her husband faced, but it certainly played a role. (She has another story on pages 282–83.)

NEEDING TO REBUILD

As most parents do, I lost freedom after my son was born, but more than I ever imagined. My son was such an eager nurser that he totally spurned the bottle. I tried pumping and leaving milk, but he wouldn't take it. I would try being gone for little longer spans of time, but he didn't like it, and we couldn't starve him by forcing him to take the bottle. So for the first year I couldn't be away and have any time by myself.

He nursed *a lot* and loved it! There was no way of letting Scott, my husband, take care of him. I remember once being a half hour late, and Jesse had been inconsolable for over an hour by the time I got home.

My husband would never blame me, but I think he was frustrated with loving a kid and not being able to comfort him, even though he was doing the best he could. The fact that I could help Jesse in a way Scott couldn't set up a difficult dynamic.

After an incident like this, when Jesse was asleep, I would come out of his room and see the anger in Scott's eyes. We could understand each other's positions, but there wasn't a lot we could do about it. And with both of us seriously sleep deprived, trying to have a discussion about something over which we felt powerless would have produced fireworks.

We were both easily distraught because we were so exhausted, like sleep-deprived ships passing in the night. And because of the exhaustion from caring for the needs of a nursing child every two hours from month to month, we didn't feel like having sex. Sex is great, but given a choice between exhaustion and sex, well, we certainly went for the sleep.

My intimacy needs were very much taken care of by breastfeeding, and my son was the love of my life for a while. We spent so much time together, and much of that time was intimate. There were moments of tenderness I can never hope to match. Now that he is three, however, my intimacy needs are *not* being met. I'm very much a huggy, kissy, connecting person. So I turn back to my husband, and he's not used to providing what I need. We've learned different patterns.

At first, I thought a lot of it was hormonal, that nursing for a little over two and a half years was driving the infrequency of sex, but I think it's more than that. Intimacy, for me, is what goes on at a daily level and that leads into something sexual. But it's hard to get that intimacy back. Suddenly we look at each other, having been on the fringes of each other's lives and sharing meals, but not being intimate. For Scott, a lot of it has to do with fatigue and feeling too many demands. He leaves the house, goes to work, comes home, has two relationships to keep up, and loves his own space.

We certainly have had great sex since our son was born, but a lot less of it. We have fun every time we do it, but the drive just hasn't been there, our energy levels are not what we'd like them to be, and I'm definitely heavier and feel less attractive, never having lost all of my maternal weight. So sex is one of the things that has fallen by the wayside. All of a sudden we realize we have to rebuild our relationship. It's just so hard to juggle personal needs, relationship needs, and loving and caring for your child. We didn't have the recipe then, and we don't have it now.

Kate Gefell, Ithaca, NY

 A CLOSER SENSE OF INTIMACY

I derived tremendous satisfaction from breastfeeding. I got a rocking chair and would fall asleep there with each baby propped up on a pillow, breastfeeding. It was incredibly sensual. I don't know anything that approximates the kind of intimacy developed and nurtured between a mother and child. I feel this is one of the reasons my kids and I are so profoundly close. I'm from a culture that is very touchy anyway, always kissing and hugging. Until they were around eight, way past the age that they should have been doing this, my daughters liked to come up and touch my breasts. I think it was the memory of that kind of intimacy.

Because I breastfed my kids for a good amount of time, I think my kids and I share a closer sense of intimacy, of physicality, which I believe children desperately need in this culture. There's so much negatively promoted about touching, sexual abuse, and violation that we tend to underplay the importance of *positive* touching. My oldest daughter has a friend who is always surprised when she comes here that we are always kissing and hugging. She told my daughter she wanted a boyfriend, and my daughter, playing psychologist, replied, "Maybe you just need to learn how to hug your dad."

Opal Palmer Adisa, Oakland, CA

Another aspect of Opal's experience appears on pages 198–99.

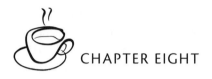

CHAPTER EIGHT

Finding Strength

STORIES OF EMPOWERMENT, RECLAMATION, & HEALING

For better or worse, bigger or smaller, in sickness and in health, breasts are wedded to our bodies and, in the best of circumstances, can offer us both pleasure and power.

Marilyn Yalom, A History of the Breast

Mother's Day sentimentality aside, society does not typically reward us for our efforts to nourish and nurture our children. In fact, we are often penalized, argues Ann Crittenden, in her compelling book *The Price of Motherhood: Why the Most Important Job in the World is Still the Least Valued.* Crittenden lays out the myriad factors that together result in an accumulative loss of income for mothers. As a result, the wage gap between women and men is not nearly as large as the gap between childless women and mothers—a "mommy tax" that adds up to over one million dollars of lost income over a woman's lifetime. "Changing the status of mothers by gaining real recognition for their work," Crittenden writes, "is the great unfinished business of the women's movement" (2001, 7).

At the same time, however, that we need to advocate for policy changes and find innovative solutions to rectify such extreme financial inequity, we are not likely to abandon our children to become more "like men," like workers "unencumbered" by the care and responsibility of children.

Breastfeeding is the perfect case in point. Remember the saying "the personal is political"? This adage from the 1960s may be thought of as a cliché, a verbal relic akin to "male chauvinist pig," but it is a concept that continues to reflect great truth.

Empowerment

Penny Van Esterik, a cultural anthropologist, breastfeeding activist, and the author of *Beyond the Breast-Bottle Controversy*, analyzes breastfeeding from a feminist perspective. Breastfeeding, she asserts, "encourages women's self-reliance, confirms a woman's power to control her own body, challenges models of women as consumers and sex objects, requires a new interpretation of women's work, and encourages solidarity among women" (1989, 69). She argues that women who aren't able to nurse because of lack of support, workplace constraints, or misinformation from formula manufacturers are oppressed and exploited (1995). Strong language, perhaps, but surely this is the case for women like Lauren (see page 176), who have to quit work in order to feed a child, or like Lacey (see pages 261–66), who are unable to obtain decent postpartum care and advice. As Rosemary Gordon, a La Leche League leader in New Zealand, asserts, "Breastfeeding can't empower women until women are empowered to breastfeed" (quoted in Liotus 1996, 39).

When women do experience the empowering aspects of breastfeeding, the energy released is palpable. What can be more empowering, at the most basic level, than to be able to produce food from one's own body?* I can't count the number of women who talked about how healthy their babies are, the awe they feel in watching their babies become chubby from their own milk, the feeling of intimacy and connectedness they hadn't experienced before, neither as a child nor with their bottle-fed children.

To have this experience when the odds are so often stacked against us can become the basis for creating positive changes in our

---

* Personal empowerment and social recognition, unfortunately, are not the same thing, and women's significant contribution of breast milk is not included in our GDP or in any U.S. national statistics concerning food production.

lives. Many of us want to go on to help others realize this transformative potential. I've yet to hear someone say, "I'll never forget that horrible toothache I had. I decided then and there to do whatever I could to prevent other people from enduring what I did. And that's when I decided to become an endodontist." But this has been precisely the experience for many breastfeeding peer counselors, lactation consultants, doulas, and others who provide breastfeeding support.

The impact goes beyond breastfeeding. Van Esterik asserts that the kinds of social changes that encourage successful breastfeeding are helpful even to women who don't nurse. To breastfeed successfully, she states, "requires that the position and condition of women be improved and that maternal health be made a household, community, and national priority" (1989, 70). And the healthier we are, the better we feel about ourselves, and the more control we have over our bodies, the better able we are to take care of our children; to stand up for what we believe in; and to advocate for ourselves, our families, and others.

The stories in this chapter come from women whose breastfeeding experience irrevocably changed them, who discovered completely new ways to think about their bodies, and who discovered that nursing has the power to heal. The stories in this first section come from women who couldn't anticipate the empowering impact breastfeeding would have on their lives.

In Their Own Words:
Empowerment

The phrase "teenage mothers" is often used derisively, as a euphemism for "irresponsible" and "ignorant" young women who have babies outside of marriage, who had the audacity to have sex in the first place. But as the next two stories reveal, such terms both deny and obscure women's reality rather than helping us understand what it means to be starting out as a young mother in a judgmental society and the strength and tenacity that requires.

Niesha relayed the following story when she was seventeen. When I last spoke with her, she was attending a charter school for pregnant and parenting teens. She hoped to have her high school diploma in two years and wanted to go on to college.

☕ A CATALYST FOR CHANGE

I got pregnant the summer after my sophomore year of high school. Before that I was a wild child. I went out every single night, had the body of a goddess, and everything was perfect. I got even wilder after I met my baby's father. I was sixteen, and he was twenty-six. (He lied to me and told me he was nineteen.) I thought I was grown up and did whatever I wanted. I was partying, smoking, drinking, and could get into older clubs. I wanted to get me a job, a car, and party, party, party!

Then the bomb hit, and I cried for two weeks. At first I told my boyfriend to give me the money. "I'm getting rid of it," I said. "I don't want to be pregnant, and I don't want to be pregnant by *you*." But I couldn't do it. I made four appointments at the abortion clinic but never went. I stopped drinking right away, but it took me a month to stop smoking. After that I stopped going to parties and hanging out with my friends. I started going back to church and stopped cussin'. I had been in a gang when I was younger, and I have a lot of friends who've brought their babies up in gangs and had them around alcohol, weed, and drugs, and I didn't want my baby in that atmosphere. I just cut it all out.

I gave my son's father a choice. I said, "Either you be in my baby's life, be a positive role model, pay your bills, and be a dad, or you leave." He left. (He went to jail four days after my son was born. I found out that my son is his fifth. He has a daughter two months younger than my son and another baby due in August.)

Alvin was born four weeks early, at six pounds, four ounces. A lot of people tried to discourage me from nursing. My younger sister said, "It's going to hurt, and you're not going to like it."

I said, "I don't care. I'm going to do it." I knew that breast milk was the best thing. My two sisters, twenty-four and twenty-five, each have five kids. Diana breastfed every last one of them, and they hardly ever get sick. And they crawled faster and did everything faster. My other sister's kids always had colds and were always constipated from the formula. So I had said, "When I have my baby, I'm going to breastfeed."

I was so determined to do it that it didn't even bother me when my breasts swelled up to the size of cantaloupes. I was *not* going to give him a bottle!

Alvin didn't eat for his first three days. I was nervous and scared, and cried because he wouldn't eat. A lactation consultant came in to help me, but Alvin was too tired. Finally, though, he latched on, and after that he had no problem.

Alvin is now four months old, and I know he is getting the best milk. I don't have to worry about him being constipated or having a lot of gas, and it's been great not having to worry about bottles and spending a lot of money.

A lot of times people say to me, "You're young and breastfeeding?" They think the two don't go together. They say, "Most teens don't want to breast-feed." And a lot of my friends are like, "Girl, please . . . I have to be in the club, and I can't be tryin' to pump no milk and havin' my breasts leakin'. If I breast-feed, I can't be goin' out every night." But after I breastfed my baby, four other girls nursed. I actually influenced my friends! It was kind of like wildfire.

I get a lot of recognition at the different programs I attend that help teen mothers. Once when I went to the WIC office, one of the ladies who works there said to me, in front of everybody, "Now this is a good example! Do you see this young mother? She is only seventeen, and she knows the value of breastfeeding! All of you young women in here should be doing exactly like her!" There were at least fifty people in the room, and it made me feel so good!

I don't really care about going out anymore. One of my friends, who I was close to before I got pregnant, had a graduation party but said there were no kids allowed. So I said, "Well, I guess I won't be there, because if it's not safe for my baby, then how safe is it for me?" That's how I look at it now.

Breastfeeding has made me more patient, more responsible. It's made me a better person. I have to take care of myself more—whatever I eat, my baby eats. Whatever I do affects my baby. And the bond between me and my baby is so strong. It makes me feel so good to know that I, with the help of God, of course, am keeping my baby alive—not some cow's milk or chemicals. This is the only source of nutrition he knows, and it's coming from *me!* That makes me feel so good inside, and I talk about that all the time.

Niesha Vann, Glendale, AZ

In her book *A Child on Her Mind*, author Vangie Bergum notes that teenaged mothers frequently assert they are mothers, just like any other moms, though they constantly have to prove to others that they are responsible and capable (1997, 106–7). Julie's story is no exception. When she finished writing her story, she was immersed in her first semester at the University of Texas, pursuing a degree in social work. "I want to send the 'professionals' who tell young moms they can't do it to the unemployment line," she writes.

☕ SHOWING HER STRIPES

I became pregnant on New Year's Day of 2000—the day the world was supposed to end. Despite being just shy of my high school diploma and the sordid details of my preconception life, I was a good pregnant woman. I ate healthily, exercised gently, gave up caffeine, and breezed through my pregnancy, bolstered by the wings of immortality and naïveté. I didn't know about all the horrible things that could go wrong, and the ones I did know about could never happen to me!

Breastfeeding was beyond foreign to most of my peer group. Still, I planned to do it, assuming the knowledge would be there instinctively once I held my child.

Walking into the hospital, I was sure the nurses and birth professionals would be just like they were on television: gentle, comforting, and possessing any knowledge or answer I might need. It never occurred to me that my age, or the absence of the former boyfriend responsible for my "condition," would alter the care I received. Only hours into motherhood, though, I was proven wrong.

After his birth, my son was taken away to the nursery for bathing and procedures that I didn't yet know were unnecessary. He was gone for an inordinate amount of time. Increasingly worried, I paged the nurse's station and left messages at the desk, my voice growing more frantic with each answerless second. I felt like a child, pointing at a burning building while tugging at mother's skirts, and hearing only, "Wait. Mommy's talking." Not until I threatened to walk down to the nursery myself, ripping out each stitch of my episiotomy (which I also hadn't known was unnecessary), did someone finally listen. A nurse from the neonatal intensive care unit came in to tell me my son had stopped breathing in the nursery. My son, in this world for mere hours, had stopped breathing, and no one had even come to tell me.

I was a bundle of jagged emotions. I was angry that no one had told me, livid that I hadn't been there, and my self-confidence was horribly shaken. Was there some clear, fundamental flaw in me? Some inadequacy I hadn't yet identified? No one in this hospital had thought I was important enough to receive answers. If I had been unnecessary during my son's scariest moment, why would I be necessary at any other moment? It's a horrible thing to feel superfluous to your child, only hours after birthing him.

To add insult to injury, the nurses had given him a bottle of formula in the NICU. My child's first food was not the special one my body had been brewing for him for nine months, but a smelly, gray, mass-produced substance created by the lowest of the corporate monsters. It felt like my fate as a formula-feeding mother was as good as sealed, due to a lack of information, support, and most important, confidence.

I was wheeled down to the NICU and introduced to the one bright spot of my seemingly eternal hospital stay, a nurse named Leon. Perhaps he was the child of teen parents, perhaps he was one himself, or perhaps he was just more understanding than most, but my age didn't seem to be an issue for him. He held my son easily in his muscled, tattooed arms and didn't give him the look I would come to know too well, the pitying one that showed they thought the baby might never be held again.

"Do you want to breastfeed him?" Leon asked.

The question caught me off guard, solely perhaps because it was a *question*. My stay had been full of brisk commands: "Lie this way." "Push." "Breathe." "Don't move." "Let me see." "Wait." For someone to actually find my opinion worth airing felt, at that point, like the highest praise. Some of that fire reignited inside of me. "Yes!" I beamed at him, my mama tiger taking a few steps out from under the brush.

After a quick lesson, I latched my son on, and he nursed hungrily. I felt proud to be doing something so "grown up" and maternal. "I'm a mom." I chanted these words over and over in my head and then offered them up out loud.

My son was put on a three-hour schedule, and I was to pump an hour and a half after nursing, in order to ensure a supply under these altered circumstances. I was exhausted, rousing myself from a dead sleep to either nurse sitting straight up in the sterile and otherworldly NICU or to latch on the tugging, intrusive breast pump.

On the morning of my third postpartum day, I awoke to the sight of breasts. It looked as though someone from plastic surgery had snuck over in the night. I had done something right; my pump-nurse-pump-nurse existence had resulted in an ample supply of sweet, squirting milk.

Tempering my high, though, was the fact that nursing was suddenly painful. Cradling my child and reverting back to my labor breathing, I felt as though I'd gone straight from the beatific honeymoon to the bitter divorce. I nursed with my toes clenched white, tears rolling down my face, smiling through gritted teeth when my son opened his eyes. I persisted, though, because this was what being a mother was about. This was what parents do. My pain was secondary because my son needed breast milk.

This little unwed teen mama was really starting to show her stripes. I was proving to my son that I would not fail him, that he could rely on me to forge ahead and give him what he deserved. I was proving to the nurses that I was a good mother, hoping to show them the irony of the "bad teen mom" who knew and cared enough to press on, while the more socially acceptable mothers were asking for formula. And I was proving to myself that I was *not* superfluous, that I was necessary and *vital*. I was showing that even if other people held my son, changed his diapers, and did all the things I wanted to be doing in my own home, I had a bond to him that was as strong and important as the umbilical cord that had connected us for nine months. I was reassuring myself that when everything else fell away, we only really needed each other.

My son and I now approach two years of nursing with an undecided number yet to come. The feelings I had in that nursery still blossom inside me, helping us to sustain the rough times and enjoy the serene ones. Passing the formula aisle at the grocery store, I often feel a surge of pride at my accomplishment. I've come to realize that nursing is not just about food, a simple transferring of calories. It is an expression, a rebellion, an acceptance, a statement, and an act of the highest, purest love. It is a validation and a vindication, a freedom and a responsibility.

Nursing has given my son and me the roots of a relationship so strong and deep that we can handle any burden, weather any storm. I can now laugh at the guilt I felt for deciding to raise a child that society told me I didn't deserve. I can applaud myself for trusting my own instincts and my ability to make decisions, and I can shrug off a decade's worth of body and self-esteem issues. I reject what society has told me about what my body parts are for, where my value as a woman lies, and what exactly I am capable of. I can sustain the life of another human being so that he flourishes, and I can do so without the help of corporations, machines, or imitations of myself.

Young mothers have a supportive and politically progressive feminist community on the Web at <http://www.girl-mom.com>. Designed and moderated by and for young moms, Girl-Mom offers various discussion forums, including those pertaining to pregnancy, birthing, and breastfeeding.

This body of mine, the same one I'd put through drug addiction, denial, and self-mutilation, is on the same side as me now. My breasts, deemed too small by me and too saggy by undeserving lovers, were perfect at feeding a newborn and became divine at nourishing a toddler. The pale stretch marks I once despised were transformed into a lacework of self-carved rivers to carry my sweet milk into the belly of my hungry child.

I made mistakes as a pregnant woman and new mother, but breastfeeding is one place where I know I did not go wrong. I'd like to revisit my former self, weeping in that NICU, and offer her some consolation, appreciation, and

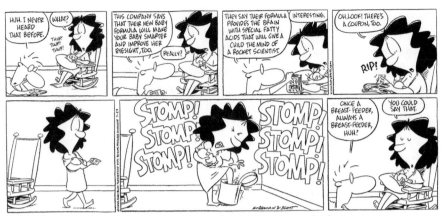

© Baby Blues Partnership. Reprinted with special permission of King Features Syndicate.

a vision of the future. She made a wonderful choice there, a selfless, maternal choice, and I want to let her know she was right.

Julie Cushing, Austin, TX

Studies of low-income women reveal that nursing successfully helped them to gain confidence and social validation (Locklin 1995). This was certainly true for Angelisa, who dropped out of school at fourteen when she became pregnant with her first son. Over the next ten years she gave birth three more times. All four were bottle-fed. Now thirty-four, Angelisa also has a sixteen-month-old son, Daniel, and a one-and-a-half-month-old baby, Joshua. A WIC recipient for all six of her children, it was only in 1995, when pregnant with Daniel, that Angelisa was given breast-feeding information and offered a free WIC breastfeeding class. Angelisa took the class, went on to nurse Daniel, and is currently nursing Joshua. When Daniel was a baby she became a breastfeeding peer counselor through the WIC program in St. Louis, Missouri. She continues this volunteer work today.

A BOOST IN SELF-ESTEEM

I wish I could turn the clock around with my first four. If I had to do it all over again and if I had the knowledge I have now, I would have breastfed all of them. My eighteen-year-old son has a friend whose fiancée is havin' a baby, and he said, "Momma, guess what? I went to a breastfeedin' class!" He said, "Momma, you're doin' a great job. That's the best milk for the baby. I wish you woulda got the chance to breastfeed me." I said, "You don't know how I think about that over and over. I wish I had a chance to breastfeed all of you." Then my daughter said, "That ain't no fair, Mom—you breastfeedin' Daniel and Joshua. You didn't breastfeed me." I said, "I'm so sorry."

But I was so young. I just couldn't see myself breastfeedin'. I didn't have any exposure to it. I bottle-fed the first four because I didn't know anything about nursing. I believed all the myths I found out later weren't true: that you weren't going to have enough milk, that your baby would be too spoiled because you would be with it all the time, that he would be clingin' to you and you wouldn't be able to go anywhere—all kinds of things.

Breastfeeding is amazing, better than I had thought. I'm plannin' on nursin' my son as long as he wants, but I would like to do it at least up to two or three years. I never thought I'd be saying that! But I know that as long as I can nurse him, the better his health will be. With my first four kids I kept runnin' back and forth to the hospital with ear infections, and they were sickly all the time with colds. I see a big difference with the two little ones.

I love all my children, but I feel closer to the two little ones than I felt with the others. I used to catch myself hollerin' a lot with my other children. I'm not now. And breastfeeding has made me feel good about myself. I had low self-esteem, and it's made me feel real proud that I'm able to help my child because I'm giving him the best thing and also helpin' myself. I'm grateful and blessed that I have a chance to experience it in my life, and I thank and praise God for that.

Angelisa, St. Louis, MO

Kim earned degrees in fashion design and fashion merchandising before working for a talent agency. While pregnant, she decided to take three months of maternity leave and then return to work. As she discovered, though, life sometimes takes us in other directions. She talks in the next story about her journey as an African American woman into the world of La Leche League, an environment often characterized as being "lily white." It began eleven years ago when she was pregnant with her first child. A woman in her childbirth class invited her to a meeting of League, an organization she'd never heard of. She never saw that woman again, but she's been involved in League ever since.

TOGETHER IN MOTHERHOOD

Even though I loved breastfeeding my daughter and wanted to help other women breastfeed successfully, I struggled with disappointment when I saw a woman bottle-feeding. I couldn't be an effective leader or counselor if I couldn't be compassionate and embrace all women's choices. I had to be able to put myself in another person's shoes, to understand where she was coming from and not look down at her. I needed a sense of balance.

Almost four years earlier, when my first daughter was about six weeks old, I had gone to my first La Leche League meeting. After I had attended a couple of times, the leader said to me, "You should think about becoming a leader. There are almost no black leaders in League, and you'd be great—you've got to do this!"

I couldn't fathom it. I felt so new to mothering that I couldn't understand why she was encouraging me. Nonetheless, I regularly attended our local meetings. Eventually I began to host them at my house and, being the social butterfly I am, invited my pregnant and nursing friends, women from all over Brooklyn, from all walks of life, and of all different colors. We started seeing a shift in the meetings where the white women were becoming the minority and the women of color were becoming the majority. It felt like we were learning from each other and seeing the commonalities in our mothering experiences, regardless of our cultural or class distinctions. Although Brooklyn is very diverse, the simple act of breastfeeding brought us together as mothers.

During this time, a woman I knew was recruiting women to become WIC breastfeeding peer counselors for a program in the Bedford-Stuyvesant section of Brooklyn, an economically impoverished community but one rich in Afrocentric diversity. She knew I was into the whole breastfeeding thing, so she invited me to participate.

When I first arrived I was shocked! Here I was, participating in a ten-week training program to become a breastfeeding peer counselor, and all the other women going through the training with me were bottle-feeding. Some of them had breastfed for only two weeks. I remember thinking, "Who do these women think they are? How are they going to be *breastfeeding* peer counselors when they are all bottle-feeding!"

As we went around the room and each woman got a chance to introduce herself and tell her story, I was humbled to my core. One woman, for example, had breastfed for only two weeks, but during a time when she was homeless and trying to leave an abusive relationship. She had been through a tremendous amount of stuff! Her baby had been nipple confused, and nobody had been available to teach her how to get through it, so, not surprisingly, she weaned at two weeks. Now she wanted to learn more about breastfeeding so she could help others. There were many stories like hers.

I began to see these incredible women in a different light. They hadn't had a lot of money, information, or support, and La Leche League wasn't in Bed-Stuy. Even if they had thought to call League, it wasn't an organization that seemed to be speaking to *them*. Amazingly enough, these wonderful ladies still came with their kids every week to learn about breastfeeding so they could *voluntarily* help others.

Our instructor was an awesome woman from Ghana, West Africa. She made sure she provided money to any woman who needed bus fare to come to the training and made sure we had a nourishing, healthy meal to eat while we trained.

I left that program feeling comfortable working with all types of women, and shortly after completing the training, I finished what I needed to do to become a La Leche League leader, as well.

Soon I was leading two or three League meetings a month, including a monthly meeting at WIC, while also working with the peer counseling program. I was one of those crazy leaders who loved to do home visits, too.

Some time before I became pregnant with my third, I began working as a postpartum doula and gained still more experience, wisdom, and insight into breastfeeding families. But after we gave birth, my husband took a new job, and we relocated to northern Virginia.

I knew League would probably be very different than in Brooklyn, but I wanted to find like-minded people. At the first meeting I went to, as I expected, I was the only person of color. Nonetheless, I fell in love with the leaders, and one of them has become one of my closest friends.

I decided, with the help of a white leader I had originally contacted, to reenergize a morning group that had fizzled out. It became very successful and still is. A lot of times, though, I'm still the only brown face, and I'm still hoping we can find a way to increase the diversity.

In my quest to find women of color who breastfeed, had homebirths, and basically did things in a nonmainstream way, I was led to a midwifery practice in Alexandria, Virginia, where one of the founding midwives is African American. I met with the two founding midwives, happily soaking up their energy. It was so refreshing, as well, to see the diverse faces in their offices, from the staff to the clients. Before I left, they gave me a copy of their newsletter, in which I saw a little ad about Mocha Moms, a support group for stay-at-home moms of color. I was elated, contacted them immediately, and went to the very next meeting they were holding in Washington, D.C.

Immediately I felt at home! It was a lot like my League experience in Brooklyn—all these different colors of women coming together, sharing their motherhood experiences, trying to do the best for their kids, and feeling validated by everyone else. And most of the Mocha Moms were breastfeeding. It was wonderful to see these black women with their progressive, open attitudes.

I knew I had to create a Mocha Moms experience for the women of northern Virginia. I had already been there for over a year and didn't really have any black women friends. I was beginning to feel very alone and misunderstood. Here in Virginia, people drive everywhere, and there aren't the same opportunities to make connections as there are in Brooklyn, where people walk everywhere. I would see black women driving in their cars and wonder where they were going, but what was I supposed to do? Follow them?

Fortunately, a black woman I had met earlier contacted me one day. When I first met her she was pregnant, going back to work, and was a little iffy about breastfeeding. I told her about the Mocha Moms group in Washington, but shortly afterward we lost touch. Now she had a second daughter, had decided not to go back to work, was breastfeeding, and doing things differently her second time around. She had contacted Mocha Moms, loved it, and was calling to say, "Let's start a group here in Reston." So we did.

For more information on Mocha Moms, visit their Web site at <http://www.mochamoms.org/>.

That was one and a half years ago. Most of the founding moms in the group belong to various playgroups where they are the only black person, so they were happy to find Mocha Moms. Since then, our group has grown by leaps and bounds, and other Mocha Moms groups have sprouted in the surrounding area. Our family potlucks are wonderfully diverse, as many of our Mocha Moms have husbands of other races. I'm an idealist. My dream is to have a place where everyone will feel comfortable, black and white, all races. And I feel like a lot of this is coming together.

Kim Durdin James, Herndon, VA

At several places in the book, particularly regarding feeding premature babies and expressing milk in the workplace, I talk about the issues that arise when we emphasize breast *milk* over breast-*feeding*. Valerie's story offers a different perspective. A thirty-four-year-old mother with two living children (her firstborn died due to a rare, genetic autoimmune disease), Valerie chose to forego breast-feeding for pumping.

THINKING OUTSIDE THE BOX

When my first child didn't latch on, everyone told me it was my fault, I wasn't doing it properly, everyone could nurse as easily as we can grow hair. But nothing worked. When Carsen was about two weeks old and I was still sleep deprived, insecure, and thinking I was a huge failure, unable to get the simplest tasks of motherhood right, a midwife came into the office and said to me, "Well, you know what the problem is? Your breasts are all wrong."

I dissolved into tears and took her word as gospel. "Forget it!" I thought. "I'm just going to pump, and the hell with everyone else." And I did what everybody told me wouldn't last for more than ten days. I set weekly goals, then two-week goals, then monthly goals. I became very proficient. I rented an electric pump from the pharmacy for thirty bucks a month and was able to pump between fifty-five and sixty ounces a day. I could pump anywhere, anytime, anyplace, even while driving—I pumped one breast at a time using an attachment for my car lighter that went into my breast pump.

I pumped until my daughter was eight months old and had a bone marrow transplant. The oncologist told me it would be more dangerous to continue giving her my milk than not.*

When I became pregnant a second time, I was a basket case. I had been in this hospital culture and couldn't visualize having a healthy child. I was a complete and total wreck.

When I was eight and a half months pregnant, I saw a lactation consultant and told her my whole story. I repeated what I had been told two years earlier—my breasts were all wrong. I was just bawling, and right away she asked, "Well, what's wrong with them?"

I was hyperventilating at this point, I was so upset. "They're all wrong!" I cried.

---

* According to Dr. Ruth Lawrence, professor of pediatrics and author of *Breastfeeding: A Guide for the Medical Profession* (1998), in order for the body to accept any kind of transplant, doctors must first suppress the body's immune system so it won't reject the transplant. Some oncologists believe that the immunoglobins in breast milk may conflict with what the suppression treatment is trying to accomplish. There is also concern that breast milk is not completely sterile unless it is pasteurized. Pasteurizing the milk will reduce the immunoglobins, but it won't get rid of all of them.

"Let me see your breasts," she said. I could barely see through my tears as I unbuttoned my shirt and undid my bra. "Look at me!" she insisted. "Look at me!" And there she was, sitting topless. "Your breasts look just like mine," she said, "and I successfully nursed six children! What stupid person told you this?"

I started laughing, she started getting dressed, and that was all I needed to hear. Seeing this woman, with her good sense and humanity, made me realize I'd been walking around for two years thinking my breasts were all wrong and I had never questioned it.

"Nugget" came out, latched on, and never came up for air. I was sore before I even left the hospital. By day four I had blisters, and by day ten I was bleeding. I went to a lactation consultant who said she had never seen breasts that sore. She told me to hang in there, it would get better. But it didn't. The kid would suck on anything. Her sucking reflex was so strong, I could have fed her through a keyhole.

I found myself making excuses so I wouldn't have to nurse. I developed such a Pavlovian response that as soon as she woke from a nap, I would start to cry in anticipation from the pain. One night when Nugget was four or five weeks old, my husband lay at the foot of the bed while I put her on my breast. When she latched on, I instantly reacted by accidentally kicking him in the face so hard that he thought I'd broken his nose. He was sitting there with his face covered in blood, I was crying, the baby was screaming, and he said, "This is ridiculous!" He took the baby from me and said, "I'm going downstairs with this screaming child so you don't hear her, and you're going to pump for twenty minutes."

"No, no, I want to be like other women!" I cried. "I want to breastfeed! I want to nurture her that way."

"There is no nurturing going on here!" he said. "You would rather empty the dishwasher!"

I was furious at him, but the next morning I realized he was right. And I happily pumped until Nugget was ten or eleven months old. I took my pump everywhere! Car trips were measured by how many boobs it was. A breast was about twelve minutes. If we were getting directions, I would ask, "How long a trip is it?"

"A boob and a half," my husband would say. Or, "Two boobs shy of half an hour."

The third child came along, and I was much calmer. If it didn't work, it didn't work. Both my other children had gotten at least eight months of breast milk, and I was sure if I could pump for eight months, I could successfully do it for a year.

I tried latching Ella on, and she did fine, but my soreness started recurring. Every time I opened my bra I ripped the scab off. Again, I had lactation consultants helping me, but at this point there was nothing they could tell me that I didn't know. Finally, I made a last-ditch effort and called another lactation consultant. She had just returned from a conference where she had heard about a glycerin patch that you tuck into your bra. It keeps a moist environment so your scabs heal, without promoting bacteria. She'd never recommended it to anyone and didn't know much about it but said, "What do you have to lose?"*

I drove one and a half hours to the hospital to pick it up, and within a few days I was fine. Within four days, I had no problems whatsoever. I nursed! Like every other normal woman. I nursed for about a year, until my daughter self-weaned.

But having a nursing relationship with a child wasn't the greatest reward. I was more excited about the fact that I was actually *normal.* I proved that I was capable of doing what other women did easily, that I was finally a member of the club. I, too, could nurse and eat salad at the same time.

Other women think of nursing as one of the highlights of their time with an infant, but it wasn't a pivotal part of my own motherhood experience. It was nice, but I felt, to a degree, it was also enslaving. People are so limited in their definition of breastfeeding, that the only way to get milk to your baby is through your breast. It's because nobody is thinking outside the box.

One of the reasons I easily embraced pumping was because I believe in egalitarian parenting, and a nursing relationship does not involve the father. I don't care how many women say, "Yes, but he goes to the bassinet to get little Johnny, and he stays up and rubs my shoulders while I nurse." I don't care. It's still not an egalitarian parenting experience. I think, in some ways, Darren is closer to Nugget because he had more infant responsibilities with her.

I actually feel that *pumping,* not nursing, has been one of the most empowering experiences of my life, and it definitely helped define me as a mother and woman. Through that entire quagmire, and in spite of what any-

---

* To date, few studies are available that consider the use of glycerin and hydrogel patches for treating sore nipples. According to Kathleen Huggins, author of *The Nursing Mother's Companion* (1995), as well as several lactation consultants who participated in a lively e-mail discussion, such patches alone are not intended to cure sore nipples, though they may speed healing. They expressed concern that using them instead of getting help could ultimately delay treatment for an underlying problem (such as poor latch-on positioning or a breast infection) and that overusing them could create a breeding ground for bacteria. As Valerie did, it is important to first try to address the underlying cause of the problem.

one said, I found what truly worked best for me and my child, not what was expected, acceptable, or the norm. As a mother, I feel that I have an obligation to provide my children with the best nutrition, and I did that. Because I was able to do something like that, against all odds, I have no hesitation to step up to the plate for what I think is the right thing for my child and me.

My breastfeeding experience was proof that I actually *can* do it my way, and the hell with anyone else. I derived so much strength from bucking the system, and I ride on that to this day. When some people are tired and overwhelmed, they might picture themselves on a beautiful beach or recite a little mantra. My kids are now five and two, and in low moments, when I'm doubting myself or questioning my actions, my pick-me-up is, "Fuck you! I did it my way, and I was good at it!" And I will continue to derive strength from that. My favorite line for my tombstone would be "She Did It *Her* Way."

Valerie Vass, Manchester, VT

Valerie is not the only woman to exclusively pump. Lactation consultant Nancy Mohrbacher found that women choose this option for a number of reasons: nipple confusion, a refusal to latch on, sore nipples, physical problems that prevent the baby from nursing, lifestyle issues, and personal unease. To be sure, exclusive pumping precludes the benefits that derive from the physical experience of nursing. Still, it remains a valid option. An excellent on-line resource can be found at <http://www.pumpingmoms.org>.

Reclaiming Ownership

Despite the many ways society sets us up to feel inadequate and insecure about our bodies, breastfeeding has the power to revolutionize how we feel about ourselves, help us restore confidence in our bodies, and reassert our power to control how we use them.

This next set of stories comes from women who found the power to carry themselves from a place of self-loathing to a place of self-acceptance, even self-love, and who discovered that breastfeeding gave them the power to transcend a culture that devalues breast milk, the nursing relationship, and the work we do to maximize our children's health and well-being. In a culture that tries to disconnect and distance us from our bodies (we shave, deodorize, hide, change, and fix them) breastfeeding asserts that we do, in fact, live in and through our bodies. "Just as women have held rallies and marches to Take Back the Night," writes anthropologist Katherine A. Dettwyler, "we can Take Back Our Breasts" (1995a, 205).

In Their Own Words: Reclaiming Ownership

Reneé is a former race-car driver and cancer survivor who now has a successful career producing and selling handblown glass beads. Since we last spoke about breastfeeding she has had a fifth child—her last.

FROM REPULSION TO PRIDE

The whole time I breastfed, my husband never really saw me do it. I never let him see my breast exposed with the baby nursing. I knew that Joe was opposed to it, though he never said, "I wish you would quit," or "This makes me uncomfortable." But if I ever complained about my blouse getting wet, for example, he would say something like, "Well, you're the one who wanted to breastfeed."

With my first three children I never even considered breastfeeding. It seemed too old-fashioned and wasn't something I wanted to do with my body or my life. I even recall feeling mildly repulsed by it.

My first child, Dustin, had been born when I was seventeen, the summer after my junior year in high school. Joe and I married when I was twenty-seven, and I became pregnant with Joey at twenty-eight. Molly, my third child, was born three months early. She weighed two pounds, four ounces. I asked the NICU nurses about the possibility of breastfeeding, not because I wanted to but because I wanted to make it clear, at least to them, that I was willing to do *anything* for this baby. And they specifically told me that breast milk was not good for preemies; they would have to supplement her anyway because breastfeeding wasn't nutritionally complete for a premature baby. This is completely untrue, I now know. They fed me a lot of bull.

With Joey and Molly, I really got into being a mother and felt I had finally found my niche. So when I became pregnant again, I decided to enjoy every single moment. My aunt gave me a book called *The Blue Jay's Dance,* by Louise Erdrich, a woman who writes of the experience of her daughter's infancy. This woman loved her baby in a way I don't think I ever had. It had such an impact on me that I decided to do this baby's infancy differently. It was to be my last, and I made the decision early on to love her with complete and total abandon, without reservation, guilt, self-consciousness, or fear.

When Alissa was born, I observed her every moment. I held her constantly and smothered her with affection. I was much more in tune with her and sensitive to her needs. Still, it was a given that I would formula-feed. When my milk came in a week after her birth, though, I suddenly felt that I should put this baby to my breast, just once, to see what it was like. It wasn't that I intended to breastfeed. I just wanted to put her to my breast once to see what happened, knowing I would never have the opportunity again.

So when a private moment presented itself, I took her back to the bedroom and offered my breast to her. I don't know what I expected to happen, but she perfectly and painlessly latched on and began nursing. I was astounded. It was so easy that I tried again later that night. The experience was incredible—poignant and sweet and right. I instantly understood why women nourish their babies in this manner, what it means to breastfeed, and why no one could ever have explained this to me. I tried it again and again and found each experience to be more rewarding than the last.

I continued to bottle-feed around my husband, though, and I'm not certain how long it was—probably a week—before I finally told him what I was doing. The weeks wore on, and despite Joe's displeasure, the bottles were fewer and fewer, and then I began to put breast milk in the bottles she did have. Gradually I realized, "*I'm* a breastfeeding mother! After four children, I'm doing this!" I felt proud.

Of course, I could talk about the health advantages of breastfeeding or about the convenience and economy of it. But these things are only icing on the cake. To tell the truth, I participated in breastfeeding for what it offered *me*. When I was breastfeeding, I felt so empowered that I could provide this physical and spiritual nourishment for my daughter. It was something that I, alone, could do for her. I felt so precious and close to her. Breastfeeding has also given me greater confidence. I feel more connected to my body and its functions, and I'm more appreciative and in awe of the *whole* reproductive miracle.

It would have been nice to have had either my husband's or my mother's approval or encouragement, but nursing felt so good and right that eventually I would have withstood any amount of criticism and disapproval. The selfish rewards were powerful enough. I'm so glad I gave myself permission to love a child this way. It has been a liberating experience and has enriched my relationship with my other children.

Reneé Holoubek, Oklahoma City, OK

❍

I went to see Sheryl Crow in concert tonight, and she was talking to the audience. She said, "How many strippers are out there?" So this very ex-

cited group of women down front was screaming, and she said, "I don't believe it until you take your shirt off!" Well none of them did so . . .

I was in the balcony, and I stood up and said, "Hey Sheryl! I take my shirt off all day long! Not only that, but my breasts make FOOD!" Then I flew down from the balcony, landed on stage, took my shirt off, and squirted breast milk all over the audience, because that's what breasts are made for, and I gave everybody an impromptu pro-breast-feeding speech, and everybody was really cool, and now they all are much less confused about the social/biological breast roles.

Well, actually that second paragraph was a fantasy . . . but if I could fly, I would have . . .

Lori Bishop, Jacksonville, FL

Leslie was a dancer until she was nineteen years old, when stress fractures forced her to quit. Over the next three or four years, she gained between eighty and one hundred pounds. Her story offers candid reflections on how body size can shape the nursing experience and how nursing, in turn, can alter one's body image.

☕ SHEDDING INHIBITIONS

The world is not geared toward an obese person. Everything from narrow aisles in clothing stores, to amusement-park rides with lap belts that don't fit, to squishy airplane and movie theater seats, to everyday things like raising and nursing a child—none of them are designed for a large person.

I shopped at a local nursing supply store, looking for nursing clothes, but the largest size they carried was a 2X, and I needed a 3X. An over-the-shoulder sling does not fit my body well because of where the padding is in relation to the baby. I tried various nursing pillows, but they didn't fit either. I ended up having to use a pillow designed for nursing twins, a huge, cumbersome thing that looked like a table.

When my daughter was first born, I struggled a lot. Everyone told me to hold her skin-to-skin, in a cradle hold or cross-cradle hold. The lactation consultant told me to turn her body in toward mine, or she wouldn't latch on properly. But because I'm overweight, with this large stomach in the way, it was difficult to do, and my daughter didn't feel comfortable like that. I had to hold her on her back, lying on my arms.

I went to a breastfeeding moms support group at the hospital and was the only extremely overweight person there. I was very uncomfortable while the lactation consultant tried to get the baby latched on. I have large, fatty breasts that just kind of hang there, and I was exposed to everyone in the room and felt terribly vulnerable.

I was even uncomfortable nursing in front of my husband. At five feet, three inches and about 245 pounds, I could never take a shower in front of him or walk around the house without my clothes on. This might sound strange, but prior to nursing, my husband never saw me naked. Never. We always had sex with the lights out, very conventional. But I needed his help to get the baby latched on and to bring me a glass of water. The nursing pajamas had an opening to nurse through, but it didn't work well with my large breasts. I ended up sitting around the house without a shirt on, and ultimately, because I was more exposed, my husband had to see me naked.

Gradually, though, I began to shed a lot of my inhibitions. I think it started with the fact that when you have a baby, you're naked and everybody sees you. All the things I had to do to get nursing established helped me to start thinking that it was silly for me to be so uptight. So as I became more comfortable with nursing, I became less concerned about whether or not people see my flab or think I'm fat.

It was very liberating for me, and sexually, it's enhanced my relationship with my husband. Feeling less inhibited, I started to do things I wouldn't have done otherwise. We've tried different positions that I normally would have thought were unflattering or would make me feel silly. I wasn't afraid of having sex during the day or with the lights on. I guess that sounds weird after being with someone for over eight years.

I remember coming home after having the baby and feeling incredibly womanly. I felt this even more after nursing. Today I feel more confident, attractive, and positive about myself, kind of like Wonder Woman or something. It's been great!

I read a statistic stating that 30 percent of obese women quit nursing in the beginning, as it's physically more difficult than it is for thin women.[*]

---

* Researchers have observed that compared to normal-weight women, overweight and obese women who initiate breastfeeding are between two and a half and three and a half times more likely to stop by the time they leave the hospital. And the rate continues to plummet over the next few weeks (Hilson, Rasmussen, and Kjolhede, 1997).

This sudden decline cannot be divorced from culture. Nutrition professor Kathleen Rasmussen notes that obese women in Denmark—where almost all women start out breastfeeding and receive much more cultural support for it—face the same mechanical and hormonal challenges that obese women in the United States face, but far fewer of them switch to formula (personal communication, 2003).

Given that, I'm really proud that I was able to nurse, and I'm glad we stuck with it. I view it as a real accomplishment. At the same time, having a baby and nursing have made me accept the fact that *this* is how I look, and I refuse to be ashamed about it anymore.

Leslie V., Phoenix, AZ

I WISHED I'D BEEN BORN A BOY

Growing up I felt it would have been better if I had been a boy. There were opportunities I felt I missed, things I wanted to do that I couldn't, subtle put-downs and denigrations only for the reason that I was a girl. I was a tomboy and loved to be rough-and-tumble. An acceptable outlet for this was gymnastics, which I loved! However, my breasts started developing when I was eleven. I loathed them because the gymnastics instructor told me I would never have a gymnast's body and I might as well give up gymnastics right then. That comment stuck with me my entire life.

I think in some ways I viewed my breasts antagonistically. I knew they were attractive to guys, and it made me kind of angry that this part of me should draw attention. In some ways, I placed all of my negative feelings about being a girl/woman on my breasts. Whenever I felt discriminated against because I was female, I remembered the comment that I couldn't be a gymnast because of my breasts. I turned that simple statement into "I can't be a . . . because I have breasts!"

Breastfeeding has made me feel that this is the reason why breasts are there. I could breastfeed my children, something no male could do, and finally I could say, "This is what a woman's body is supposed to do." Breastfeeding was healing, in a way, and it made me glad I was born a girl. It has made me feel more feminine, more womanly, more connected to women.

Arlene Jacobs, Montgomery, AL

A WISDOM ALL OUR OWN

I grew up in the 1970s and 1980s, in what I regard as the heyday of feminism. It seemed like there were constantly battles of the sexes, women proving that they could do things as well as men could and maybe better—the whole Billy Jean King versus Bobby Riggs kind of thing.

Despite having grown up with such a prevalence of what I consider to be mainstream feminist thought, never did I hear that birthing is empowering, that it takes strength, that a woman's body is beautiful and resilient. Never did I hear anything about breastfeeding, that a woman's ability to produce this incredible liquid is miraculous and should be honored and revered. We can pump iron and build up our muscles, but the strength of our bodies and the unique things a woman's body does aren't acknowledged. Our bodies are somehow pathological.

When I got into college I had this idea that men and women were equal. But then I took some women's arts and women's theater classes and found that the artistic things women do are referred to as *craft,* not as art. I started realizing that many of these wonderful things women had been doing were not acknowledged. We weren't meeting that male standard.

I think back to my biology and physiology classes, and I don't recall hearing any of the benefits of human milk, any of the risks of *not* giving your baby human milk, anything about the primary function of breasts being to make milk. I never heard that breast cancer and osteoporosis rates are higher for women who don't breastfeed. It's another example where we see that women's contributions are overlooked and devalued unless they are like men's.

I think feminists have done a lot of work on the sexual exploitation and violation of women's bodies, but I would like to see breasts less sexualized. I'm not uptight, and yet I felt more comfortable in college, doing nude modeling for art classes, than I initially felt breastfeeding in public! When you go into a figure-drawing class, everyone knows there's going to be a nude woman or man in the class, and we all accept that it is not about sex, it's about figure drawing. I had total control over the positions, and no one could ever touch me. The boundaries were clear. With nursing in public, you don't have control over who is around you, and it's not something expected to happen. Sometimes you can't control how covered or not covered you are. And as comfortable as I have been with my body, I wasn't sure what people would think. I was on guard.

Then I thought, "This is stupid! I'm not exposing my breasts in any kind of a sexual fashion. Why should I feel uncomfortable when this is the most natural thing in the world?" Just as our arms serve a purpose and our liver serves a purpose, our breasts happen to make milk. It's a function of the female body. I think, because it's been oppressive to us, there's a reluctance to look at a woman and define her in any way, shape, or form based on her biology. But while I don't think a woman should be solely defined by her biology, she certainly has that as part of her repertoire of power.

Birth and breastfeeding have empowered me in ways that no career or educational experience has done. Giving birth taught me that my body has a wisdom all its own and has strength and resilience. Breastfeeding has taught me that I can make this incredible fluid that makes my babies grow at an incredible rate for the first few months. This is soooo amazing to me, and I am still in awe when I see the milk drip out of my breasts. I think, "I made that! I did it without really trying in the 'masculine' sense. I simply *was*, and my milk simply *was*, and because of this, my baby *thrives*."

Petra, Denver, CO

Other aspects of Petra's experiences appear on pages 33–34.

Healing

When I was four months pregnant with my second child, I was away for the weekend at a women's retreat. On Saturday evening, a dozen of us gathered in a dimly lit room, giving voice to different women we wanted to honor, women who devoted their life and work to helping others. Despite having given birth in a hospital with top-notch *nurse*-midwives, I decided to honor direct-entry or "*lay*" midwives, who, in today's medically powerful and litigious birthing environment, believe in giving women the choice to birth at home. I introduced the subject by sharing a recent dream:

> I was at a hospital in labor when suddenly I was holding my baby. I realized, to my horror, that I could recall little about the labor and nothing about the delivery. I couldn't understand why. My health care provider in the dream was an obstetrician, represented by a real-life doctor I know who treats his patients with a certain amount of paternalism and disregard. I asked him about this complete absence of memory, but he dismissed my question. It was then that I realized I had been rendered unconscious. "Why did you do this to me?" I demanded to know. He informed me that I'd been talking too much and making too much noise, so they drugged me to keep me quiet. I began yelling at him and pounding his chest with my fists: "How could you do this!" I demanded. "You robbed me! You stole my birth experience from me, and I can never have it back!"

As I was coming to the end of describing my dream, a young woman who had been sitting silently across the circle slowly curled her body into a fetal position and began to weep—deep, heaving sobs. "You described my birth," she later revealed. "I, too, felt violated, raped, by my doctor. I thought I was over it, but I guess I'm not."

Unfortunately, her experience is not unique. Women in labor are often disrespected; denied support, compassion, and the ability to have a fully informed active role in their labors; powerless to object; psychologically and emotionally harmed; and in many cases robbed of an authentic birth experience. Naomi Wolf's book *Misconception: Truths, Lies, and the Unexpected on the Journey to Motherhood* (2001) provides an infuriating look into her own experience. After researching why so many women become subservient to the fetal monitor, indeed almost superfluous to the experience itself, Wolf concludes that what we experience are "ordinary traumas" resulting from "ordinary bad births."

Wolf asserts the importance of speaking about the darkness as well as the light on the journey to motherhood; that we need to understand the full spectrum of stories to honor the victories involved "in the tough, sweet work of making ourselves into mothers" (2001, 10). Breastfeeding, for some of us, is the light after the darkness. It can help us heal not only from disempowering birth experiences but from other forms of violation and loss.

Breastfeeding is seldom discussed with relation to death and grief, though sadly the two are sometimes intimately connected. Women who have lost a child may still lactate. In some cases, expressing milk can offer women an opportunity to heal from loss and emotional pain. This is seldom acknowledged in the literature available to help grieving parents. For example, in *Empty Cradle, Broken Heart: Surviving the Death of Your Baby*, Deborah L. Davis gives advice about how to alleviate the discomfort of engorged breasts but nowhere acknowledges that continuing to lactate may be another way of coping with grief (1991, 20–21).

The stories in this section reveal the myriad ways that breastfeeding can help heal our minds and spirits and move us forward in our lives.

In Their Own Words:
Healing

Mary's words, here, are only one version of her story. When she heard about *The Breastfeeding Café*, she contacted me, eager to share her experience. Injured from an auto accident, she rose early every morning for an entire summer and wrote and wrote—hundreds of pages. "I completely stepped back and examined my life in a way I never had before," she said. "At the same time that my body was healing from the accident, I healed my spirit." Here are excerpts from her story.

THE GOLD RUSH

My newborn nestles at my breast. It is springtime, and I'm thirty-three, nursing my firstborn, Kayley. We are soaking in the beauty and sunshine of northern California wine country through my bedroom window. There is a profound simplicity of the moment—a pure joy of just being together skin-to-skin, heart-to-heart. I gaze at my daughter and begin to wonder what she's like on the *inside*. What kind of person will she evolve into? Will I be able to provide what she needs from me?

Born under the southern California sun, I was raised and ripened in a middle-class Catholic family, the youngest of five girls. I grew up with Barbies, bikes, the Beach Boys, and betrayal. At age four, I was molested. On more than one occasion my friend's father lured me into his cold, dark den, grabbed me, put his hands down my underpants, held me down like a predator capturing his prey, and robbed me of my innocence. Then he threatened me never to tell. I didn't. I kept the shame, the secret, the hurt, in dark storage for many years.

Growing up I had all the basics but felt disconnected, lonely, and longed for connection. I was constantly striving to earn love from my parents. They never intended to hurt me, yet I never felt their intention to bond with me. They were always too busy, distracted, wounded from their own untold stories. My father existed in his own world, and my mom was usually angry, retaliating for her own unmet needs and expectations. On a rampage, she would tear through our house yelling, screaming, pouncing on myself and my sisters. I remember the sound of neighbors closing their windows. There was no way to jump far enough, fast enough, or high enough. Burnt, bruised, broken from all that hoop-jumping, I failed miserably. And it was my fault. And my sisters', too.

Consequently, I never learned how to protect myself or develop an assertive presence. As a twenty-one-year-old senior in college, I fell down at work. The hands I put myself into for help with my injury turned out to be those of a sick physician who violated me and reopened my painful past. Fortunately, I broke his restraints and got away before he finished raping me. Yet the emotional rape and his threats warning me not to tell echoed for a long time. But despite having him threaten and stalk me, I did tell. I told a therapist, the police, the insurance authorities, the San Diego American Medical Association, and finally the California Medical Board. I told them all. They filed reports, yet he's still in practice. And I am too. Practicing telling, which is exactly where I started out as a nurse.

In 1994 I launched my nursing career by working with and advocating for abandoned and abused children. Standing up for these children gave me the strength and courage to face my own painful past.

Twenty-seven years after being molested, I went to the police and turned in the perpetrator. I wasn't the only one. Child Protective Services, which confirmed that there were many more child victims, slapped a restraining order on him preventing him from being alone with any more children.

But this didn't completely mend me. That would require the help of a healer, my obstetrician. After a few years of infertility and a miscarriage, I felt like a complete failure and was totally discouraged. My husband and I wanted to share our love with a child and were trying everything to conceive. Dr. Drexler acknowledged my grief, encouraged me, and offered further treatment options. His intent was to heal, not harm. One day during a transformative moment in his office, he looked me in the eye with strength and conviction and said, "It sounds like you blame yourself for not being pregnant. I don't know why you're not pregnant, but I do know IT'S NOT YOUR FAULT. IT'S NOT YOUR FAULT. IT'S NOT YOUR FAULT . . ."

A skilled surgeon, Dr. Drexler used his sharp scalpel to cut away the layers of blame, shame, and pain of infertility, of insults and injuries as a woman, a teen, a child, and helped me to connect to myself in a way I never had before. A future emerged from the dark into light, from the slippery to the solid. And my baby, Kayley, was born warm and wet, received into the safe hands of Dr. Drexler.

Within minutes of her birth, I was nursing her. Tears of hurting became tears of happiness. I felt so lucky, so blessed. Breastfeeding became an important part of our relationship, and I connected with her through constant feedings around the clock. And on a deeper level, we were bonding through singing, talking, holding in a way I had never experienced with my own mother.

No longer broken or living in fear of being abandoned or devoured, I was healing myself of wounds that didn't have to get passed on from generation to generation. Instead, milk from my body was nourishing my high-spirited yet gentle Kayley.

Eight months later, while still nursing, I began growing another. Christopher came into the world cheerful, cuddly, and constantly nursing. But along with the joy of nursing him I became overwhelmed with exhaustion and fatigue trying to be the "perfect" mother meeting my family's needs. The reality of how challenging motherhood is hit hard and fast.

But while nursing Christopher, all the chaos and responsibilities of cooking, laundry, house cleaning, bills, and the phone had to wait. Everything became still and calm with Christopher at my breast and Kayley at my side. My children didn't care if I accomplished my daily tasks "perfectly." They only cared about our time together, which nursing always provided.

My life was full with two dear children and one good man. From half to whole, hopeless to hope, empty to enough, more than enough. I had a need to give back, to return some of the richness I was receiving.

My milk was cascading out of me through double pads, nursing bra, and t-shirt. So I decided to donate some. Sara, a neighbor I'd never met, was planning to adopt a baby and had a strong desire to give him human milk. A kindhearted nurse and coworker introduced us.

Sara's intentions touched me deeply. She wanted to provide the best for her baby, and that included breast milk. So over the next four months I pumped 345 ounces of gold, golden milk for baby Jeremiah, born August 12th, my birthday, my *best* birthday.

I was nursing a one-year-old, potty training a two-year-old and a puppy, sustaining a marriage, and maintaining a part-time position as a nurse. It was a full-time, round-the-clock life with little sleep and lots of laundry. I had little energy, yet it couldn't have been more convenient or comfortable to pump milk for baby Jeremiah.

I would sit at the kitchen table while my children napped and set up my pump. Plugged in, cups on, brain off. The whole process of my Gold Rush got me to slow down, take a deep breath, and collapse in release and relief. In those quiet moments I became closer to myself, my children, my husband, Jeremiah, Sara, and her husband, Tim.

The birth of a baby, friendship, and awareness. Milk from my own breasts helped form connective tissue that has tied together my life with the lives of others. Now we're on solid food and solid friendship built on trust and mutual understanding, bonding without bondage or bruising. From hole-life to whole-life, from powdered milk to pure milk, this flow of mine is a deep vein of richness that rewards in its receipt and in its giving.

Written by Mary O'Brien, Sonoma, CA

In her foreword to *Of Woman Born*, Adrienne Rich writes, "I believe increasingly that only the willingness to share private and sometimes painful experiences can enable women to create a collective description of the world which will truly be ours" (1986, 16). The next three stories contribute to this, centered around the painful experiences of loss. The first comes from Arlene, the child gymnast.

BREASTFEEDING MADE HIM MINE

My first son, Kevin, was born without a functioning immune system. It's a genetic defect I can pass on to my sons. He died when he was eighteen months old. Three months before he died, I became pregnant. I was too preoccupied caring for an extremely ill child, I didn't want the baby, and I was terrified when I found out he was a boy. I didn't think I could go through it again if he had the same condition as Kevin. We tried to have him tested in utero, but the testing was unsuccessful.

As soon as Jeffrey was born, he had to have extensive blood work done to make sure his immune system was functioning. It was terrifying. He was tested again two days later. Since immunities are passed in breast milk, breastfeeding would have masked the immune-system testing they were doing on him. We wouldn't have known whether the immunities showing up in the tests were mine or his. Instead of my milk, he was given completely sterile formula in tiny, premade bottles with nipples from hermetically sealed packages. Every time he got a bottle, I pumped so my milk was on the same schedule he was.

After three days, we received a phone call telling us that Jeffrey was normal. I can't believe how happy we were! My husband opened a bottle of champagne, and I sat down in the rocking chair near the window and immediately put my son to my breast. I knew he was hungry because it was getting close to the time to feed him. I remember holding him in my arms and looking at him. His mouth was open, ready for the bottle. I turned his head to my breast and put my nipple in his mouth. He raised his eyebrows, opened his eyes wide, and looked up at me, like, "Wow! This is good stuff!"

I didn't realize it then, but I hadn't bonded with him until we got the word he was healthy. He wasn't *mine* until I nursed him. Breastfeeding made him mine.

Arlene Jacobs, Montgomery, AL

Breastfeeding has put me in touch with myself as a woman. I've had endometriosis, laser surgery, and infertility workups, so I associated menses and everything else as being painful and inconvenient. I viewed the bio-logical rhythms of being female as problems to be overcome. Then I had a C-section. Breastfeeding my son was the first part of the reproductive process that went the way it was supposed to.

Laura Hankins, Charlotte, NC

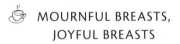

MOURNFUL BREASTS, JOYFUL BREASTS

The doctor, head of obstetrics at the Long Island hospital, called us into her office to try to talk us out of having a natural childbirth in a birthing room.

"Why would I do less to get *this* baby off to a good start than I would do for a baby I was going to keep?" I said to her and to the only midwife we could locate in the area.

"People who are gonna give the baby away *never* do that," she said.

Of course, what she meant was, how could I possibly open myself so wide to that baby and then not keep her? But at that point in my life, I lived more by youthfully zealous moral imperatives than by my feelings, at least about things that involved others—in this case, getting the baby off to what I felt would be the best possible entry into life. I did what I had to do and dealt with the feelings later.

And so I have. Sometimes the feelings are brought on by some definite thing—such as October 8 or seeing kids her age—and sometimes they arise seemingly spontaneously, crashing like huge, unheralded waves, born out of the fabric of an everyday day.

And Brendan, eight weeks old and breastfeeding now, even as I write, reaffirms my sorrow that the little girl we gave away didn't get to breastfeed for more than her first two and a half days. I feel this way, even as my conviction that I couldn't have parented *then* is strengthened by this *present* experience of feeling ready, desirous, able to mother.

Then, twelve and a half years ago, my *breasts* mourned her leaving much more than I was consciously able to mourn her absence. My milk came in as we drove in to the Manhattan adoption agency. By the time we'd been sent downtown to a pediatrician to have "our" little girl checked out and then returned uptown to meet her new parents and give her to them (we'd refused to allow the customary forty days in a foster home), my breasts were engorged, full, ready to nourish in a way that the rest of me wasn't. And it hurt, literally. My body felt about to split open. That first night after she was gone I could barely touch my breasts to express the milk. And in the ensuing weeks as I weaned myself off the pump, I would overflow, my breasts weeping for the child who wasn't there, while my eyes remained dry. It was just what I had to do, and I did it.

In the years since then, the shape of my life has changed a lot. I have finally learned how to take care of and mother myself, a kind of nurturing my father didn't understand and couldn't teach or give, as he raised four kids alone. I have found myself living in a more stable place, from which I can go back and sort out all the blurred years of confused feelings and events. Little by little I have let myself feel the loss and wonder about my daughter, where, how, and who she is.

Still, I was overwhelmed by the torrent of feeling for her that came during my pregnancy and after Brendan's birth eight weeks ago. Now I am breastfeeding again, this time through and *beyond* colostrum, taking this present joy and the promise of a full life with Brendan and integrating with it the physical and repressed emotional surges of over a decade ago, as well as the sense of appropriateness I felt breastfeeding our little girl, giving her what I *could:* colostrum with love, a natural birth, carefully chosen parents, and no foster home to attach to and then detach from.

These days if I even look at Brendan as he sleeps, waves of love for him well up at the same time that my milk lets down, almost painfully spurred not just by physical stimulation but by the overflow of love I feel in being with him.

All my past condenses now into a readiness to mother Brendan. And someday, I hope to meet the daughter I couldn't mother.

Written by Larkin Brigham, Spencer, NY

 FULL BREASTS, EMPTY ARMS

Malaika would have been two months old today if she had been born alive, and I have been feeling brittle all day, as though I would break if handled roughly or moved too quickly. My poor husband, David, told me he spent yesterday on the verge of tears. He doesn't cry much, and he has already had two big sobbing sessions over Malaika. My heart went out to him, and I wished I could spare him some of the pain. He had completely let down his guard and opened his heart to his little girl, which made him more vulnerable to greater pain than perhaps at any other time in his life. And the gamble didn't pay off, so will he ever have the courage to gamble again? Of course, that applies to both of us.

Malaika was our first child. We lost her at forty weeks gestation due to a knot in her umbilical cord. She was perfect and beautiful. I miss her so much, and I never imagined that these little ones could be snatched from us so soon.

I expressed milk for a month and donated it to the milk bank at Georgetown University. It was a way of helping myself deal with my devastation at my daughter's absence, and I found it comforting that some baby, somewhere, benefited from all that work, even if it could not be Malaika.

I took the second and final batch of breast milk to the milk bank today. I'm not sure why, but I have been putting off the trip for a whole month now. Perhaps I was waiting for the symmetry of taking it to the bank two months after she was born. I seem to create impromptu rituals for all sorts of things these days, both consciously and unconsciously. The milk filled half the large freezer compartment in the refrigerator. We needed the space, and the frozen bags slipped all over each other, escaping regularly and bombarding my feet when I would go seeking peas for dinner.

Finally this morning I decided to go, and David loaded two canvas grocery bags full of rock-hard frozen plastic bags and tubes of milk. I dropped him off at the Metro and drove to Georgetown University Hospital. The bags, perhaps weighed down with our broken dreams, felt even heavier than the objective weight of their contents. A tall, blond, professional-looking woman stood when I entered the crowded little basement room that the lactation consultants and the milk bank use for offices, storage, breast pump rentals, and all sorts of things.

I explained my errand. After asking me if I had been screened as a donor and after labeling the containers with my name, we silently transferred the semitransparent milk briquets from the canvas bags to the supercold giant freezer.

For the last several days I thought I would like to see the tiny babies who will get Malaika's milk, but I wondered if the staff would find that a strange request. I couldn't find the words to ask, so I turned to leave. As I opened the door, I felt the inspiration to introduce myself to the woman and shake her hand. She said her name, and I recognized it from the milk-bank phone recording as that of the nursing supervisor—a person with the authority to take me to the nursery if she wanted. I gathered my courage and told her my baby had died. I asked if I could see the newborn intensive care unit with some of the babies who might benefit from the milk I had brought. Her eyes got moist, and she walked past me, signaling that I should follow her. I felt relieved that she hadn't turned me down.

I recognized the NICU from our tour, many months ago, and shuddered at my smug confidence that I would not need those particular services. The nursing supervisor spent quite a bit of time with me explaining how the preemies develop and when and how they get fed once their systems can handle it. Apparently, about 60 percent of moms there with preemies express breast milk for their babies. Some of the other infants can handle specialized formulas. They use donated milk for babies who can't tolerate formula but whose mothers aren't providing milk for whatever reason.

Standing on the outside of that glass, trying to get a glimpse of a baby, made me realize that what I really wanted was to hold one, but they are much too fragile and vulnerable for strangers to wander in and hold, so I didn't ask. It was hard. I cried almost the entire time I was there. I certainly didn't mean to do that, but I'm glad I asked to see those tiny people. All I could really see were a couple of blanket-covered bundles in Isolettes with blue bilirubin lights on them, but I knew they were there fighting for their lives, and I felt glad to help them. The nursing supervisor started to cry with me when I told her I was glad that some baby would benefit from my having been pregnant. She assured me that many babies would get my milk because from the first and second donations combined, I had given them over six hundred ounces. It seems that a preemie only takes an ounce or two a day, depending on the size.

On the way out of the hospital I still had tears streaming down my face. I stopped at a tiny garden outside the door and asked Malaika to look after those babies and help them grow up as she couldn't do. I hope she heard me. I couldn't help thinking that if she had been premature (my worst fear at the time because of my previous miscarriages), she could be alive today. Instead she stuck around and grew big and strong but tightened that knot as she moved into position for birthing. Funny how things work out.

There is precious little out there on postpartum recovery for mothers with empty arms. The little material I have found generally amounts to a paragraph buried inside a lengthy chapter on infant needs and behavior. I found sifting through all of that quite painful, but I wanted to know what to expect from changes in my body, so I did it. I think bereaved mothers of neonates need to know that expressing and donating milk is an option.

Written by Jacqueline Hamilton, Washington, DC

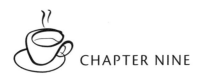

CHAPTER NINE

_____

Moving On and Letting Go

STORIES OF WEANING
& OTHER MILESTONES

We have to believe in the value of our own experience and in the value of our ways of knowing, our ways of doing things. We have to wrap ourselves in these ways of knowing, to enact daily ceremonies of life.

Bettina Aptheker, Tapestries of Life

In *Having Faith: An Ecologist's Journey to Motherhood*, Sandra Steingraber writes about trying to help her toddler learn how to fall asleep without nursing. She describes walking along an ocean beach with her daughter in a stroller, hoping to transfer some of her daughter's connectedness from her to the natural world, hoping that the motion, waves, and sound of seagulls would lull her child to sleep. "It occurs to me," she writes, "that there should be some kind of ceremony for the commencement of weaning, as there is for birth, marriage, and other rites of passage. So I whisper a little prayer of commemoration. *Sleeping girl, I release you from my breast into the world, where the tides run with fish and berry bushes flutter with migrating birds*" (2001, 283).

As I read her words that recognized and honored this important transition, I was struck by the discrepancy between her appreciation of weaning and the approach of the dominant American cul-

257

ture. Medical recommendations notwithstanding, many Americans still think of breastfeeding beyond six months as a long time. Family members, friends, even strangers feel it is within their right to question this deeply embodied, highly personal relationship between a mother and her child. (One woman was even cautioned that if she nursed her son into toddlerhood he would grow up to be obsessed by breasts—unlike all of today's men previously formula-fed, I'm sure!) In worst-case scenarios, women actually have been charged with abuse for nursing their children into toddlerhood and beyond, and extended nursing has been used against women in court battles over child custody (Dettwyler 1995b, 56).

Rather than allowing weaning to unfold naturally, most women are encouraged to wean prematurely and have to process their jumble of feelings within a culture that fails to understand the U.S. emphasis on early weaning as a cross-cultural anomaly, one that often places the values of independence and self-sufficiency—even in infants—above the values of empathy and nurturance.

Among those who may pressure us to wean are our pediatricians. In the foreword to *Breastfeeding: Biocultural Perspectives*, Edward Newton, physician and son of the late, renowned breastfeeding researcher Niles Newton, asserts that the medical community plays a greater role in determining how long women nurse than it does in influencing whether or not we initiate breastfeeding (Stuart-Macadam and Dettwyler 1995, x). But many American pediatricians have little experience or knowledge regarding extended nursing and fail to provide women with accurate information about what is "normal," instead relying on what constitutes "typical" behavior in the United States today. "When her pediatrician is known for expressing the view that, 'Any women who nurses an infant beyond the age of six months is doing it for her own sexual pleasure,'" asks anthropologist Katherine Dettwyler, "how can the mother of a nursing toddler turn to him or her for advice on any aspect of infant feeding?" (1995b, 57).

Lost in the brouhaha is the larger picture, and our narrow cultural lens fails to place weaning in any sort of cross-cultural, historical, or biological context. Dettwyler points out that in most traditional societies around the world, children are weaned between the ages of two and five years. Moreover, her own research on weaning behavior among nonhuman primates, our closest relatives, suggests that the natural age of weaning based on biology without cultural modification would be somewhere between two and a half and seven years, depending on the biological and developmental milestones studied (e.g., a quadrupling of birth weight, arrival of first permanent molars, etc.) (1995b, 39). From a biological perspective, then, the breastfeeding recommendations from the American Academy of Pediatrics, the Surgeon General, and the World Health Organization are not progressive but conservative.

But the judgment works both ways. Even though many of us feel pressure to wean *before* our children—and we—are ready, some women feel pressure to nurse *longer* than we would like. "One thing that bugs me," said one woman, "is an attitude from some people that you should nurse your kid for as long as you can, no matter what. My neighbor told me that she only nursed her youngest for nine months but she had nursed her first two for over a year. I told her I thought it was great that she did it for nine months and she should be proud of herself!"

In short, no matter what we choose, misconceptions, discomfort, and judgment seem to pervade the cultural climate surrounding weaning. Overshadowed is the emotional intensity both we and our children may feel and the issues that arise for us. How we feel about weaning, how we approach it, and why we initiate it vary greatly. But most of us likely feel a jumble of mixed emotions as we enter the next stage of our parenting journeys: joy, relief, disappointment, and sorrow. Despite this ambivalence, a Boston-area pediatrician once told me: "It is the rare person who says, 'I nursed too long.' I tend to hear, 'I wish I had nursed him longer.'"

The stories in this chapter—many of which involve weaning toddlers, preschoolers, or older children—speak to this important time, from the perspective not of our babies' development but of our own. They come from women who weaned after a long and successful nursing relationship, as well as from women who weaned because circumstances made it too difficult, if not impossible, to continue. Thus, to consider the reasons why nursing comes to an end for some of us, we must first go back to the beginning.

Constrained Choices

The first three stories belong to women for whom nursing was a disappointment, who reluctantly weaned due to inadequate support, information, and assistance. But remember the "mommy wars" that began to flare up in the 1980s between employed mothers and "at-home" mothers? Similar hostility rages today between breast-feeding mothers and mothers who use formula.

While many nursing mothers feel frustrated by being around people who push formula and devalue nursing, bottle-feeding women may resent breastfeeding enthusiasts. "There is so much peer pressure, at least in my community, that women who have a tough time with breastfeeding are made to feel like failures and rotten mothers," writes Gilah, of Washington, D.C. "I had to keep reminding myself that my breasts were not failing me—they were doing the best they could, and that would have to do."

Some women end up directing their frustration and anger at breastfeeding advocates, rather than at the ways society has failed them. Lactation consultant Nancy Mohrbacher, IBCLC, refers to this as a breastfeeding backlash. "Although on the face of it, these women are very unsupportive of breastfeeding," Mohrbacher asserts, "under the surface, they are grieving for what they and their babies have lost (personal communication, 2003)."

Staci Carlson, a mother in Nebraska who operates a Web site for "the women in this world who are not breastfeeding," agrees. "What many don't realize," she explains, "is that when a woman fails after wanting so badly to succeed at breastfeeding, she is literally going through a phase of mourning."

Susan, for example, who spent three grueling months trying to establish breastfeeding, reflects:

> In early August, when my son was about three months old, my husband and I were eating in a cafeteria, and I had just given Sam a bottle. A woman sat down near us and proceeded to nurse and eat lunch at the same time. I lost it. I had to go to the ladies' room, where I sat crying, bent over my baby, saying, "I wish it could have been us." Breastfeeding is the way to go if you can do it, but there has to be compassion and understanding. My husband and I were taken aback at how affected and sad I was by the whole experience. It's amazing how long these feelings last.

Regrettably, some breastfeeding enthusiasts let their *passion* override their *com*passion. Staci shared several representative comments she has received from hundreds of breastfeeding mothers who have accused her of being an irresponsible or "bad" mother. "You are feeding your child crap in a can," wrote one woman. Another added, "I hope your child dies from the crap you are shoving down her throat."

"It concerns me," says Mohrbacher, "that there is in-fighting going on among mothers, when we should be joining forces to try to correct our society's issues about breastfeeding."

Adds Staci, "It's incredibly hard to respect other people when they do nothing but disrespect you."

Ultimately, we all need to give each other the benefit of the doubt and work toward creating a society in which all women who want to nurse are able to.

In Their Own Words:
Constrained Choices

Sometimes we don't know why we aren't able to breastfeed well. This was the case for Lacey. A more effective pump would probably have helped, and a skilled helper most definitely would have. But whatever the underlying reason, her story, like so many others, is one of tenacity and commitment in the face of professional disinterest or ignorance.

A single mother/waitress/student living in the East Bay area of California with her daughter, Madison, Lacey has wanted to be a writer all her life. "My writing has flourished since my daughter was born," she says. "She gives me an opportunity to see life with a fresh eye and to feel my experiences more deeply."

BUTTONS

My breasts have never defined me. They were as important as any other body part in the matter of functions and as unimportant cosmetically as the millions of other parts that make up my physical being. After all, I never worried about the size of my fallopian tubes, so I held my breasts to the same expectations.

And they came through for many years. They were evident enough to prove I was not a boy when I wore my hair shaved a quarter inch from my skull. They stood up proudly when I decided to get my nipples pierced. They offered me tingly sensations during sexual stimulation. And when I became pregnant with my daughter, they grew to a joyous B cup. I never asked for much from my breasts, and they never let me down. I thought we had a pretty decent relationship.

It was a summer afternoon in my late pregnancy when I first realized I was sporting a pair of swinging udders. I thought sweat had formed a trail into my bra, leaving a sticky puddle, but on investigation, the sweet and sour smell and milky texture proved to be my first experience with leaking. Feelings of glee washed over me, knowing that this was the beginning of small miracles I was to experience.

At eight and a half months pregnant, I grasped those hard little water balloons firmly in my hands. I aimed and squeezed to shoot plentiful streams of creamy breast milk clear across the room! I was bursting with excitement! I woke my partner up, for I'd been shooting my breasts off at two thirty in the morning. He grumbled and asked what in the hell I wanted now. "Okay. Stay there. Watch!" I stood in the entranceway and aimed. Splat! I got him right on the cheek! Of course, he found this more disgusting than miraculous, but the worth of his opinions had already begun to decline in my book.

In fact, I left him within months of my daughter's arrival, after he kicked me out four months into the pregnancy and then took me back at seven. After he told me I needed therapy to change the things he didn't like about me. After he refused to tell his mother about the forthcoming baby. After I fell out of love with someone who didn't love me for *me*. I came to the conclusion that I could marry this fool, but I would hate myself, hate my life, and resent him. So I chose to do it on my own. I chose to raise my daughter in an organic, harmonious atmosphere full of dedication and happiness. No one said it would be easy. But when is anything worthwhile ever achieved through ease?

Earth mother. Hip mama. Attachment parenting. Not only was I about to become a mother, but—in a world that exists outside of Martha Stewart ideals—I was going to be the best mother that ever lived. I didn't have a college education, a husband, or a dog named Spot, but I did have a scorching determination to give my child every gift of life she was entitled to. From emotion to imagination, nurturing to nutrition, I had everything I needed inside of me.

On August 2, 2000, I gave birth to my beautiful daughter at the county hospital. She was all peaches and cream, wrinkles and sparkling blue eyes. As the doctors and nurses took her Apgar scores and cleared the mucus out of her throat and nose, I reminded them, as I had stated in my birth plan, not to give her a bottle, that I wanted to breastfeed as soon as possible. I wanted to hold her. I'd waited nine months, let me see her! Now, damn it!

Ah, little fresh baby with her heavenly baby scents, wrapped tight in a hospital print blanket, a tiny knit cap pulled over her soft skull. Little sweet baby girl with those wise, tired eyes. I marvel and weep and coo. And then I breastfeed. Little sweet baby girl's teeny mouth clamps on with the suctioning power of a Hoover, but is still gentle. She feeds like an old pro, like she had been practicing her part for the last nine months. Nurses flutter around, outside my tunnel vision, making sure I am holding her right. She is suckling correctly, and they leave us be, satisfied that we are up to par. See me—sweaty, oily, hair frightening. See me—after the most awesome, liberating, empowering moments of my life. See me bursting with my first rush of maternal pride.

On day three I returned to my apartment like a triumphant warrior clutching my prize. I was eager to show off to my father, brother, and favorite aunt what a natural mother I was and how easy a baby my sweet Madison was, when Madison decided to show them another side. She began wailing and never seeming satisfied. Every few minutes I unclasped my maternity bra and attempted a feeding. She would greedily suckle for a few seconds, then spit out the nipple and scream. I'd switch sides, and she'd do the same. I assumed she was feeding. I checked her diaper, changed her clothes, and tried to burp her. I couldn't figure out what was wrong and felt my cheeks burn red. This was my first experience of helplessness as a mother. My aunt gently pointed out that she hadn't wet her diaper in over two hours. Maybe she wasn't getting any milk.

Instantly panicked that my three-day-old daughter was on the brink of starvation, I ran to the cupboard for some formula. All of a sudden the whole dream of the breastfeeding champion mother fell aside as the only important thing to me was feeding Madison. Of course, as the fable goes, the cupboards were bare. But this was my own engineering, as I'd blissfully tossed every formula sample that had come my way from wicked "do-gooder" companies wanting to foil my game and sway my decision with their promises of convenience and ease. My aunt walked to the corner store and came back with a little can of the enemy: Enfamil.

Madison energetically emptied the first four ounces and cried for more, confirming two things: (1) my aunt had been right—she was hungry; and (2) I had essentially failed my first mothering goal. My breasts were not holding up to their end of the bargain.

Once I was alone and Madison was sleeping with her full belly, I called La Leche League. The counselor suggested a multitude of exercises to get my

The WHO/UNICEF International Code of Marketing of Breast Milk Substitutes

Lacey referred to free formula samples she received in the mail. This is in direct violation of the International Code of Marketing of Breast Milk Substitutes. Known in breastfeeding circles as the Code, its purpose is to serve as a minimal set of voluntary guidelines for the ethical marketing, promotion, and distribution of breast milk substitutes. It includes ten main provisions:

1. *No advertising of breast milk substitutes.*
2. *No free samples of breast milk substitutes to mothers.*
3. *No promotion of products through health care facilities.*
4. *No company mothercraft nurses to advise mothers.*
5. *No gifts or personal samples to health workers.*
6. *No words or pictures idealizing artificial feeding, including pictures of infants, on the labels of the products.*
7. *Information to health workers should be scientific and factual.*

(continued)

milk production going again. And they assured me that my past piercings weren't the problem. Once her father returned from work I sent him back out to purchase a breast pump. He came back with a manual one. I hastily put the contraption together and went to work. After a few healthy squirts, I got nothing. When Maddy woke up I tried to feed her again. Same reaction. I was astounded. There had been no problems in the hospital, and milk had leaked from me at the end of my pregnancy. Were my breasts slyly trying to betray me, now that we were out of reach of the nurses and doctors who could have suggested solutions? I laid her on my lap and held her hand, trying to get the old hormones stimulated while I fruitlessly pumped away. After a week of this I had incredible hand muscles, but not much else had changed.*

We took turns, the bottle and me. I begrudgingly bought countless cans of formula with my WIC vouchers, hating that they were producing more milk than I. WIC might have offered me some type of support or counseling had I been honest with my problems. By this time I had heard, "Don't worry, it will happen," so many times that I believed it. Though I was aggravated, I was also ashamed. So when I sat in the WIC office politely answering questions about my voucher preference, and they asked, "Are you breastfeeding?" I would exclaim, "Oh, absolutely." I let them believe we were using formula as a supplement by choice, lest I should humiliate myself further and let others know of my failure. They were satisfied.

I finally went to see the doctor, in early October. My prenatal care at Planned Parenthood was incredible, but my postnatal was severely lacking. Planned Parenthood only does one follow-up visit; then I was switched to

---

* See page 168 for a discussion of the limitations of manual breast pumps.

the crowded, unventilated city clinic as patient number 4936. My doctor was underpaid, overworked, and had no answers for me. She asked a series of questions, including, "What do you think about when you're breastfeeding?" and "Are you under any stress?"

No, Doc, I'm a twenty-two-year-old single mom just this side of the poverty line, and my breasts aren't fulfilling their womynly obligation—I'm not stressed at all!

She felt me up briefly and said, "There is nothing wrong with you. Just relax and keep trying. Next."

Well, she was wrong.

My breasts were broken. They were hardly producing milk at all. Everything I read and tried was fruitless, annoying, and unhelpful. All the wussy advice I got like, "Don't worry so much, you'll work it out," made me angry and snappy.

"Yeah, fuck you, your breasts aren't broken."

"Come on, breasts!" I pleaded. "You didn't give me an hourglass figure, you didn't give me cleavage, I never spited you for it. Could you do the one important thing you were made to do? Could you give me milk so I can feed my daughter?"

But by four months I was back waiting tables, and the bottle was more my adversary than ever before. I couldn't even pump an ample amount to store and give to the friend who ran the home day care in which we placed Madison. We dropped down to only feeding at night when she'd wake up, and I'd roll over to her, eager to get it right, to stimulate the milk production, to be the perfect mom.

Then the day came every mother hopes for—but the night I dreaded. Madison slept through the night. And after that, it was all over. She stopped breastfeeding altogether.

The WHO/UNICEF International Code (continued)

8. *All information on artificial feeding, including the labels, should explain the benefits of breastfeeding and the costs and hazards associated with artificial feeding.*
9. *Unsuitable products, such as sweetened condensed milk, should not be promoted for babies.*
10. *All products should be of a high quality and take into account the climatic and storage conditions of the country where they are used.*

These standards were adopted in 1981 by the World Health Assembly, a part of the World Health Organization, and the United States was the only one of 122 member countries to cast an oppositional vote. In 1994, the United States withdrew its objections to a resolution then being considered and thus, by default, fell into consensus agreement.

The Code does not have force of law, however, and regulations do not exist in the United States to restrict direct marketing to new mothers. Nor does legislation prohibit promotion via the healthcare system (Walker 2001, 7).

My daughter will be two next month. She drinks whole milk from regular cups and will eat everything in sight from sugar cookies to tofu. I look back on my story and still feel regret that I couldn't breastfeed longer, more efficiently. I'm sorry that my shame kept me from actively seeking more help.

But I laugh at the thought that I failed as a mother. I know there's a large group of people who want to label me the scourge of society because I am a single mom and assume I'm a white-trash welfare leech on crack. But I know that being a single mom means being fucking strong and powerful and blessed. And tired. But a contented tiredness.

After almost two years I have finally, truly embraced the fact that there is no perfect mother. I have days where I excel as the patient, caring, earth mother. And I have equal days when I am a worn-out, tired, twenty-four-year-old hag who does not want to watch another episode of *Blue's Clues* or be the in-home jungle gym. Overall, though, I am a great mother. And my daughter is as lucky to have me as I am to have her. She is not damaged or lacking. She is exceptionally bright, energetic, and blows my mind and makes me proud every day. As much as I wanted to breastfeed, as dire as it was to me, as important as it is to a child to have the nourishment of breast milk, I did my best. I did what I could. Then I forgave myself, and I moved on. My breasts still don't define me, not as a womyn and certainly not as a mother.

Written by Lacey Reneé Graham, Concord, CA

J. Hollander's story emerges out of a dysfunctional childhood characterized by emotional and sexual abuse. The middle child of an upper-middle-class family, she was ignored and neglected and, in a "not said out loud but we're thinking it" way, somehow blamed for her brother's cancer. While ultimately it was a lack of information that caused her to wean, her family and her first two husbands illustrate some of the challenges new mothers face when they themselves are not nurtured.

WHEN WINGING IT DOESN'T WORK

About three weeks after my daughter was born, we went to a formal wedding, and the baby stayed with Betty, a close friend of my husband's family. My daughter had already been sleeping through the night, so I guess I thought she'd sleep until morning. I came home at two or three A.M., and my breasts were full and painful. I was going to wake the baby, but Betty said,

"That baby woke up screaming at eleven P.M. I went down to the drugstore, bought bottles and Enfamil, and now she's sleeping soundly with a full belly."

So when I woke up the next morning at about nine A.M., I was torpedo tit, rock hard, hot to the touch, and sore. I tried hand expressing but couldn't get any milk out. I was so engorged that my daughter couldn't breast-feed and started screaming. Betty put a bottle into her mouth, and that was pretty much the end of it. I tried to breastfeed for another two weeks, sup-plementing with bottles, but it was all over. My daughter was no longer in-terested.

I went through torture drying up. Andy, my husband at the time, was pissed at me because he had visions of everything being all natural. He was very much into the image of being "different" and "bohemian." Of course, he didn't do a thing to help, but I didn't know any better.

Our relationship was horrendous. He was handsome, sophisticated, and urbane, but also cool, sinister, and steely. All during my pregnancy he told me I was fat and ugly. Within days of giving birth he wanted me to go on a starvation diet. He couldn't believe I could even live with myself.

That day after the wedding we went out for brunch with Betty before heading home. I was engorged and really sore. And Andy somehow hit me in the breast—I don't think it could have been an accident. It hurt so much. I can't believe that it still brings tears to my eyes. During the brunch he was making fun of me for eating because he thought I was so fat. Betty just looked at him and said, "How can you say that to her? She just had your baby!" I was devastated.

J. Hollander eventually divorced her husband, moved to New Hampshire, remarried, had another two children, and divorced again. She is now married to her third husband. None of her breast-feeding experiences was positive or well supported. Each time she supplemented early, her milk supply began to dry up immediately thereafter, and she was unable to express milk to rebuild her milk supply. She reflects on what happened.

I always think I might have been able to breastfeed successfully if I could have filled a bottle with some goddamn milk. After my second child, I bought a motorized pump but still couldn't express anything. I think if I could have *seen* some milk coming out, I would have known they were getting some.

The only time I ever saw milk was after I'd had my third child—she had stopped breastfeeding, but I just kept dripping.

I have been winging it my entire life. Breastfeeding was something I just couldn't wing. With what I know now I would have gotten some advice, stood on my own two feet a little more, and done a little more research.

Maybe if I'd had a supportive, well-meaning mother (or someone acting like a mother) to guide me through it, things would have been different. Maybe I thought something was wrong with my breasts because of all the mixed sexual messages I got growing up. Or maybe I had so much angst associated with boobs that there was no way something as natural as breastfeeding would work. I just don't know.

                                                                    J. Hollander

For those of us who have enjoyed a mutually satisfying nursing relationship, weaning is seldom as straightforward as it may seem. Some of us wean by choice; others have to wean *before* we are ready. The next two stories shed light on some of the reasons we bid our nursing bras adieu, even when it is something we don't want to do.

Emma conceived her first son after a year of undergoing fertility treatments. After spending her last ten weeks of pregnancy on bed rest for preterm labor, she gave birth to a five-pound baby who didn't latch on or suck well. She talks about the hard work of getting him to nurse and the painful process of having to wean him when he was six months old.

☕ A BIRD IN THE HAND

It took us four weeks until our son was able to nurse. We had schedules taped to the bedroom door of when to pump, when to feed him, and when he had wet and dirty diapers. His bedroom seemed more like a human milk factory than a nursery, with breast pump attachments, shells, shields, SNS's that we couldn't get to work, and breast pads everywhere! Between what I had to do to get the milk out of me and what my husband had to do to get it into him, every feeding was a two-person job.

I became increasingly desperate to nurse my tiny son. Every time someone would raise the issue of why I was killing myself, why I would get up every two hours to pump milk, why I would do oral-motor stimulation exercises with my finger in his mouth to help him develop a stronger suck and better latch, I would be reduced to tears. But at four weeks, on the verge of conceding defeat, I put him to my breast to cuddle, and he did it! It was like somebody had turned on a light switch for him. It was one of those "Eureka!" moments, and I knew then that everything would fall into place.

After that, things went relatively smoothly. I could finally feed him by myself and feel like I was *his* mom and not the pump's. Our nursing relationship fell into a nice rhythm during my last four weeks of a three-month maternity leave, after which I returned to work, pump in hand. Our nursing relationship adapted, and my son thrived.

My plan from the beginning was to nurse for six months. I was thirty-seven when he was born, and we didn't want him to be an only child. It had taken us a year to conceive, and we had no idea how long it would take us to conceive again. My infertility doctor had said, "Don't even think of coming back to me until three months after you quit nursing."*

I began to wean him according to our plan. Each week I cut out one feeding and pumping session. Then I gave up the morning feeding, and the last thing that went was the nighttime one.

So there I was, my last week of nursing. I had worked so hard to get my son to nurse, and everything was going so well. "Why rock the boat?" I thought. "I'm enjoying it, my son is thriving, and expressing my milk at work makes it easier for me to be away during the day." I just wasn't psychologically ready to quit. I loved nursing him, perhaps more so because of our initial struggle. Before he was born, I ate and drank and could feel him grow and develop inside me. Now I ate and drank and could watch him grow and develop in front of my own eyes. It was amazing.

All of this seemed reason enough to change the original plan. Besides, our nursing baby was "a bird in the hand." There would be no guarantee that the second child would ever come to be. My son and I could pay this price, give up our nursing relationship prematurely, and get no little brother or sister in return. My husband was more optimistic. I think he was less able to understand the joys nursing brought me or the pain weaning was causing me. But in the end, we agreed to stick with the plan.

---

* It is well-known that breastfeeding lowers the likelihood of becoming pregnant. In fact, some women rely on it as a temporary form of birth control. Known as "the lactational amenorrhea method," or LAM, it is most effective for women who have not yet resumed their periods, whose baby is less than six months old, and who are exclusively breastfeeding day and night. Although formula-feeding mothers can ovulate as early as three weeks postpartum, mothers who meet the criteria listed here have less than a 2 percent chance of ovulating (Vekemans 1997).

I had always nursed my son before bedtime. After he fell asleep in my lap, I would hold him for a while and then move him to his crib. After a week of feeding him only before bed, I knew this was the last time. I could tell you the exact date. I wanted to savor those ten or twenty minutes, but I was so sad. I just sat there and wept through the whole feeding. I was so upset for not being able to enjoy it. My son is now five, and even though I know the happy ending to my story, I still can't talk about that feeding without crying.

I spent the next three months depressed. Much of it had to do with the pressure to wean him, and I was all too aware that we might not be able to have another child. All the awful stuff we'd gone through during that year of fertility treatments came pouring back to me. It was a miserable time.

Eventually, though, we went back to the reproductive endocrinologist. I got pregnant right away, and it felt like a miracle. I said, "This baby is nursing until he's ready to stop or until *I* am. There isn't going to be any artificial timetable."

Unlike my first pregnancy, this one was uneventful. My son was bigger and stronger and didn't have a sick mother when he was in utero. I remember sitting in the delivery room, nursing him, and just weeping. Not only did I have another baby, but he was healthy and nursed immediately, just like in all the books.

Again, I went back to work when he was three months old and expressed milk until he was a year. At fourteen months, he suddenly weaned himself. Before putting him to sleep one night, I tried to nurse him, as I usually did, but he wasn't interested. The next morning he still didn't want to nurse. I continued to offer for a week, and then I finally got the message that he wasn't interested anymore. It felt less awful than when I so artificially weaned his older brother, but it caught me by surprise. I had anticipated natural baby-led weaning to be a more gradual process, and I missed it.

To her surprise, Emma went on to have a third child, another boy, who was born prematurely and was not able to nurse exclusively until he was six weeks old. He was sixteen months old and still nursing when we spoke, but getting him to nurse was very challenging. (See her story on pages 110–12.) In reflecting on nursing her three sons, Emma, a medical doctor, says:

I'm a well-established, professional woman with a successful career. I never considered not going back to work, but I grossly underestimated how physically taxing and psychologically hard being a working mother would be. I also think that when one goes through fertility treatments there are a lot of psychological issues involved in wondering if your body is failing you, issues involving your femininity and womanhood. Nursing my babies put those concerns to rest and helped me begin to make peace with that experience.

If you were to ask me today what my biggest life accomplishment has been, I'd say it's having nursed my babies. Five years ago, I couldn't have imagined that anything in the realm of nursing or motherhood would even be on that list.

Emma, Brooklyn, NY

In this next story, Elizabeth talks about her daughter's sudden refusal to nurse. Nursing strikes are usually a baby's way of communicating that something is wrong, that he or she is unhappy, in pain, or bothered by something. While it is easy to interpret this behavior as a desire to wean, weaning typically happens gradually, whereas nursing strikes come on suddenly. Lasting anywhere from a couple of days to as long as two weeks, nursing strikes can happen for many reasons. A good how-to breastfeeding book will contain helpful suggestions for how to understand and, hopefully, overcome them. (See, e.g., La Leche League International's *The Womanly Art of Breastfeeding*, [2004].)

JUST WHEN IT WAS GETTING GOOD

After six months or so, just when I was beginning to enjoy breastfeeding, my daughter went on a nursing strike. She'd been sleeping well, but one night she woke up several times. I tried to nurse her, but she didn't want to. I gave her a pacifier and rocked her back to sleep. The next morning she still refused to nurse. I waited a while and tried again. She refused. We went to the doctor later that day, thinking maybe she had an ear infection, but she had absolutely no health problems.

For two days, she didn't eat. She wasn't used to taking a bottle, and she refused to nurse. I'd never heard of a nursing strike, and this just hit me out of the blue. I received lots of different advice. For two or three days we tried feeding her out of a cup, but she wasn't getting enough to eat. I worried that she was going to get dehydrated. And it felt like I was withholding food from her until I could break her spirit to get her to nurse again. Eventually, I de-

Relactation

Although it is not common knowledge, women who have weaned can often relactate. Motivations vary, explains Nancy Morhbacher, IBCLC. Some women do so for the milk itself; others care less about their output than they do about the breastfeeding relationship. For a helpful article on relactation, see "Can There Be Breastfeeding after Weaning?" at <http://www.artofbreastfeeding.com>.

cided against fighting her. I went to a bottle and ended up pumping until she was a little over a year. For about a week I was pumping every two hours around the clock to get my supply back.

I hated pumping. Her refusal to nurse felt like a huge rejection, and having to pump all the time was a reminder of it. It was even harder for me because she quit just when I was starting to enjoy nursing. I cried for many days, and it still makes me sad. It's funny. I think I'm okay, and then when people ask questions I realize I still have issues about it. It was just a shock. Not knowing what was going on made me feel like someone had died. I really went through a grieving process.

Elizabeth Butler, Westminster, CO

My Child, Myself

Early on in this book's development, I gathered half a dozen women—none of whom were still breastfeeding—to write about our breastfeeding experiences. After an hour of writing, we read our pieces aloud. I was struck by how emotional two of the women became. One of them, through her tears, couldn't get through it and asked me to take over. Thinking about this makes me realize how little time and space women take to reflect on what nursing has meant for us. It affects us profoundly.

From the moment we give birth, we begin the poignant process of differentiation and separation. Weaning, of course, is part of this. We know that the natural and healthy road our children must take means they become increasingly independent of us, and assisting them along that path is one of our main responsibilities. But at the same time, we may be reluctant to let go of that never-to-be-repeated time when we share such an embodied intimacy, when our very bodies meet their deepest needs.

In this next group of stories women reflect on the impact of weaning, not simply for their children but for themselves. Some are written by women still nursing and others by women looking back. Some come from women who *actively* weaned, others from women who practiced child-led or natural weaning—that is, who trusted their children to know when they were ready to move on. The commonality linking these stories is an understanding of weaning as an ongoing process—sometimes two steps forward and one step back—but ultimately arriving at the same destination.

In Their Own Words:
My Child, Myself

Susan, a high school guidance counselor, speaks to the embodied, physical relationship that breastfeeding creates, even when our nursing days are behind and our children no longer remember how to nurse.

☕ CONFESSIONS OF AN EX-NURSER

Nursing was Cody's first love. "I pledge allegiance to my tit," we imagined him saying. Yesterday his dad watched him slowly wake up, sucking away, as if he were still nursing, his lips moving bunny-like, puckering in and out. Often at night when we check on him we hear little sucking, smacking sounds.

Last week, Cody, getting close to his third birthday, wanted us to reenact his birth for him, something we've done many times. We'll be cozily reading a book together, and he'll snuggle up and say, "I want to go back in your belly." I'll lift up my shirt, and he'll crawl underneath. "Tell the story," he says, so we do.

"Your mommy and daddy were so excited they were going to have you. As the nine months went by, you grew bigger and bigger, and in the middle and later months I could feel you inside me—sometimes moving like a fish (there is swimming going on under my shirt), sometimes kicking (Cody is kicking under my shirt), sometimes resting (a few fidgets). You grew bigger and bigger, and then on November 9th you were ready to be born. We went to the hospital. Luke's mommy was there, and so were Judy and Tammy. We were so excited. On the way out, you got a little stuck, and the doctor helped you out, and we all said, "'It's a boy!'" (Cody emerges from my shirt all excited and sweaty and then tells how Daddy cut his umbilical cord and he got weighed and washed up and then he got to nurse, at which point I usually try to distract him and explain that my milk is gone.)

Last week he really wanted to try to nurse, so we did. He stopped at one point and said, "I'm really nursing!" and continued until I said that was enough. Cody then asked if he could nurse on the other side and proceeded to do the same. Again, I told him that was enough. The next day I walked around with tender nipples, almost like they had been at the beginning of nursing, from my not-so-little nurser, who wishes he could still nurse and wasn't up for distractions until I told him it was his turn to nurse his bear. He gently picked it up but then started yelping in frustration: "Mommy, I can't find my nipples. They're gone!"

I explained that he still had them, they were just smaller. He nursed his bear on one side of him, then turned him to the other side and decided to let the bear suck on his belly. "Mommy, when I grow up, my nipples are going to be as big as yours. No, they're gonna be bigger!"

If I could do it all over again, I'd nurse for longer. Seventeen months was too short a period for my little guy. Was that trip to Zydeco Cajun Land Louisiana really worth it?

Written by Susan, Trumansburg, NY

Each of my children has helped me better follow my instincts in terms of when, how much, and how often they need to eat. I weaned my first child at seven months. He bit me, so I quit. I broke that bond way too early. He's almost nine, and I still struggle to remain close to him. I nursed my second for nine months. I'm embarrassed to admit this now, but it was summer and I didn't want to have him on me when it was so hot. My third child nursed for about nineteen months. He seemed ready to quit and didn't notice when I took away that last nighttime feeding. My fourth child nursed until she was about two, when I weaned her because I was already pregnant with my fifth and was having severe digestive problems. I felt that my body needed to be done nursing so I could concentrate on the new baby. This baby, now, I'll nurse until I get pregnant again or until she's ready to stop.

Amy Snyder, Sardis, OH

Barbara is one of many women who expressed the ambivalence that often accompanies nursing. An assistant professor of environmental engineering, she recounts the carefully implemented strategy to wean her son.

MY BABY IS WEANED

My baby just turned three years old. I know it's time to admit he's not really a baby anymore, but in my heart he always will be. It's also time to admit that he is weaned. Frankly, I never thought I would manage to wean him. He's a determined child and extremely persistent about trying to get what he wants. But nursing had become less enjoyable, and with a new baby on the way and feeling that I couldn't simultaneously handle nursing, a demanding full-time job, and pregnancy, I felt it was time to wean.

We started by giving Andrew four pennies each day, which he could exchange for nursings, and we told him he could put any leftover pennies into his piggy bank, which he loves to do. The first day, he nursed twice and put two pennies into his bank. I was devastated, thinking he was going to wean right away, and I didn't feel mentally prepared yet. I had expected that weaning might bring some mixed feelings, but the intensity of it was a surprise. I needn't have worried, though, because after that he was burning every penny he had. Only one more ever found its way into the bank. The thing that amazed me, though, was that once his pennies were gone, he fully accepted that there would be no more "mama" for the rest of the day.

We were astounded! Andrew has never been one to gracefully accept waiting even two minutes for his precious "mama"! (This has often gotten us funny comments from people when he would shriek, "I want mama! I want mama!" and people would say, "She's right there!") I must admit that I did feel a bit cheap, but since the system was working I put up with feeling like a hooker for a while. Fortunately, Andrew didn't understand the concept of money well enough to feel that he was actually "buying" his mama. To him, the pennies were just tokens, and exchanging them when he wanted gave him some power over the weaning process.

Andrew's first nursing was usually before we got out of bed, after which he usually went back to sleep. Not wanting to wake him up more, I never fussed with the pennies for that session. I just told him he'd already used up one penny and gave him three when he got downstairs. After about two weeks, I chose a morning when he hadn't woken up to nurse in bed and still gave him only three pennies for the day. He never seemed to notice that he was getting fewer nursings. Two weeks later, I again chose another morning without nursing in bed and cut him back to two pennies a day. Again, no complaint.

I knew that going to one penny a day would be tougher because his wake-up mamas were like his morning cup of coffee. He often nursed once in bed, went back to sleep, and then nursed again when he woke up for good. Again, I chose a day when he didn't nurse in bed and had no trouble cutting him back to one penny.

The next day, though, after he used his only penny in bed, the shit hit the fan when he woke up for the day. I brought him downstairs and tried to distract him with kids' early-morning television shows. This worked like a charm until a commercial came, when Andrew would start yelling, "I want mama! I want mama!" until the next episode came on—not a parenting scene I remember with pride. Eventually he accepted some water, and I went off to get ready for work. Each morning got a little easier until he eventually gave up nursing in bed so he could have his mama when he woke up for the day.

The next challenge was for him to give up that last nursing. We waited until I had a three-day trip. On the morning I left, after Andrew's last nursing, I came downstairs in tears, knowing it was probably his last, ever.

The first day after I returned, Brian got him out of bed, and he never even asked to nurse. We optimistically thought weaning might be easier than we had thought, but the second day he wanted it, and he wanted it *now!* It was a repeat of the yelling scene during television commercials, but again we got through it. Each day got easier, and eventually he stopped asking for it at all.

Two weeks after Andrew's last nursing all those emotions came storming into the open when we were singing "Happy Birthday" to him and I couldn't stop crying. I'm still crying as I write this. I tend to hide my emotions and think I'm doing fine until something triggers them to come swarming out.

Despite the fact that my husband stays home with him, I have always been the one Andrew comes to for comfort and support. I attribute that to breastfeeding. He never had a blanket or a stuffed animal for comfort, just mama. Even the name he chose, mama, epitomizes how wrapped up his nursing is in our relationship. I fear that we may become more distant. He's never been particularly affectionate, and his nursing sessions were one of the few times he had for cuddles.

Lately, though, Andrew has been asking for "snuggles" when he would have asked for mama. He sits in my lap with his knees tucked under his chin, and I wrap my arms around him and rock him gently. I find it immensely satisfying, in some ways more so than nursing, since he doesn't fidget or bite like he did.

I suppose if Andrew had eventually self-weaned I would have had the same fears and emotions—they just would have surfaced later. It's all a natural part of children growing up and slowly moving away from us.

Written by Barbara Spang Minsker, Urbana-Champaign, IL

LISTENING TO HER DAUGHTER

My daughter, Hannah, was almost three the first time she promised to wean on her birthday. Well, her birthday came and went that year—and the

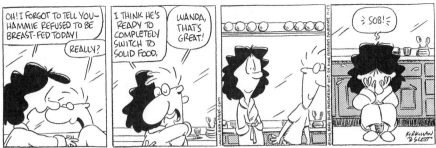

© Baby Blues Partnership. Reprinted with special permission of King Features Syndicate.

next—without her losing interest in having "na-na." As she became more verbal, we had a number of discussions about why she wanted to continue and when she would wean. She taught me about what it meant to her, so I decided not to make her stop before she was ready. Each year when I reminded her of her promise to stop, she convincingly conveyed to me how important it was to her and asked if it was okay to continue. I let her.

Weaning was very gradual. As Hannah grew from three to five, she developed a larger and more secure repertoire of coping mechanisms. She learned to deal with her upsets by talking them out, acting them out in play, etc., and didn't need to be comforted at the breast as much. Still, nursing was like a magic formula (pun intended!) for being able to comfort an upset, overtired, cranky four-year-old and for dissolving tears, whining, and grouchiness.

Eventually I wanted Hannah to stop because nursing had become unpleasant. She began to get careless with my breasts, engaging in annoying acrobatics with my nipple in her mouth and generally treating me with disrespect. So despite my commitment to "child-led weaning," I decided it was time for Hannah to stop. About three months before her fifth birthday, I started talking with her about giving up na-na when she turned five. She agreed. I also felt that it was important for her to learn to keep her word.

On the day before her birthday, we made a little fuss over her last nursing and took some pictures. The next day, she asked to nurse in the evening. When I reminded her of our agreement, she whined and complained for about five minutes, then seemed to accept that I was going to hold her to her word. She complained again each night for two more nights. In the three months since then, she has not asked to nurse and hasn't expressed any disappointment. I feel proud of my daughter, first for having stuck to her guns and making me recognize her need to continue, and second for letting go of it when she didn't need it anymore.

J. Rachael Hamlet, Falls Church, VA

The theme of continuity, of nursing as a way to maintain the physical, tangible connection with our babies, emerged even for women who weaned long ago. It is as if having nursed them, our relationship is forever altered. Kathleen, who nursed in the 1970s (see her story on pages 16–20), reveals that weaning is a never-ending process.

AFTER ALL THESE YEARS

Lately, I've been dreaming a lot about my son, Ian. He's twenty-six and living in Manhattan. He's a drummer and, like a lot of performers and actors, supports himself by waiting tables and with other service-sector jobs. I spoke to him on the telephone recently, and there was a question about him having enough money. I was wondering whether or not I should offer to give him something; he doesn't like to ask, and he sometimes refuses when I offer. I didn't want to hurt his pride, but I remember hanging up and feeling as if I should have been a little more forceful about it. That was on my mind when I went to bed and had this dream:

> I'm holding a baby, a boy with a sweet, round face and intelligent eyes. I suddenly realize this is *my* baby and I forgot I had him. I am startled, almost frightened, as I wonder, "Who's been caring for him? Who's been feeding him?" I ask Jack, my husband.
> "I've been changing him and things like that," he says.
> "But have you been feeding him?" I ask.
> "No. Haven't you?" he answers.
> "No. I've forgotten. I forgot to breastfeed him!"
> Immediately I bare one breast. I can feel the pull and tingle. The baby sucks for a few minutes, then stops. He releases the nipple and looks at me, confused. "I don't think he knows how to nurse," I say to Jack. I keep trying. One breast, then the other. Each time the baby nurses for only a minute or two. I wonder if I have any milk. Maybe it dried up. I try to express the milk, and a little spray appears. I am relieved. I think if I nurse the baby a lot now, the supply will increase, but he won't nurse except in that start-again, stop-again way.
> As I'm holding him, I can feel how light he is, and he's getting lighter and lighter in my arms. His little hand when he curls his fingers around my finger is shriveling. His face is puckering, his round cheeks thinning. His eyes, nose, and mouth are bunching together like a

dried-apple doll's face. I tell Jack to call the doctor. While he looks for her name in the phone book (since neither of us is sure of it) I think about going to the health-food store and buying baby food. Even in this emergency, I'm aware that I don't want to give it to him. I think of the first solid food of some nursing babies—mashed banana—and I'm distraught to realize that we don't have any.

Jack is still leafing through the phone book. Suddenly I'm aware there is another child in the room. It is our son, Ian, who, in the dream, is seven or eight. I carry the baby in the crook of my arm and wander around the house talking with Ian. I notice many surprising things about our house, especially the furnishings. I hate all these changes, but somehow I know it won't matter what I say and that I'll just have to get used to them being there.

I go to a back door, mostly glass, and realize there is snow and frost caking the inside and all around the frame. Still balancing the baby, who is limp and silent, I try to scrape the snow off the door. I clear one long stripe of glass to see outside. Then the door swings open, and I see Jack and Ian outside on the lawn with a sled. Ian is saying he's afraid. Jack is trying to encourage him: "Here. I'll do it first," he says. He does a belly-whopper on the sled—pushing himself forward down the slope, hard, with his feet. I see that the slope is only partly covered with snow. There is bright green grass and thick brown mud, and Jack's sled grinds to a halt before it reaches the bottom. Ian is watching silently from the top of the little slope. I look on from the open door, the baby still limp, silent, and small in the crook of my arm. And then the dream ends.

I'm no expert on dreams, but I think nursing is such an interesting metaphor for supply. Like many parents, I worry about my children's ability to provide materially for themselves in today's economic climate. I worry about them having enough—because they struggle—and I sometimes feel that it is my responsibility to provide for them, and I feel conflicted about that. When do I offer? How much is enough? The questions are the same now as they were about breastfeeding, all those years ago.

I wonder if it's any harder for a mother who has provided complete physical sustenance for her infant to let go of feeling responsible for continuing to provide some kind of support. I don't know. Probably not. It's probably hard for any parent.

Kathleen Kramer, Newfield, NY

While the next story is not about weaning per se, it speaks profoundly to the depth of the nursing experience. It is almost as if nursing represents the true heart of mothering.

 ## TRANSCENDING MEMORY LOSS

I went with my husband's family to visit his aunt in a nursing home. Since there were a lot of us, we took turns, and there were some extended periods of time during which we waited in the front visiting room. A resident of the nursing home, who must have been in her eighties, came and sat down beside me. She pointed to a woman next to her and whispered to me, "I don't know who this woman is, but she's very nice and comes to visit me."

So this other woman tucked her hand around, held it out to me, and said, "Hello, I'm Margaret. I'm her daughter." She then put her hand on her mother's shoulder and said, "I'm Margaret. I'm your daughter. Remember me?"

The woman nodded. A moment later, though, she turned back to me and said again, "I don't remember who this woman is, but she's very nice."

I asked her how many children she had, thinking if I could get her to reach into some deeper memories, she might remember her. She told me she had three children. I then asked if she had breastfed them. I believe breastfeeding memories are very strong, very powerful.

She replied, "Oh, yes. I nursed all my children. I didn't think my last little one, Margaret, would ever wean. She must have been three or four. We lived on a farm, and she would come running out to me when I was milking the cow and ask to nurse, and I would stop to nurse her. I would be hoeing in the garden, and she would come running out for milk, and I would stop and nurse her." She gave me a couple more examples that I can't remember.

I looked up, and there was her Margaret, tears streaming down her face. Her mother couldn't remember who she was, but she had wonderful memories of nursing her as a child.

I think this is such a wonderful illustration of the power and impact breastfeeding has in a woman's life, so powerful that it even transcends memory loss. There are very few things that can do that. Our culture just doesn't realize how valuable it is to us.

Cathy Liles, TX

Honoring a Milestone

Birthdays and graduations, confirmations and bar/bat mitzvahs—all are publicly recognized milestones and opportunities for celebration. But too often in our busy lives, we fail to honor the less public moments and transitions, less showy, perhaps, but no less meaningful and important. Weaning falls into this latter category. Nursing had been so central to my relationship with my first daughter that when I weaned her at three years and four months, I felt I had to find a way to put closure on this significant era in our lives. I was five months pregnant, and Emily was about to become a big sister, but I didn't know how to mark this important change in our relationship.

One afternoon I wandered into a small gift shop. I was gazing at the jewelry when I saw a pendant so perfect that I found myself in the embarrassing position of trying to hide my tears from the salesclerk. It was an abstract representation, in silver, of a mother bent over her child, as if she were nursing. Less than an inch around, it touched my heart, and I knew instantly I had to have it.

But buying the necklace wasn't enough. I decided not to give myself permission to wear it until I wrote Emily a letter. Back home that evening, I sat down and wrote about our nursing relationship, from the difficulty of getting her started to the difficulty of getting her to stop. It was filled with anecdotes, memories, and reflections on who she was and who she was becoming. I acknowledged the changes that were happening and shared with her my hopes for her future. I wrote nine pages. Then I read it over, had a good cry, sealed it, and put on the necklace. Someday, when Emily is grown up and hopefully has a child of her own, I will give her both the letter and the necklace.

Three and a half years later, when I weaned Rachel, I again felt the importance of acknowledging her growing independence. But our nursing relationship had been less central, less sensual. And having nursed for a total of almost seven years, I was not weaning with ambivalence. I didn't feel the need to *process* in quite the same way. I would write her a letter and find an appropriate memento on another occasion. Instead, I took her to a local bakery to celebrate. Ironically and humorously appropriately, I thought, she chose a cookie shaped like a cow. She called them "moo-cow cookies."

These last stories acknowledge the passing of an era. They come from women who found ways to help their children celebrate their growing independence and honor their changing relationship. The possibilities are endless, and I hope they will be inspirational, helping us all to rethink the ways in which we honor and recognize the value and worth of our experiences.

MOTHER'S DAY, 1996

I had sort of targeted three years as the time to wean. I believed in nursing on demand and did that until Jesse was about one and a half, but because of various health problems I was having, I decided to wean him at two and a half. A friend of ours, who had weaned at age four, had a "bye-bye tittie party." So we decided to have a "bye-bye ba party" since his name for breast was "ba." It was the whole idea of making it celebratory: "Boy, you've grown, and growing up means all these great things."

At the time, Jesse was typically nursing three times a day—morning, nap time, and evening. First we gave it up at nap time by putting on tapes and trying to get him to gentle down in a different way. Then I said, "When babies grow up, they don't nurse anymore. Imagine Mommy still nursing with Grammy. Imagine Daddy nursing with Nana." He thought that was funny. So I said, "We're going to pick a day when it will be bye-bye ba, but first we'll pick a date to give up one nursing."

Jessie chose to give up the morning. He continued to come into our bed and ask to nurse, but we would say, "No. No more. We agreed not to." He complained a little, but then we would tickle or cuddle him or toss him in the air. Even though it was sometimes too early and we weren't awake, we tried to make it a good time for him.

Two or three more weeks went by until the final "bye-bye ba." Even though Jesse didn't know anything about dates, we looked at the calendar together, and I let him pick the date, believing he needed to be part of family decisions that affected him. He happened to pick May 12. Mother's Day. So bittersweet. I was sad about this, I really was. I don't want it to sound like it was so mechanical, because it wasn't. It was heartbreaking.

We tried to think of something that would signify a passage or coming-of-age ritual. My husband says it was more for me, but I think on some level Jesse understood that growing up means *leaving* things but also coming into things and abilities. So we decided to get him a tricycle. I drew a calendar. He wanted cupcakes, so I added those, and we'd count down the days by putting X's on them. The day before, he said eagerly, "Tomorrow's "bye-bye ba day!" Our kid had become excited about it! We'd made it into a big, fun thing.

During that night, that last nursing, he was all excited about "bye-bye ba" day. He had done such a good job, and there I was weeping all over him!

When I left his room, it was like closing the door on something so beautiful that you never can go back to. I wrote in my journal for a long time. Pages.

So we had "bye-bye-ba" day, and weaning was successful in that it wasn't traumatic for him. This was a kid who loved nursing yet never asked to do it again. But the significance of it was unbelievable—such clarity that we are on separate roads. Who knows who he'll be? He's just on his way, wherever he's going.

But of course I want that closeness back. I never had with my husband the degree of intimacy, that deep-soul connection that I had while nursing. It's a look into a human connection that's precious, rare, and brief. The selfish part of me would love my son to be a baby forever. But I realize it's important for him to have his independence, and I'm glad he's on his road.

Kate Gefell, Ithaca, NY

Kate, who did go on to have a second child, a girl, has a related story (see pages 221–22) about the changes and challenges of intimacy.

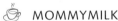

I realized my daughter wasn't going to stop nursing unless I did something about it, and I was getting social pressure to stop. I figured I had to choose a day, so I chose Independence Day. I said, "Honey, this is it. Mommy's milk is drying up, and we have to choose a time to stop nursing. This seems like a good day. It's Independence Day, and from now on you will be independent of me."

Bara Hotchkiss, Trumansburg, NY

☕ MOMMYMILK

Since my first baby latched on to my breast, more than nine years ago, we have always called it "mommymilk." It has been a part of our household and vocabulary for so long that it was a startling thought to me that at some point we might rarely use the word again. I wonder how many words are like that: used for a certain time in one's life and then no longer needed.

One day, there I was, efficiently starting to defrost the freezer, when I was suddenly taken aback by the sight of six Baggies of frozen mommymilk stored in the freezer door for more than a year, for those just-in-case times when Mommy might have to rush out and someone might need to eat. They had been there so long I no longer noticed them when I reached in for frozen corn or peas. Yellowish, hardened, long lumps. Dates written on the side in black marker. Closed with green and white striped twisty ties. Lined up next to the cans of frozen apple juice.

I felt paralyzed. I closed the door, leaned against it, and could not go on with my job. I thought about the tiny mouths that had once cried for that milk: toothless, hungry mouths; open like baby birds' beaks waiting for their worms. I recalled the minutes I had spent hand-expressing it, amazed at the fountains that poured into the measuring glass I usually used. I remembered once counting the sprays and finding ten tiny spouts in my nipple that released the milk. Amazing. I sat down against the freezer and reflected on the ways those three babies decided, all very differently, that they were done with mommymilk.

My daughter, Julia, initiated me into the world of mommymilk. What a magical place. I loved that I fed Julia with myself, that I produced and stored and offered the food and that she knew, from the first moment, how to take it. What a perfect arrangement. My breasts became regulated: they filled, I ached, Julia cried and emptied them. My body became both a clock and a prison. My connection with Julia was binding: I loved that she needed me; I hated to have to be there at her whim.

Julia stopped nursing at fifteen and a half months. One night she asked for mommymilk, bit my nipple, squeezed my breast with her hand, and cried. Was she angry with me because she was becoming aware of how much she needed me? For several nights afterward, I'd put her to my breasts, she'd nurse a bit, then bite and cry. Was I not making enough milk anymore? Other than in the evenings, Julia seemed fine, but I felt very upset. I wasn't ready to stop nursing! I felt guilty that I had cut out other feedings and hadn't let her wean herself: was she punishing me? I wasn't ready to let go of her as my baby, as someone who needed me in this special way, of our alone time every night, of my ability to soothe and comfort her. Suddenly I was just like my husband: just one of her two parents. It was like losing the use of a limb: my breasts grew smaller, and I knew that soon my milk would be gone. How could I let this resource dry up? I felt I should go feed starving babies somewhere. I could remember when I was so heavy I ached and dripped milk; soon I would have just breasts.

An entry from my journal:

You play, experiment, pull up my shirt and touch a breast and say, "Ma Ma!" delighted by your game of "Baby": you open your mouth and play, closing but not latching on, licking, pretending, then "No!" and onto another toy. It breaks my heart. And yet I know there could be no better way to wean: you decided, you took control, you chose independence. I respect that. I miss my baby.

Weeks later, I still had milk. I kept squeezing and getting milk and wanting to wail.

Less than two years later, two little boys arrived, and I was once again wealthy beyond measure. Ezra was voracious, chewing insanely on his fists and panting, wild-eyed, when he saw me; his brother, Noah, was sleepy, accepting milk when it was offered and perfectly content to do other things if he needed to wait a bit. In the wee hours of the morning, all alone with two babies, I once again had that intimacy like no other: just us, in the dark and quiet living room, their mouths attached to my body.

I was their life force.

They grew. They nursed together in football positions on my half-circle nursing pillow, their little fists against my breasts, heads touching one another. They grew some more. The passionate one slowed down in his hunger but clung to me, content only when I was within his view. The dreamy one giggled at the world and accepted any and all offers to entertain him, even if it meant missing nursing. After a few years, they almost always nursed in the same position: Ezra lying across my lap and Noah laying his head on Ezra's lap. Ezra often stroked Noah's hair as they nursed, and frequently one would stop nursing for a moment to tell the other something or to ask if he would shift a bit to make things more comfortable.

Noah gradually lost interest in nursing, and by age two and a half, his was a perfunctory sip, an I-don't-want-to-be-left-out gesture. He found nursing pleasant—he got to lie there while his head got stroked—but it wasn't a life-or-death thing for him, like it was for Ezra, who had always nursed with full concentration, intensity, and relish.

Before bed, Ezra would call, "Noah, it's momo time!" Noah, building a tower or enthralled by a book, would answer, distractedly, "I'm coming . . ." but make no move, so Ezra would latch on and nurse alone, completely content. He was always looking up at me, and when he'd smile, he'd break his latch-on and I'd spurt milk all over. Then he'd get right back on.

Ezra stopped nursing at thirty-eight months. When he stopped asking for momo, I felt torn. Because he was old enough to talk about it and because it had been such a meaningful activity for us, I wanted to find a way to mark this incredibly significant transition in both of our lives. And yet that felt like it was my need and not his. How did I expect him to stop? A strong, "No!" like his sister? A preoccupied "I don't want momo" like his brother? I felt shaken by Ezra's unconsciousness. I worried that he would be devastated to suddenly realize he couldn't go back.

An entry from my journal:

Sweet Ezra in my arms. I said to you, "Ez, I noticed that you haven't had momo for a while—it seems like you're done."

"No," you said, " I'm not." Sucked, hardly any milk. "I think you're getting to be so big that there are other things you're interested in. There are other ways to be close to Mommy." Put you on the other breast. Sucked. Afterwards I asked, "Was there much milk left?"

"No."

"Maybe this will be your last momo, Ez?"

"Yeah." A beat. "No. I will have momo other times."

"Okay, Ez. You can have some more other times."

And my milk dries up. Crackles. I kiss you, and you giggle. Then I run into my room to cry because you are so sensitive to my moods that I wouldn't want to confuse you with my tears. They are about me, about letting go. My milk stops flowing, and the tears take their place. My breasts weep salt tears.

I stood up and opened the freezer. After I finished the defrosting, I lined up the Baggies again, next to the frozen juice.

That night I told my ever-sensitive husband about the forgotten mommy-milk and how I had felt unable to throw it out. "Would you like to do a ceremony with the Baggies?" he asked. I told him I could not imagine a ritual that would speak to the ache, the emptiness I felt, knowing these were the last Baggies of my mommymilk ever. The milk in my breasts was gone. There was no need to say the word "mommymilk" ever again. The subject was dropped.

Some months later, we found ourselves talking with friends about my dilemma, joking about it but also expressing the depth of the feeling and exploring possibilities. What about thawing it and pouring it out while we talked about our children growing up? What about watering flowers? Maybe we could grow a particular plant using it as fertilizer, as some people do with their placenta. There must be some way we could find to honor the end.

It was after many ideas, some very wild, that my husband conceived of it. It seemed funny at first and met with a lot of laughter, but it began to grow, to blossom, in my mind. Yes, I said. I'm not kidding. Yes.

And so we created a sourdough starter. Sugar and flour and dry yeast topped off with Baggies of mommymilk. As anyone who is familiar with bread starter knows, the most special part about it is that the original batch can be handed down, literally, from generation to generation, because a small part of the very first batch will always be present in every other batch. You never finish it up; you just divide it and add on. And aren't our children the same, with mommymilk as their starter? All of us are living organisms that keep breaking into new parts.

We call it our mommymilk starter. I know now that there is no reason to banish the word from our home, because we will never reach a time in our lives when we no longer need such a life-sustaining, nurturing, special word. I love the idea of someone, someday, saying, "Oh, that bread? These pancakes? Those muffins? The recipe? Well, actually that was made from the sourdough starter with my great-great-great-grandmother's mommymilk."

How essential the legacy is, will be, to us all. And what delicious bread.

To Make Your Own Breast Milk Starter

2 ½ cups warm (110 degrees) breast milk
1 package (1 tablespoon) active dry yeast
2 cups all-purpose flour
1 tablespoon sugar

In a glass or ceramic bowl, soften the yeast in ½ cup breast milk. Stir in the remaining 2 cups breast milk, flour, and sugar. Cover loosely with a dish towel, and let stand at room temperature until bubbly. This may take up to ten days—the warmer the room, the quicker the fermentation. Stir two to three times a day. The starter will develop a strong sour odor as it ferments. When fermentation has occurred, refrigerate the starter until needed.

To keep the starter going: After using 1 cup of starter, add to the remaining ¾ cup water or breast milk, ¾ cup all-purpose flour, and 1 teaspoon sugar. Stir well. Let stand at room temperature until bubbly, at least one day. Cover and refrigerate. If not used within ten days, stir in 1 teaspoon of sugar. Repeat the addition of 1 teaspoon of sugar every ten days.

Written by Anjelina Citron, Bellingham, WA*

---

*A version of Anjelina's story originally appeared in *Mothering* 84 (Fall 1997).

Where Do We Go from Here?

Women lament the lack of narratives of women's lives, yet women's stories are all around us. We don't hear them because our perception is shaped by a culture that trivializes "women's talk" and devalues the passing down of female lore and wisdom.
Naomi Ruth Lowinsky, Stories from the Motherline

Imagine giving birth in a country where 99 percent of new mothers start off breastfeeding. Your baby does not receive supplemental formula in the hospital, and when you go home there are no samples in your discharge pack. In fact, formula advertisements are unheard of, and supermarkets only stock a limited supply because the demand for formula is so low.

Once home, you have a few concerns, so you open your phone book and locate a company called Breastfeeding Help. They give you the help you need.

Breastfeeding is going well, so you get together with two other nursing mothers at a local café. You enjoy your decaf latte, and no one asks you to nurse in the bathroom. No one even looks askance. It is simply a common assumption that if you have a baby, that baby nurses. You and your friends enjoy the camaraderie, meet for lunch often, and because you have ten months of maternity leave at full pay, you don't worry about how to pay for your meal.

Six months after giving birth, you are happily nursing, as are 80 percent of new mothers.

Now imagine that fewer than thirty-five years earlier, in this same country, breastfeeding was invisible, devalued, and rare. Bottle-feeding was the modern, hip feeding method, and doctors and formula companies promoted it heavily. Yet somehow, this huge cultural transformation had taken place in one or two generations.

This scenario is not my fantasy of a dramatic turn of events in the United States. (Well, it is, but that's beside the point!) Nor is it a utopian ideal that could never happen. In fact, it is an actual description of what took place in Norway beginning in 1970 (Alvarez 2003). To be sure, Norway has a highly educated, homogenous population with a government that provides high-quality social services. But it wasn't the government that initiated these changes—it was one mother, Elisabet Helsing, who set the ball rolling. As Margaret Mead once said, "Never doubt that a small group of thoughtful, committed citizens can change the world; indeed, it's the only thing that ever has."

So where do we start? After all, creating a true breastfeeding culture in the United States will involve nothing less than revolutionary change, change that will affect not simply breastfeeding but all of motherhood. But most mothers would gladly forego any number of pink, sentimental Mother's Day cards for true expressions of maternal value.

In her book *Misconceptions: Truth, Lies, and the Unexpected on the Journey to Motherhood,* feminist author Naomi Wolf concludes with a "Mother's Manifesto," a platform of broad goals to underlie a movement that would honor the realities of mothering. She argues for real flextime for mothers and fathers, family leave with pay, changes in federal benefits and policies to recognize and support the work of parenting, on-site day care, an overhaul of the birthing industry, and a push to bring children into the world of adults so women don't have to choose between family and earning a living (2001, 283–87). No simple agenda, but one clearly worth working for.

All of these changes would facilitate the right and ability to breastfeed. Until recently, however, and still today, breastfeeding has only flickered on the feminist cultural radar screen. Bernice L. Hausman, author of *Mother's Milk: Breastfeeding Controversies in American Culture* (2003), explores how various feminist scholars have argued that breastfeeding has become a criterion of good mothering, a social mandate that doesn't take into account women's diverse life circumstances. Indeed, one only has to read Barbara Ehrenreich and Deirdre English's *For Her Own Good: 150 Years of the Experts' Advice to Women* (1978) to understand why some women distrust and resent the expectation that they should alter their behavior to meet the latest scientific research findings.

But rather than thinking of breastfeeding as a medical imperative telling women what they *must* or *should* do, the fundamental issue is really that women should have the *right* to do it. Of course, one-size-fits-all advice is inappropriate and counterproductive. And clearly women should not be *coerced* to breastfeed nor sequestered from the public sphere to do so. But as long as we have the right to bear a child, we should have the right to nurse that child without apology, not simply because it matters to our babies and children but because it also matters to *us* and to the kind of parent-child relationships we want to create. Some of us are fortunate to live in communities where health care professionals are well-informed, nursing is common, and attitudes are open. But these conditions should extend beyond liberal college towns, progressive coastal cities, and other pockets of social acceptance.

Some of us can also afford private lactation consultants and have the wherewithal to be particular about our health care providers. But our ability to breastfeed should not depend on our income or investigative abilities. Nor should it depend on whether or not we have a private office.

There is a great need to challenge both the circumstances and the messages that surround mothering and nursing. Why can't we be sexual and maternal at the same time? Why can't we nurse for our own pleasure and not just that of our babies? Why should we have to choose between an income and our children's health? Besides, would it be so terrible if we leaked at the office? If someone heard the sound of our pump? If our suckling baby made ecstatic, guzzling sounds in public? If we nursed until our child was ready to stop?

The only way to create a breastfeeding culture is to take matters into our own hands. People don't *receive* rights; they fight for them. And we can do so on many fronts. One of the best places to begin is to help restore the links among pregnancy, childbirth, breastfeeding, and early parenting. For example, we can:

- Encourage local health care facilities to become designated as mother- and baby-friendly.

- Support midwives in their efforts for professional autonomy.
- Work to reverse trends that undermine breastfeeding, particularly the high rates of C-sections, epidurals, and in-hospital supplementation.
- Advocate for hospital-based policies that don't separate mothers and babies.

We can direct our efforts toward better and more accessible breastfeeding support and information. For example, we can:

- Educate health care providers who push formula and dispense poor information.
- Lobby insurance companies to pay for breast pumps, doula services, and lactation consultants.
- Join or create coalitions to establish milk banks in local communities.
- Help create breastfeeding drop-in centers where women can find professional support and other nursing mothers.
- Advocate for and participate in peer counselor programs.
- Volunteer to help support teen parents.

To improve women's ability to continue to nurse after going back to work, we can:

- Educate employers about corporate lactation policies and help to create them.
- Work for extended maternity leaves, better flextime options, and the creation of on-site nurseries.

Our efforts are limited only by our imagination and dedication.

Through it all, of course, we talk and share our experiences. In *The Myth of the Bad Mother,* Jane Swiggart asserts that without someone to listen and understand us, we feel devalued, silenced, and ignored: "This excruciating experience for mothers, of feeling unimportant and unseen, is much like the experience of infants whom no one loves, cares for, or mirrors. If no one is there to validate a child's deepest emotions and inner life, that child will not receive the feedback necessary for a sense of reality and a strong sense of self. The same is true of mothers" (1991, 12).

"When I was a child," adds Rachel Naomi Remen, author of *Kitchen Table Wisdom*, "people sat around kitchen tables and told their stories. We don't do that so much anymore" (1996, xxvii). This is not just a way of passing time, Remen explains, but a way to pass along wisdom. This is a real loss. Telling and listening to each other's stories can be healing. We realize we are not alone, that we have company as we travel along our parenting journeys.

Telling our stories is an act of power, of taking control of our own life, of helping other women in theirs. It is, above all, a starting point. My hope is that the stories in *The Breastfeeding Cafe* will give women the courage and permission to dispel myths, reveal secrets, and be honest. Diana Greer, whose story appears earlier in this book, talked about how difficult it is to explain parenting to her single friends. "How do you describe the color orange to someone who is blind?" she asked. So it is with nursing. May we all contribute to this overall description of the color orange.

Support and Information
on the Web

Shortly before this book went to press, I entered "breastfeeding" on google and got 1,700,000 hits. Overwhelming? Just a little. In addition to the index of sites and organizations listed on page xiii, the following sites are good places to start.

Articles, Advice, Encouragement, and Support

Breastfeeding Resources. The site of a breastfeeding mother who has put together a well-organized, comprehensive collection of over one thousand links to pretty much everything related to breastfeeding, including working and pumping, common problems and special circumstances, extended breastfeeding, weaning, parenting, advocacy, and much more. See <http://www.marie.org/bf/>.

Breastfeeding.com. Information, support and attitude. A collection of articles, features, and information and a good place to learn about pumps, nursing clothing, and more. The site also has a national directory of lactation consultants, a breastfeeding answer center, many breastfeeding-related message boards, advocacy links, and a sense of humor. See <http://www.breastfeeding.com>.

Australian Breastfeeding Association. A well-respected source of information for women (regardless of nationality!). See <http://www. breastfeeding.asn.au/>.

Promotion of Mother's Milk, Inc. (ProMom). A highlight of this site is the number of breastfeeding-related discussion forums. See <http://www.promom.org>.

Common Sense Breastfeeding Topics. Thoughtful, insightful handouts from lactation consultant Diane Wiessinger. See <http://www. wiessinger.baka.com/bfing/index.html>.

The Militant Breastfeeding Cult. A site for breastfeeding enthusiasts and activists, with many breastfeeding stories and an active forum. See <http://www.militantbreastfeedingcult.com>.

San Diego County Breastfeeding Coalition. Offers a collection of articles for families, as well as professionals, with information also available in Spanish and Chinese. Great links, too. See <http://www. breastfeeding.org/bfarticles.html>.

Other Helpful Sites

National Center for Chronic Disease Prevention and Health Promotion. Information about government programs, services, and policies that support and promote breastfeeding at federal and state levels. See <http://www.cdc.gov/breastfeeding>.

National Women's Health Information Center. Provides a wealth of health-related information, with a special section on breastfeeding. Text is also available in Spanish and Chinese. See <http://www. 4woman.gov/Breastfeeding/index.htm>.

References

AAP Work Group on Breastfeeding. 1997. Breastfeeding and the Use of Human Milk (RE9729). *Pediatrics* 100 (6): 1035–39.

Alvarez, Lizette. 2003. Norway Leads Industrial Nations Back to Breast-Feeding. *New York Times* (October 21).

Angier, Natalie. 1999. *Woman: An Intimate Geography.* Boston: Houghton Mifflin.

Apple, Rima D. 1987. *Mothers and Medicine: A Social History of Infant Feeding, 1890–1950.* Madison: University of Wisconsin Press.

Aptheker, Bettina. 1989. *Tapestries of Life: Women's Work, Women's Consciousness, and the Meaning of Daily Experience.* Amherst: University of Massachusetts Press.

Arms, Suzanne. 1994. *Immaculate Deception II: Myth, Magic, and Birth.* Berkeley: Celestial Arts.

Avery, Melissa D., Laura Duckett, and Carrie Roth Frantzich. 2000. The Experience of Sexuality during Breastfeeding among Primaparous Women. *Journal of Midwifery and Women's Health* 45 (3): 227–37.

Baumslag, Naomi, and Dia L. Michels. 1995. *Milk, Money, and Madness: The Culture and Politics of Breastfeeding.* Westport, CT: Bergin and Garvey.

Behrmann, Barbara. 2003. Reclamation of Childbirth. *Journal of Perinatal Education* 12 (3): vi–x.

Bergum, Vangie. 1989. *Woman to Mother: A Transformation.* Granby, MA: Bergin and Garvey Publishers.

———. 1997. *A Child on Her Mind: The Experience of Becoming a Mother.* Westport, CT: Bergin and Garvey.

Blakely, Mary Kay. 1994. *American Mom: Motherhood, Politics, and Humble Pie.* New York: Pocket Books.

Blum, Linda M. 1993. Mothers, Babies, and Breastfeeding in Late Capitalist America: The Shifting Contexts of Feminist Theory. *Feminist Studies* 19 (2): 291–311.

———. 1999. *At the Breast: Ideologies of Breastfeeding and Motherhood in the Contemporary United States.* Boston: Beacon Press.

Bove, C. F. 1996. Sociocultural Environments and "Ways of Knowing" as Breastfeeding Determinants in Socioeconomically Disadvantaged Women. PhD. diss., Department of Nutrition, Cornell University, Ithaca, NY.

Bronner, Y. L., et al. 1996. Influence of Work or School on Breastfeeding among Urban WIC Participants. Abstract of the 124th annual meeting of the American Public Health Association. New York: American Public Health Association.

Brownmiller, Susan. 1984. *Femininity.* New York: Simon and Schuster.

Burck, Frances Wells. 1986. *Mothers Talking: Sharing the Secret.* New York: St. Martin's Press.

Cadwell, Karin. 2002. *Reclaiming Breastfeeding for the United States: Protection, Promotion, and Support.* Boston: Jones and Bartlett Publishers.

Cardozo, Arlene Rossen. 1986. *Sequencing: Having It All but Not All at Once . . . A New Solution for Women Who Want Marriage, Career, and Family.* New York: Atheneum.

Coalition for Improving Maternity Services. 2003. The Risks of Cesarean Delivery to Mother and Baby: A CIMS Fact Sheet. Ponte Vedra Beach, FL.

Crittenden, Ann. 2001. *The Price of Motherhood: Why the Most Important Job in the World Is Still the Least Valued.* New York: Henry Holt and Company.

Davis, Deborah L. 1991. *Empty Cradle, Broken Heart: Surviving the Death of Your Baby.* Golden, CO: Fulcrum Publishing.

Davis-Floyd, Robbie E. 1992. *Birth as an American Rite of Passage.* Berkeley: University of California Press.

Declercq, Eugene, and Kirsi Viisainen. 2001. The Politics of Numbers: The Promise and Frustration of Cross-National Analysis. In *Birth by Design: Pregnancy, Maternity Care, and Midwifery in North America and Europe,* ed. Raymond Devries, Cecilia Benoit, Edwin R. Van Teijlingen, and Sirpa Wrede. New York: Routledge.

Dettwyler, Katherine A. 1995a. Beauty and the Breast. In Stuart-Macadam and Dettwyler 1995.

———. 1995b. A Time to Wean: The Hominid Blueprint for the Natural Age of Weaning in Modern Human Populations. In Stuart-Macadam and Dettwyler 1995.

———. 2000. Weaning the Breastfed Baby. In *Breastfeeding Annual International 2000,* ed. Dia L. Michels. Washington, DC: Platypus Media LLC.

Devries, Raymond, Cecilia Benoit, Edwin R. Van Teijlingen, and Sirpa Wrede, eds. 2001. *Birth by Design: Pregnancy, Maternity Care, and Midwifery in North America and Europe.* New York: Routledge.

Dr. Lennart Righard's Delivery: Self-Attachment. 1992. Sunland, CA: Geddess Productions.

Eagan, Andrea Boroff. 1985. *The Newborn Mother: Stages of Her Growth.* Boston: Little, Brown.

Ehrenreich, Barbara, and Deirdre English. 1978. *For Her Own Good: 150 Years of the Experts' Advice to Women.* New York: Anchor Books.

Ensler, Eve. 1998. *The Vagina Monologues.* New York: Villard Books.

Flower, Hillary. 2003. *Adventures in Tandem Nursing*. Schaumburg, IL: La Leche League International.

Freed, Gary L., and Jacob A. Lohr. 1995. National Assessment of Physicians' Breast-feeding Knowledge, Attitudes, Training, and Experience. *Journal of the American Medical Association* 273 (6): 472–76.

Furman, Lydia. 1993. Guest Editorial: Breastfeeding and Full-Time Maternal Employment: Does the Baby Lose Out? *Journal of Human Lactation* 9 (1): 1–2.

Gaskin, Ina May. 2003. *Ina May's Guide to Childbirth*. New York: Bantam Books.

Goer, Henci. 1995. *Obstetric Myths vs. Research Realities*. Westport: Bergin and Garvey.

———. 1999. *The Thinking Woman's Guide to a Better Birth*. New York: Perigee.

Gordon, Mary. 1991. Having a Baby, Finishing a Book. In *Good Boys and Dead Girls and Other Essays*. New York: Viking.

Gromada, Karen Kerkhoff. 1999. *Mothering Multiples: Breastfeeding and Caring for Twins or More*. Schaumburg, IL: La Leche League International.

Hale, Thomas W. 1999. *Clinical Therapy in Breastfeeding Patients*. 1st ed. Amarillo, TX: Pharmasoft Medical Publishing.

———. 1999–2000. *Medications and Mother's Milk*. 8th ed. Amarillo, TX: Pharmasoft Medical Publishing.

Hausman, Bernice L. 2003 *Mother's Milk: Breastfeeding Controversies in American Culture*. New York: Routledge.

Hrdy, Sarah Blaffer. 1999. *Mother Nature: Maternal Instincts and How They Shape the Human Species*. New York: Ballantine Books.

Hilson, J. A., K. M. Rasmussen, and C. L. Kjolhede. 1997. Maternal Obesity and Breastfeeding Success in a Rural Population of Caucasian Women. *American Journal of Clinical Nutrition* 66:1371–78.

Hodnett, E. D., S. Gates, G. J. Hofmeyr, and C. Sakala. 2003. Continuous Support for Women during Childbirth (Cochrane Review). *Cochrane Library*, no. 3. Oxford: Update Software.

Huggins, Kathleen. 1995. *The Nursing Mother's Companion*. Boston: Harvard Common Press.

Hurst, Nancy. 1996. Lactation after Augmentation Mammoplasty. *Obstetrics and Gynecology* 87:30–34.

Kendall-Tackett, Kathleen. 1998. Breastfeeding and the Sexual Abuse Survivor. *Journal of Human Lactation* 14 (2): 125–30.

Kroeger, Mary, with Linda J. Smith. 2004. *Impact of Birthing Practices on Breastfeeding: Protecting the Mother and Baby Continuum*. Boston: Jones and Bartlett Publishers.

Ladd-Taylor, Molly, and Lauri Umansky, eds. 1997. *Bad Mothers: The Politics of Blame in Twentieth Century America*. New York: New York University Press.

La Leche League International. 2004. *The Womanly Art of Breastfeeding*. Schaumburg IL: La Leche League International.

La Leche League International. 2003. Annual Report. Schaumburg, IL. Available at <http://www.lalecheleague.org/ed/PeerAbout.html>.

Lang, Sandra. 1997. *Breastfeeding Special Care Babies*. London: Bailliere Tindall.

Lao Human Rights Council, Inc., and the United Hmong International, Inc., in the United States. 2001.

Lawrence, Ruth A. 1998. *Breastfeeding: A Guide for the Medical Profession.* 2d ed. St. Louis: C. V. Mosby.

Lerner, Harriet. 1998. *The Mother Dance: How Children Change Your Life.* New York: HarperCollins Publishers.

Liotus, Betsy. 1996. More Than Milk. *New Beginnings* 13 (2): 36–39.

Locklin, Maryanne P. 1995. Telling the World: Low Income Women and Their Breastfeeding Experiences. *Journal of Human Lactation* 11 (4): 285–91.

Love, Susan. 2000. *Dr. Susan Love's Breast Book.* Cambridge: Perseus Publishing.

Lowinsky, Naomi Ruth. 1992. *Stories from the Motherline.* Los Angeles: Jeremy P. Tarcher.

Luddington-Hoe, Susan M., and Susan K. Golant. 1993. *Kangaroo Care: The Best You Can Do to Help Your Preterm Infant.* New York: Bantam Books.

Maloney, Carolyn B. 2001. Foreword to *Breastfeeding Annual International 2001,* by Dia L. Michels. Washington, DC: Platypus Media LLC.

———. 2002. Breastfeeding on a Worldwide Scale: How the United States Lags Behind Its International Counterparts. Available at <http://www.house.gov/maloney/issues/breastfeeding/worldwide.htm>.

Marin, Lynda. 1994. Mother and Child: The Erotic Bond. In *Mother Journeys: Feminists Write about Mothering,* ed. Maureen T. Reddy, Martha Roth, and Amy Sheldon. Minneapolis: Spinsters Ink.

Maternity Center Association. 2002. *Listening to Mothers: Report of the First National Survey of Women's Childbearing Experiences.* Executive Summary and Recommendations. New York: Maternity Center Association.

Maushart, Susan. 1999. *The Mask of Motherhood: How Becoming a Mother Changes Everything and Why We Pretend It Doesn't.* New York: New Press.

McKenna, James J. 1995. Babies Need Their Mothers Beside Them. Available at <http://www.naturalchild.com/james_mckenna/sleeping_safe.html>.

McKenna, James J., Sarah S. Mosko, and Christopher A. Richard. 1997. Bed-sharing Promotes Breastfeeding. *Pediatrics* 100 (2): 214–19.

Michels, Dia L., ed. 2001. *Breastfeeding Annual International 2001.* Washington, DC: Platypus Media LLC.

Neifert, M., A. DeMarzo, J. Seacat, D. Young, M. Leff, and M. Orleans. 1990. The Influence of Breast Surgery, Breast Appearance, and Pregnancy-Induced Breast Changes on Lactation Sufficiency as Measured by Infant Weight Gain. *Birth* 17:31–38.

Nommsen-Rivers, Laurie. 2003. Guest Editorial: Cosmetic Breast Surgery: Is Breastfeeding at Risk? *Journal of Human Lactation* 19 (1): 7–8.

Olsen, Tillie. 1995. I Stand Here Ironing. In *Points of View: An Anthology of Short Stories,* ed. James Moffett and Kenneth R. McElheny. New York: Mentor.

Oxenhandler, Noelle. 2001. *The Eros of Parenthood: Explorations in Light and Dark.* New York: St. Martin's Press.

Palmer, Gabrielle. 1999. *Politics of Breastfeeding.* London: Pandora Press.

Reddy, Maureen T., Martha Roth, and Amy Sheldon, eds. 1994. *Mother Journeys: Feminists Write about Mothering.* Minneapolis: Spinsters Ink.

Remen, Rachel Naomi. 1996. *Kitchen Table Wisdom: Stories That Heal.* New York: Riverhead Books.

Renfrew, Mary, Chloe Fisher, and Suzanne Arms. 1990. *Bestfeeding: Getting Breastfeeding Right for You.* Berkeley: Celestial Arts.

Ribbens, Jane. 1995. *Mothers and Their Children: A Feminist Sociology of Childrearing.* Thousand Oaks: Sage Publications.

Rich, Adrienne. 1986. *Of Woman Born: Motherhood as Experience and Institution.* New York: W. W. Norton.

Righard, Lennart, and M. O. Alade. 1990. Effect of Delivery Room Routines on Success of First Breast-Feed. *Lancet* 336:1105–7.

Rodriguez-Garcia, R., and L. Frazier. 1995. Cultural Paradoxes Relating to Sexuality and Breastfeeding. *Journal of Human Lactation* 11 (2): 111–15.

Ryan, Alan S., Zhou Wenjun, and Andrew Acosta. 2002. Breastfeeding Continues to Increase into the New Millennium. *Pediatrics* 110 (6): 1103–9.

Sears, William. 1999. *Nighttime Parenting: How to Get Your Baby and Child to Sleep.* Schaumburg, IL: La Leche League International.

Semple, J. L., S. J. Lugowski, C. J. Baines, D. C. Smith, and A. McHugh. 1998. Breast Milk Contamination and Silicone Implants: Preliminary Results Using Silicon as a Proxy Measurement for Silicone. *Plastic Reconstructive Surgery* 102:528–33.

Small, Meredith. 1998. *Our Babies, Ourselves: How Biology and Culture Shape the Way We Parent.* New York: Anchor Books.

Smith, Linda. 1996. Why Johnny Can't Suck. Available at <http://www.bflrc.com>.

Souto, Glaucia C., Elsa R. J. Giugliani, Camila Giugliani, and Marcia A. Schneider. 2003. The Impact of Breast Reduction Surgery on Breastfeeding Performance. *Journal of Human Lactation* 19 (1): 43–49.

Statistical Abstract of the United States. 2001. 121st ed. Washington: GPO.

Stearns, Cindy A. 1999. Breastfeeding and the Good Maternal Body. *Gender and Society* 13 (3): 308–25.

Steingraber, Sandra. 2001. *Having Faith: An Ecologist's Journey to Motherhood.* Cambridge: Perseus Publishing.

Stuart-Macadam, Patricia, and Katherine A. Dettwyler, eds. 1995. *Breastfeeding: Biocultural Perspectives.* Hawthorne, NY: Aldine de Gruyter.

Swiggart, Jane. 1991. *The Myth of the Bad Mother.* New York: Doubleday.

Turner-Maffei, Cindy. 2002. Overcoming Disparities in Breastfeeding. In *Reclaiming Breastfeeding for the United States: Protection, Promotion, and Support,* ed. Karin Cadwell. Boston: Jones and Bartlett Publishers.

Umansky, Lauri. Breastfeeding in the 1990s: The Karen Carter Case and the Politics of Maternal Sexuality. In *Bad Mothers: The Politics of Blame in Twentieth Century America,* ed. Molly Ladd-Taylor and Lauri Umansky. New York: New York University Press.

Van Esterik, Penny. 1989. *Beyond the Breast-Bottle Controversy.* New Brunswick: Rutgers University Press.

———. 1994. Guest Editorial: Lessons from Our Lives: Breastfeeding in a Personal Context. *Journal of Human Lactation* 10 (2): 71–74.

———. 1995. Breastfeeding: A Feminist Issue. WABA Activity Sheet 4, World Alliance for Breastfeeding Action.

Vekemans, M. 1997. Postpartum Contraception: The Lactational Amenorrhea

Method. *The European Journal of Contraception and Reproductive Health Care: The Official Journal of the European Society of Contraception* 2 (2): 105–11.

Vincent, Peggy. 2002. *Baby Catcher: Chronicles of a Modern Midwife.* New York: Scribner.

Visness, Cynthia M., and Cathy I. Kennedy. 1997. Maternal Employment and Breast-feeding: Findings from the 1988 National Maternal and Infant Health Survey. *American Journal of Public Health* 88 (7): 1042–46.

Walker, Marsha. 2001. *Selling Out Mothers and Babies: Marketing of Breast Milk Substitutes in the USA.* Weston, MA: National Alliance for Breast-feeding Advocacy, Research, Education and Legal Branch.

Weiner, Lynn Y. 1994. Reconstructing Motherhood: The La Leche League in Post-War America. *Journal of American History* 80:1357–81.

West, Diana. 2001. *Defining Your Own Success: Breastfeeding after Breast Reduction Surgery.* Schaumburg, IL: La Leche League International.

Wiessinger, Diane. 1996. Guest Editorial: Watch Your Language! *Journal of Human Lactation* 12 (1): 1–4.

Wolf, Naomi. 1991. *The Beauty Myth: How Images of Beauty Are Used against Women.* New York: Anchor Books.

———. 2001. *Misconceptions: Truth, Lies, and the Unexpected on the Journey to Motherhood.* New York: Doubleday.

World Health Organization, Division of Child Health and Development. 1998. *Evidence for the Ten Steps to Successful Breastfeeding.* Geneva, Switzerland: World Health Organization.

Yalom, Marilyn. 1997. *A History of the Breast.* New York: Knopf.

Zimmerman, Susan M. 1998. *Silicone Survivors: Women's Experiences with Breast Implants.* Philadelphia: Temple University Press.

Index